4

CARE OF
THE SURGICAL PATIENT

CARE OF
THE SURGICAL PATIENT

A Textbook for Nurses

Shirley Graffam, R.N., M.Ed.
Assistant Professor of Medical-Surgical Nursing
School of Nursing
University of North Dakota
Grand Forks, North Dakota

The Blakiston Division

McGRAW-HILL BOOK COMPANY, INC.

New York   Toronto   London
1960

Dedicated to my mother and father

FOREWORD

This text for nurses aims at a new approach to patient care—the development of the subject matter in terms of the care of selected patients. The patients are composites of those for whom the author has cared or about whom she has written in some detail. For the most part, those sections of the text in which the care of specific patients is portrayed involve actual patients. They serve richly as examples and as illustrations.

Among the major emphases in the text is one of special significance. It has to do with teaching the student not only the "what" and "how" of nursing, which are important, but also the "why," which is paramount. In teaching the "why," the author strives to ensure a deep appreciation and understanding on the part of the student of the needs of patients, whether physical, psychologic, spiritual, emotional, or social. She specially emphasizes the development of psychologic and social skills essential in reassuring patients. These and other interpersonal skills, as viewed by the author, are of value in relationships not only with patients and their families but also with associates, other members of the health team, and all who are involved in providing care for the patient.

Another feature of unique interest to students and faculty is the discussion of the nursing care of surgical patients from the point of view of a "generalist." No specialist is the author in her presentation! She visualizes, for example, the care of a patient with thoracic surgery or abdominal surgery. She may refer to these major fields by citing specific examples, as, for example, cancer or ulcer, but by and large she uses a general approach.

The author has arranged her material in four parts: Part One presents the basic concepts every student should possess; Parts Two, Three, and Four deal with abdominal surgery, neck and chest surgery, and surgery of the extremities. This order is much the same as that in which students tend to encounter these subjects.

It is intended that this text should primarily serve undergraduate basic professional students in both the degree and the diploma programs. It should also serve as a source book for graduate nurse students in the clinical field of surgical nursing and should be of real value to nursing education and nursing service personnel with teaching, supervisory, and administrative responsibilities for the care of surgical patients.

The author's preparation and experience have specially prepared her for the writing of this kind of text. Her basic preparation was at the Cook County School of Nursing, a school providing unusually comprehensive clinical resources, particularly in the area of surgical nursing. In addition to her nursing education program at the University of Minnesota, Miss Graffam completed a minor in the teaching of sciences in schools of nursing. She draws richly upon this broader scientific knowledge throughout the text. Since 1949 Miss Graffam has been an instructor in surgical nursing. During this period of almost a decade she has experimented with every method described in the text and has tried out repeatedly the types of instruction she has felt to be most effective. It was primarily her evaluation, in cooperation with students, of her methods of instruction that led her to select the case-method type of presentation utilized so extensively in this text.

KATHARINE J. DENSFORD

PREFACE

The aim of this textbook is to help students of professional nursing to learn how to evaluate and meet the needs of adult surgical patients. This aim is threefold: (1) to help the student to learn the basic principles of surgical nursing care, (2) to encourage her to function as a health teacher, and (3) to assist her to develop some understanding of the dynamics of human behavior in relation to surgical intervention and nursing care.

The application of these three inseparable components of surgical nursing is demonstrated in seven major presentations of patients, illustrating how to develop plans for care and teaching based upon individual needs. The areas of need which are considered include socioeconomic, spiritual-psychologic, and physical. Chapter 8, dealing with the preoperative and postoperative care of Betty Marrow, is purposefully detailed to show how needs are identified and evaluated, how a plan for care and teaching is evolved from this evaluation, and how such a plan is carried through. Other chapters present patients when special needs are pointed out. No effort has been made to complete each case description; the reader is urged to do this in her own thinking. For complete and realistic learning, each patient discussed is a composite of many; all names are fictitious, but the problems are real. Emphasis is placed upon the fact that the surgical patient is a person who has a medical condition requiring surgical intervention.

Considerable emphasis has been placed upon health teaching. Chapter 2 is devoted entirely to a presentation of the general principles and methods of teaching applied to specific patients. Throughout the text the special teaching needs associated with surgical conditions are identified, and the student is encouraged to assume her role as a health teacher.

Furthermore, the student is helped to view surgical care not as a series of procedures or isolated facts, but rather as a dynamic nurse-patient relationship. Health guidance and the effecting of constructive interpersonal relationships are inseparable. The nurse is encouraged to establish channels of communication through which patients' needs can be expressed and met.

Meeting the spiritual needs of each patient is emphasized. This is an area of nursing which merits more formal attention in curriculum planning than is generally given. The patient's faith in a Supreme Being, or his lack of it, is a deciding factor in his recovery from surgical procedures, or from any illness. The nurse must be able to encourage the patient in his faith and to assist him in his religious practices. No attempt has been made to discuss theologic doctrines, but patients representing major religions, or professing none, are presented to point out the religious needs of each and how the nurse meets these needs.

This textbook has been organized into four major units. Part One presents the basic concepts of care and teaching which are necessary in the treatment of all surgical patients. The last chapter of this unit is designed to help the student to formulate these concepts into a correlated whole by considering the preoperative and postoperative care of Betty Marrow, who undergoes a laparotomy. The care of patients undergoing abdominal surgery is presented in detail in Part Two. Part Three deals with the care of a patient who requires a thoracotomy. Part Four considers the care needed by patients with vascular surgery and burns, conditions commonly, but not necessarily, involving the extremities.

The text was organized in this manner because it was felt that this is the order in which students are generally introduced to the care of surgical patients. There is merit in retaining this order because each unit builds upon the preceding material and technical words are defined in context when first introduced. However, there is no reason why Parts Two, Three, and Four can not be taken out of sequence for use in a surgical nursing course. The detailed contents, index, and cross references permit this to be done without sacrificing learning.

Part One is basic not only in content but also in the method of presentation. Principles are clearly identified, and thought-provoking questions are raised in context. Subsequent units are based upon principles, but the principles are less obviously identified, so as to encourage the formation of more mature study habits. The student should seek to identify basic principles independently. She should study with a dictionary at hand, since all words unfamiliar to her may not be defined in this text. In her study of terminology, the student should continue the practice illustrated in Part One of breaking down a word into its constituent parts. Each chapter has a summary, and provocative study guides and bibliographies are furnished to assist the student in broadening her understandings and in applying the material to her own situation.

It is the author's feeling that many classes and textbooks present the

student with a barrage of facts about many conditions in an effort to
furnish a complete background. This tends to confuse the student and
encourages blind memorization of disconnected facts. Therefore, no effort
has been made in this textbook to describe every surgical condition the
student may meet. Rather, broad concepts of care required in surgery of
the major anatomic divisions of the body are presented. The material on
each major area of general surgery includes a discussion of diagnostic
methods; symptoms, pathology, and indications for surgery; anesthesia
and surgical technic; rehabilitation—all correlated with the principles of
nursing care and teaching. For conditions not included, the student and
instructor should refer to current literature and, by a process of active
problem solving, should formulate the plan for care and teaching.

In this period of medical-surgical growth it is of little value to mem-
orize a given body of information. Students must develop an analytic
viewpoint and skill in evaluating reference material as well as their own
experiences. A textbook can do little more than set the stage. Each student enters onto that stage with her own insights, health team, and patients.

Throughout this text, every effort has been made to select those practices most widely accepted in surgical care. Medical-surgical practices
vary markedly, depending upon the patient's needs, geographic location,
hospital policies, and the surgeon's preferences and abilities. On the basis
of the general principles of surgical nursing care and teaching presented,
local adaptations are left to the thoughtful consideration of the reader.

For simplicity only and with full recognition of the fact that both men
and women contribute actively to the professions of medicine and nursing, the masculine gender is used in reference to physicians and the
feminine to refer to nurses. Either gender may be used in reference to
patients.

In the process of writing a textbook, an author becomes indebted to
many persons. Many surgeons, medical specialists, and nurses have
freely given their time, ideas, and encouragement. Authors and publishers have graciously granted permission to use materials, many send-
ing notes of encouragement which were truly appreciated. Specific contributions from the following persons are gratefully acknowledged: Katharine J. Densford, University of Minnesota School of Nursing, Minneapolis, who contributed the foreword and who has been a continuous
source of inspiration to the author throughout her nursing career; Dr.
Frank Caporale, Augustana Hospital, Chicago, who reviewed substantial
portions of the manuscript; Dr. William Grove, Research and Educational
Hospitals, University of Illinois, Chicago, who reviewed all of Part Two
and Chapters 18 and 19; and Mrs. John Coe, University of Minnesota
School of Nursing, Mary Reglin, Cook County School of Nursing, Chi-

cago, and Rena Boyle, United States Public Health Service, who gave many helpful suggestions. Especially time-consuming reviews of certain chapters are credited to the following persons: Dr. George Milles, Augustana Hospital, and Mrs. Edith Wolf, Memorial Center for Cancer and Allied Diseases, New York City, Chapter 4; Carole Connaughton, formerly of Research and Educational Hospitals, Chapter 13; Dr. Oliver Renaud, Augustana Hospital, Chapter 14, Neck Dissection; Dr. Hiram Langston, Chicago State Tuberculosis Sanitarium, and Wilma Phipps, University of Illinois College of Nursing, Chicago, Chapter 16; and Drs. Ormand Julian and Nicholas Cotsonas, Research and Educational Hospitals, and Dr. Robert Trout, The Glover Clinic, Philadelphia, Chapter 17. Chapter 7 was reviewed by Gloria Blado, Cook County Hospital, and by Dr. Richard Lyons and Sagrid Johnson, Augustana Hospital.

Bernice Fash, Cook County School of Nursing, by sharing her own writing experiences, helped in the motivation and preparation of the author for this project. She has been a staunch support and helpful adviser throughout the writing of this textbook.

With fond affection and with sincere appreciation, the author acknowledges the help of her mother, who skillfully typed and retyped the entire manuscript, giving freely of both time and encouragement from the inception of this textbook.

Students in nursing have lent enthusiastic support to this venture and method of teaching and have helped to clarify the study guides. Grace Whyte, formerly of Mount Sinai Hospital School of Nursing, Chicago, was helpful in initially stimulating the author's interest in the development of effective nurse-patient communication.

The drawings were made by Angela Bartenbach, medical illustrator, Veterans Administration Research Hospital, Chicago, and by Ramona Morgan, Assistant Instructor in Medical Art, Illustration Studios, University of Illinois, Chicago.

To all others who have lent support and suggestions throughout the writing of this text the author is indeed grateful.

SHIRLEY GRAFFAM

CONTENTS

Part Three: Care of the Patient Undergoing Surgery of the Neck and Thorax

Part Four: Care of the Patient with Surgical Conditions of the Peripheral Vascular and Integumentary Systems

Part One

BASIC CONCEPTS IN SURGICAL CARE

1

THE PERSON WHO IS THE SURGICAL PATIENT

Who is the surgical patient? How does he resemble or differ from one whose condition is medical? What special needs does he present because he is considered a surgical patient? How does he view his surgical treatment? How have the changing concepts of surgical care and treatment affected the patient who goes to surgery in this age? These are vital questions which must be considered by nurses if the patient is to benefit from care designed to meet his needs.

WHO THE SURGICAL PATIENT IS

The surgical patient is a person who has a condition requiring operative intervention. This condition is usually medical. For example, cholecystitis, inflammation of the gallbladder, is a medical condition which is cured by removal of that organ, cholecystectomy. For the convenience of discussion and treatment, diseases which patients have are classified as medical or surgical, or they are further subdivided into specialties, such as dermatology; urology; neurology and neurosurgery; eye, ear, nose, and throat; gynecology; orthopedics. This classification risks the impression that each patient has different basic needs. Actually the needs of all patients are fundamentally the same. The surgical patient has the same needs as a medical patient for nutrition, fluids, elimination, correction of deficiencies, the combating of infection, and reassurance. Therefore, one may say that the preoperative and postoperative management is medical. However, the surgical patient differs from the strictly medical patient in that he must usually elect to undergo operative technics which will make him temporarily more acutely ill. Usually the medical patient is first treated in an acute episode of his illness—pneumonia, for example—and therefore welcomes treatment which affords relatively prompt relief from symptoms. The surgical patient, on the other hand, may be acutely ill, as with appendicitis, but in order to gain relief from symptoms he must

3

elect to undergo surgery which will effect his recovery but which will also prolong his discomfort for a time.

Like the medical patient, the one who is considered surgical is a person who has left a familiar part of the community to enter the hospital, which to him is unfamiliar and which in many ways may threaten his sense of security and self-esteem. He has left temporarily not only the familiar places in his community but also the persons with whom he interacts and plays definite roles. These roles may include those of father, husband, employee, friend. Each role requires certain behavioral characteristics and attitudes from this person and also gives him a way of meeting his needs. In the hospital new roles are created to which the patient reacts on the basis of previous patterns of behavior. The nurse can guide the development of constructive interpersonal relationships with this patient more effectively if she takes time to learn what roles he has been playing and what their significance is to him.

CONCERNS OF THE SURGICAL PATIENT

Fear of the unknown is accentuated by the experiences through which the surgical patient must pass: diagnostic procedures, preparation for surgery, anesthesia, the operation itself, the postoperative period, and rehabilitation. General anesthesia, while it has granted release from pain for surgical patients, may be more dreaded by patients than the actual surgery.

The desire of every human being to be physically whole cannot be lightly overlooked in a consideration of how a patient views his surgery. Fear of mutilation is strong in all patients, especially those awaiting amputation of a part. In a sense, all surgery involves some mutilation, and patients react with varied feelings.[1] Some are depressed, some are angry, while others may be anxious and confused. The nurse can be most helpful if she will encourage the patient to express his concerns. In this way fears can be viewed realistically, misinformation can be corrected, and the patient can build confidence in his recovery and in the health team.

The nurse must help the patient develop a healthy attitude toward his surgical experience. The patient's reaction will be strongly influenced by the reason for the surgery. If surgery is *curative* in aim and successfully accomplished, the patient and his relatives can anticipate a relatively prompt recovery leading to health. However if surgery is performed for *diagnostic* purposes, there is generated a fear of the unknown—of the diagnosis and what it may mean to future health. When surgery is performed for *palliation*—i.e., to relieve symptoms, such as

[1] B. Bird, Psychological Aspects of Preoperative and Postoperative Care, *Am. J. Nursing*, pp. 685–687, June, 1955.

pain due to cancer—but not to cure, the patient will appreciate the temporary improvement in his condition; he may even think for a time that he is cured. But his optimism is usually short-lived; as his symptoms recur, both he and his relatives may be profoundly depressed. If surgery is *reconstructive*, i.e., to improve appearance or function, there may be a great deal of anxiety about the anticipated results. For example, a rhinoplasty, surgical revision of a nose, profoundly alters a person's appearance; the patient may or may not like the results of surgery; he is bound to have an emotional adjustment to make.

Surgery usually means relief from symptoms and a return to health. Sometimes a patient will seek to have an operation because he has strong guilt feelings, and surgery to him represents punishment which vindicates these feelings. Patients are usually not aware of these deep psychologic motives for seeking surgery, but the attitudes each has toward surgical treatment greatly influence his recovery. Patients vary considerably in their completeness and rate of recovery, and unusually long periods required for convalescence are not always attributable to surgical complications. A psychologic evaluation was made of a series of patients who were to have elective surgery. It was found that the majority of those who were poorly adjusted emotionally (as ascertained by history and psychologic testing) had a recovery period significantly longer than did those patients who were undergoing similar surgery but were better adjusted.[2] The nurse will learn to detect excessive dependency feelings in patients by observing their behavior and comments. For example, the young man who is extremely reluctant to turn and get out of bed after an appendectomy may have more fear of recovering and resuming independent status as a working member of the community than of the pain he admits to fearing. The nurse must be alert to detect attitudes and motives which are detrimental to the patient if she is to help him develop a positive outlook upon his surgical experience. The nurse should remember in handling such problems that she is a member of a health team which can help her meet the needs of her patient.

Also to be considered is the effect upon the patient of the length of time allowed to pass between the recognition of the need for surgery and the actual performance of the operation. Surgery may be *elective*, i.e., the condition for which the operation is being performed does not immediately jeopardize life. There is ample time to prepare the patient optimally for surgery. On the other hand, surgery may be *emergent*, i.e., the jeopardy to life requires the operation to be performed as soon as the patient can be prepared adequately enough to withstand the pro-

[2] R. A. Schneider, J. S. Gray, and C. U. Culmer, Psychological Evaluation of Surgical Patients, *Bull. Univ. Minnesota Hospitals & Minnesota M. Foundation*, vol. 20, pp. 201–211, Dec. 10, 1948.

cedure. Emergent surgery precludes much preoperative teaching and many procedures, but there is always time to reassure the patient. The need for reassurance is increased when an emergency has suddenly disrupted the patient's living pattern, forcing him to undergo surgery without thought or planning on his part.

CHANGING CONCEPTS IN SURGICAL CARE

Also to be considered are the effects of changing concepts of surgical treatment upon the patient's adjustment. Within the past generation many contributions have been made to medical science. The sciences of microbiology, anatomy, physiology, chemistry, and anesthesiology, to mention only a few, have contributed toward safer, more extensive surgery for patients and toward a more comfortable, shorter, postoperative period. Emphasis is now placed upon more intensive preoperative preparation, which includes such measures as correcting deficiencies, combating infection, and attaining adequate fluid and electrolyte balance. This preparation complements the newer methods of anesthesia and allows the surgeon to operate in a more leisurely way, i.e., to emphasize deftness rather than speed.

The postoperative period, influenced strongly by the practice of early activation of the patient, is now shorter and beset with fewer complications than could previously have been hoped for. There is now more emphasis upon rehabilitation of the patient so that he can achieve the greatest degree of health his condition allows. The concept of rehabilitation has changed in recent years from one concerned primarily with restoration of function following impairment due to injury, surgery, or disuse to one directed toward the prevention of the loss of any resources the patient has. Such a program must involve total patient needs and must begin for both medical and surgical patients with admission to the hospital. Injurious habits, such as poor posture due to faulty positioning and prolonged bedrest, are not allowed to develop. Efforts are made to correct erroneous attitudes which are detrimental to the patient's welfare and to medical progress. The nurse must exercise good judgment in allowing the patient to go as far in rehabilitation as it is wise for him to go.

Moreover, the adult patient may not have been made aware of these changing concepts. His views of surgical treatment may be strongly influenced by the ideas prevailing at the turn of the twentieth century, when the mortality rate for surgery was high and little attention was given to the preventive measures commonly practiced today. Therefore, the older patient may fear a blood transfusion or intravenous infusion, not only because the equipment seems strange to him, but also because such treatments were once performed only as lifesaving measures. Today these procedures have prophylactic, as well as therapeutic, value, and the patient must be helped to understand this changed concept which has influenced his care. This same patient will be reluctant to turn, cough, and eat because he remembers, and expects, the prior pattern of therapy, which advocated absolute bedrest, tight binders, and markedly restricted diet for several days postoperatively.

SUMMARY

The surgical patient is a person who has a condition requiring operative intervention. His basic physical and psychologic needs are similar to those of the medical patient. Both have feelings, attitudes, and motives which tremendously influence recovery and which, therefore, demand recognition by the nurse and the rest of the health team. In addition, the surgical patient is markedly affected by the reason for his surgery and the nature of the procedure, i.e., whether it is curative, palliative, diagnostic, reconstructive, and whether it is elective or emergent. The patient and his relatives must be helped to understand changed concepts of surgical care and rehabilitation. Surgical care will continue to change as the health team moves forward to new understandings and discoveries. It will continue to be a richly rewarding, challenging, and stimulating experience for the nurse who endeavors to meet the needs of the surgical patient.

2

HEALTH GUIDANCE OF THE PATIENT

If the reader will reflect upon her own experiences in learning nursing care and technics, she will remember that the principles of caring for the patient had to be presented to her repeatedly and in varied ways before she really understood how to apply them. She will also recall that her own health and attitudes influenced her learning and that much of her own experience was necessary before the information became a functional part of her. Why, then, do nurses so often tell a patient all at once how to care for his wound, what foods to eat, how much activity to assume—and expect the patient to assimilate the information so that he is capable of self-care?

Teaching of patients is a vital part of nursing. Nurses frequently feel pressed to give bedside care and may omit teaching because they feel they have insufficient time. Yet failure to instruct a patient properly too often results in his return to the hospital in an acute exacerbation or with a preventable complication of his illness. His care then requires more time than his teaching program would have originally taken.

Then, too, teaching of patients may be neglected because physician and nurse each thinks this role is being filled by the other. Actually, total care of the patient, which includes teaching, is a responsibility shared by a professional health team. The physician heads this team and directs what he wants the patient to know. He also prepares the patient for learning and helps his adjustment to the future by discussing with him the diagnosis and prognosis to the degree deemed necessary. Other members of this team, in addition to the nurse, are the dietitian, physical therapist, occupational therapist, clergyman, and social worker. Each has a distinct contribution to make to the care of the patient. The well-prepared nurse is in a strategic position to evaluate a patient's need for health guidance and to carry through a teaching program designed to meet the needs imposed by his surgical condition and by his general health concept.

Nursing care once implied primarily bathing and feeding the patient, but now nursing is much more involved. It extends beyond the patient's ambulation and discharge from the hospital to prepare him to function to the best of his capabilities in the broader community outside the hospital. This concept of professional nursing necessitates a more extensive interpretation and program of teaching patients than is commonly practiced. It requires that the patient be taught methods of caring for his physical condition and in addition that he be helped to gain a sense of his own important role in attaining the health goal which he and the health team have decided upon. Such mutual understanding is essential before a cooperative program of rehabilitation can be carried out. The patient who feels that he needs to learn to care for himself and that he really wants to will carry out more conscientiously the health practices learned in the hospital. His hospitalization will truly have been a learning experience if motivation toward a positive health goal was basic to the teaching program.

Before the principles and methods of teaching patients can be presented, one must first consider what learning actually is. Learning is more than the acquisition of skills and the memorization of facts. It is primarily a change in a person's behavior and attitudes effected by experience and training.[1] Learning is complete when a person grasps the idea of a solution as a whole and understands the essential relationships of all aspects of the situation.[2]

PRINCIPLES OF PATIENT TEACHING

A person tends to repeat behavior patterns until helped to gain new insights. This applies to a person's own health concept and habits. Sometimes these patterns of behavior are detrimental to a person's welfare. Unless his hospitalization is an educational experience for him, he will tend to perpetuate habits which may have led originally to his illness. This principle is illustrated by the following description of a patient who is reluctant to undergo surgery.

Helping Mrs. Erickson Accept Surgery

Mrs. Erickson has had two severe attacks of acute cholecystitis with cholelithiasis, inflammation of the gallbladder with stones, prior to this admission to the hospital with the third attack of biliary colic and vomiting. Each time her doctor has relieved her symptoms but has emphasized

[1] Arthur I. Gates, Arthur T. Jersild, T. R. McConnell, and Robert C. Challman, "Educational Psychology," 3d ed., The Macmillan Company, New York, 1948, p. 288. (Adapted with permission of The Macmillan Company.)
[2] *Ibid.*, p. 323.

the need for keeping to her diet and undergoing surgery to effect a cure. Each time during her distress she promised to follow orders and to have surgery, but when relief came she could see no need for an operation or a diet. Now in the hospital with another attack, even more severe, she may repeat her procrastination of surgery unless she is helped to see the need for it as basic to her comfort, health, and future happiness.

Mrs. Erickson illustrates the need a patient has for (1) understanding and accepting her diagnosis and prognosis, and (2) being helped to face her problem realistically, i.e., to gain new insights. She needs to realize the advantages of undergoing surgery to regain health, and the alternatives that may ensue by refusing to have this operation. This involves helping Mrs. Erickson establish a health goal for herself which she can work through with the cooperative efforts of the health team.

A person must be ready to learn. Usually a patient is concerned with his future and the adjustment he must make because of his condition. He is, therefore, in an acceptive frame of mind for learning. However, if he rejects his diagnosis or future, he must first be helped to accept his condition and to overcome feelings of hopelessness before he can learn to care for himself adequately. This attitude of rejection is common with patients who have surgery which they consider mutilating, such as a colostomy or amputation of a part. The nurse can help the patient view his problem realistically and convey a feeling of optimism by her own attitude and by skillful conversation with the patient. She can also arrange to have the patient visited by a well-rehabilitated person who has overcome the same type of problem.

The patient must feel motivated to learn. The reasons for learning must bear real meaning for the patient. No one can be motivated to learn by the teacher; motivation must come from the person learning. However, a person will want to learn if he realizes that he will gain thereby. This principle is related to the one immediately preceding.

Influencing Mrs. Erickson's Motivation

Mrs. Erickson (see page 9) illustrates this principle. She followed doctor's orders temporarily because she was in pain and sought relief from her symptoms. Once she was symptom-free her motive for following a diet or undergoing surgery was no longer effective. She needed to realize the value not only of being free from discomfort but also of achieving a health goal. The nurse would have to help Mrs. Erickson understand what cholecystitis with cholelithiasis is, how it is cured, and why she experiences relief from symptoms only temporarily. The nurse would have to draw out from Mrs. Erickson through discussion what her acute episodes mean to her and why she fears surgery. This instruction is shared with the rest of the health team.

Teaching must build upon the patient's present fund of knowledge and range of experience. No two patients can proceed in learning from the same point. Individual differences must be considered, as illustrated in the following descriptions of two patients who have the same disease but very different learning needs.

Considering What the Patient Already Knows

Mrs. Romano was admitted to the hospital in diabetic acidosis. She had controlled her diabetes fairly successfully for 8 years with insulin and diet therapy. However, she had been ill with an acute gallbladder attack for 1 week prior to her admission; during that time she had taken neither insulin nor food regularly. Her teaching program, therefore, must emphasize means to avoid complications and need not start with methods of administering insulin and the simple rules of diet. However, she must be made to understand that in the absence of food intake, the body uses its own stores and that some insulin is therefore necessary even in fasting.

On the other hand, Tommy Jones, a 14-year-old, has been admitted to the hospital for an appendectomy and has been discovered to be diabetic. His teaching program must include all aspects of diabetic care.

Teaching must be carried out on the patient's level of comprehension. In order to gain a patient's cooperation and avoid confusion, terminology must be such that the patient understands what is expected of him. Avoid "talking down" to patients; it may cause resentment. Mrs. Romano and Tommy illustrate this principle.

Choosing the Level of Teaching

Mrs. Romano graduated from an Italian university with a degree in music. She came to the United States following her graduation 10 years ago. She has a language difficulty; in addition, she understands no medical terminology other than the few terms she has learned during the 8 years in which she has had diabetes. Her teaching program must be based upon a consideration of this problem in communication and must be designed to meet her needs; it must not, however, be based upon the assumption that Mrs. Romano cannot learn.

Tommy, on the other hand, was born in the United States. He has no language barrier, but his experience is limited. His teaching program must be much more basic and must be geared to his level of comprehension. It must also be planned to meet the special needs of an adolescent.

Teaching must be complete to avoid erroneous notions. It is not enough to tell a patient to irrigate his wound, for example. He must know when, how, why, and with what solution and equipment. A patient who is inadequately instructed may do more harm than good in attempting to apply information, as is illustrated by the following incident.

Supplying Missing Information

Mr. Youngreth, a clinic patient, was instructed to take a high enema. He was not told that "high enema" means that the fluid should reach the ileocecal valve and that this is best accomplished by holding the enema container approximately 8 to 12 in. above the level of the buttocks. He therefore suspended the container several feet above the level of his buttocks. The result was a painful overdistention of the rectum without the therapeutic value of a high enema.

The teacher must consider the patient's home environment, social roles, and economic status. The health habits which the patient learns must be compatible with his daily activities and responsibilities, i.e., they must be capable of fulfillment. This principle is illustrated in the following description of Mr. Smither.

Designing a Practical Teaching Program

Mr. Smither has had a *colostomy* (an operation in which a loop of intestine is brought to the exterior through the abdominal wall to allow for evacuation of stool when the distal loop of intestine is obstructed) in the treatment of cancer of the sigmoid. The surgeon has ordered daily irrigations through the colostomy opening to facilitate the patient's control of defecation. The nurse who teaches Mr. Smither how to carry out these irrigations must consider the following factors:

1. Where does Mr. Smither live? Does he have a private bathroom where he can carry out the irrigations without hurry or interruption? Or does he live in a boarding house where he must share the bathroom with many people?

2. What time of day is best for Mr. Smither's irrigation? This depends upon his habits of elimination, when he leaves for work, and what his usual routine is.

3. Who lives with Mr. Smither? Do his relatives know of his condition? Are there small children in the house?

4. What equipment does Mr. Smither have at home that can be used for his irrigation? No unnecessary economic burden should be placed upon the patient by teaching the use of hospital equipment only.

The physical condition and strength of the patient must be considered in planning his teaching program, since the concentration span decreases with fatigue. This principle is illustrated by the following description of Mr. Jones, who has been considerably weakened by surgery and a complicated convalescence.

Considering the Patient's Strength

Mr. Jones, who has a draining wound, had a difficult night but rested well in the morning of the day he was to start to learn to dress his own wound. His nurse allowed him to wait until afternoon when he was not too tired and planned his first lesson so that it was in keeping with his strength. This first time Mr. Jones dressed his wound he applied the dressings after the nurse cleansed the area and explained the need for keeping the area clean. As he gains strength he can be expected to dress his wound entirely by himself.

Learning is facilitated by judicious repetition. In teaching, it is important that the instruction be repeated in various ways so that the patient can view all aspects of the problem. This principle is illustrated in the following description of dietitian and nurse working together to teach a patient how to follow a therapeutic diet.

Repeating Information in Varied Ways

A dietitian was assigned to teach Mrs. Jorgenson how to plan her diet, which was to be high in carbohydrate, protein, vitamins, and minerals, but low in fat. The dietitian first interested Mrs. Jorgenson by explaining the principles of her diet as it was served at lunch. She gave her a list of foods and encouraged her to make out sample menus. Cooperating in this teaching, the nurse clarified this instruction and gave the patient opportunities to discuss problems about her diet and questioned her to be sure that she understood how to manage her diet at home. In this way the original teaching was reinforced, and the patient was helped to understand all essential aspects of her diet.

METHODS OF TEACHING THE INDIVIDUAL PATIENT

Before any method of teaching can be selected for a particular patient, the nurse should employ the art of listening. In this way she gains a knowledge of teaching needs and estimates the learning capacity of the patient and the type of teaching necessary. While she strives to meet the major teaching needs of the patient, the nurse should also be alert to detect erroneous health concepts. For example, a patient may incidentally remark that she is opposed to an immunization program for her three preschool children. The nurse should accept the responsibility of learning why the patient holds this view and of helping her to understand the value of immunization.

To ensure the success of any method selected the patient must be an active participant and must really want to learn. Sometimes a patient's resources, such as ability to see, hear, manipulate, or remember, may be impaired; in such a case the nurse may need to teach a relative or friend. Whoever the student is, the same principles of teaching apply. It is well to remember that some patients tend to want to be dependent and will prefer to have a relative care for them. The nurse must first help such patients accept a health goal of self-care compatible with their capabilities. Real rehabilitation is goal-directed toward independent status.

The Conference

The conference is an informal discussion, or conversation with a purpose, in which the nurse may both give information and also evaluate how well the patient is learning. Participation of the patient must be encouraged lest the conference become a lecture, a formal method which does not lend itself so well to the teaching of one patient but which may be effective in the teaching of several patients with the same condition, as in a clinic. Implementation of the conference method may well be carried out in the course of bedside care and treatments. Some of the uses of the conference method are:

1. To introduce the patient to the problem at hand; to arouse interest
2. To teach principles of care
3. To detect further areas in which the patient needs instruction
4. To evaluate patient progress in learning
5. To detect detrimental attitudes and inaccurate concepts which the patient may have about his condition, and to help the patient view his problems realistically

Demonstration and Return Demonstration

A procedure can best be taught by demonstrating how to carry out each step and requiring the patient to repeat or return the demonstration. The nurse demonstrates each time she carries out a treatment, e.g., a dressing. The patient should gradually participate more actively in each performance that he must learn to do at home until he gains a feeling of self-assurance and skill, as illustrated in the following description.

Teaching Mr. Smither to Irrigate His Colostomy Opening. Mr. Smither's teaching program began preoperatively when he was taught the principles of his diet and was introduced to the idea of defecation through an abdominal outlet. He learned to irrigate his colostomy opening by gradually imitating or repeating the steps of the procedure after observing the nurse. The first few times he watched intently and helped where he could by introducing the catheter and applying the dressings. Gradually he assumed greater responsibility for his irrigation so that he was able to carry through with this procedure under the supervision of the nurse. Before his discharge from the hospital he was able to irrigate his colostomy opening effectively and without fear as he sat at the toilet using the equipment he would use at home.

Question-and-answer Period

This method is allied to the conference and is valuable in evaluating learning. Indirect questioning is usually as effective as direct; some patients resent direct questions, but others, especially children, like this method, which may remind them of school and familiar routines.

Assistance from a Well-rehabilitated Person

Encouragement from a successfully rehabilitated patient aids a patient who is discouraged but who is trying to face reality. Seeing another person who has succeeded in handling a problem similar to one's own tremendously boosts morale. Rehabilitated patients may also know practical helpful hints that have proved effective in their own care. They are often valuable as liaison between patient and nurse. This method depends for its effectiveness upon the patient's "readiness" to make his adjustment, for without this he may feel a comparison instead of a challenge.

Visual Aids

Visual aids designed for lay use are helpful in lending interest and clarity to teaching. Aids such as the following have been found helpful:

1. *Illustrations* which may be drawn by the nurse or taken from pamphlets are helpful in teaching.

2. *Pamphlets* which may be obtained from insurance companies, pharmaceutical houses, national and local agencies, private organizations, state health departments, and surgical supply houses, or which may be written by the hospital personnel summarize essential teaching points. The nurse must review these pamphlets, however, to be certain they are accurate and appropriate for her patient.

3. *Scrapbooks* made by the patient as a learning device are helpful, especially in teaching general hygiene and diet.

4. *Posters,* especially those showing principles of care and diet, are often effective.

5. *Lists or written directions* for detailed information should be given the patient for study and reference at home.

6. *Films and filmstrips* are helpful in teaching groups.

7. *Magazines* such as *Today's Health* are an authoritive source to use in teaching patients.

8. *Prosthetic* devices, if needed, should be obtained and their use demonstrated before a patient is discharged.

CONCLUSION

The nurse must avoid teaching the patient highly technical material, such as pathology and the course of a disease. The nurse's guide in the selection of how much to teach should be, "What does this patient need to know in order to make a satisfactory adjustment?" The nurse is reminded that she must consult with the physician and the other members of the health team in order to plan a program of health guidance.

While each patient presents individual needs which influence his particular teaching program, there are over-all needs which patients present with each condition. Therefore, a teaching program for health guidance is most effective if it is planned to meet these general needs, with allowances for individual variations. The major aspects of care which patients need to be taught for each condition should be decided upon by the health team in each hospital and then written out for accessible reference. This might be done in the form of cards or a notebook. Such a planned program eliminates haphazard teaching, which may overemphasize some aspects of care and neglect others entirely; it is realized that the teaching program will not be carried out entirely by one nurse. It is also suggested that a record of teaching be kept. This may be in the form of a teaching record on the patient's chart or in a card file. Such a record helps in planning and carrying out the teaching program by showing the health team what instruction has been given and what remains to be taught.

SUMMARY

Guiding the patient in the selection and attainment of proper health goals is an important part of nursing. Teaching of patients is a cooperative venture undertaken by the entire health team and based on the individual needs of the patient.

The following principles of teaching can be applied in a program of health guidance:

1. A person must be helped to gain new insights lest he repeat unsatisfactory behavior patterns.

2. A person must be "ready" to learn.

3. The patient must feel motivated to learn.

4. Teaching must build upon the patient's present fund of knowledge and range of experience.

5. Teaching must be carried out on the patient's level of understanding.

6. Teaching must be complete, to avoid erroneous notions.

7. The teacher must consider the patient's home environment, social roles, and economic status.

8. The physical condition and strength of the patient must be considered in the planning of his teaching program, since the concentration span decreases with fatigue.

9. Learning is facilitated by judicious repetition.

Methods effective in teaching the individual patient are as follows:
1. Conference
2. Demonstration and return demonstration
3. Question-answer period
4. Encouragement from a successfully rehabilitated patient
5. Use of visual aids

A HEALTH–GUIDANCE PROGRAM IN CONNECTION WITH APPENDICITIS

Mrs. Brown, a neighbor, calls to say that her son Jimmy, age 12 years, has a severe stomach-ache and asks what to do for him. She further states that Jimmy awoke with pain in his abdomen and vomited once.

This is not an uncommon problem for a nurse to meet. People will ask for her advice in countless situations, and it is important that she realize her responsibilities and limitations. In considering which needs of Mrs. Brown and Jimmy the nurse must meet, some of the principles and methods of teaching presented in this chapter can be applied in review.

Initial Needs and Responsibilities Identified

Mrs. Brown needs to be instructed in the first-aid treatment for un-diagnosed abdominal pain. She needs, before this information is given, however, a great deal of reassurance if she is to be prevented from conveying her own apprehension to Jimmy. She should be encouraged to follow these instructions:
1. Call the physician.
2. Put Jimmy to bed.
3. Give him nothing by mouth.
4. Give him nothing by rectum.

The nurse must realize her legal and ethical limitations in giving advice in situations like this.
1. The nurse must instruct Mrs. Brown to call the physician.
2. The nurse must review the definition of *first aid,* which is "the immediate and temporary care given the victim of an accident or sudden illness until the services of a physician can be obtained." [3]

Subsequent Needs and How Met

Mrs. Brown reports later that the doctor has advised hospitalization of Jimmy because he feels the diagnosis is appendicitis. Mrs. Brown is apprehensive and asks:

[3] American Red Cross, "First Aid Textbook," Doubleday & Company, Inc., New York, 1957, p. 1. (Reprinted with permission of the American Red Cross.)

1. "Will they operate?"
2. "What will happen if I keep Jimmy home?"
3. "What is appendicitis?"
4. "How does the doctor know Jimmy has appendicitis?"

Mrs. Brown needs reassurance that Jimmy will be well cared for in the hospital and that her doctor's decision is competent and should be followed.

Jimmy needs reassurance that he will get better more rapidly in the hospital and that he will be home again in a week or so.

Mrs. Brown needs to have her questions answered adequately:

1. "Jimmy may have an operation if the doctor finds he has appendicitis. Much of the danger has been removed from this operation because of modern methods of care."

2. "If you keep Jimmy home, he may have a ruptured appendix and will then be much sicker. Early surgery can prevent rupture."

3. "Appendicitis is a condition in which the appendix, a small pouch off the intestine and serving no known useful purpose, becomes sore and festered."

4. "The doctor suspects appendicitis when the patient is 'sick to the stomach' and complains of abdominal pain which usually shifts later to the right side. In the hospital he can perform a blood test to help him be more sure of the diagnosis."

Much of the teaching of Mrs. Brown can be done in conference. She must feel free to question and discuss what she is worried about while you, the nurse, listen and help her view the problem realistically.

Another effective method that can be used to convey information about appendicitis is the use of a pamphlet. Such pamphlets are available from state public health departments and insurance companies.

BIBLIOGRAPHY

PEARCE, E. C.: "Nurse and Patient," 1st American ed., J. B. Lippincott Company, Philadelphia, 1953, pp. 3–60.

PEPLAU, H. E.: Themes in Nursing Situations (Power), Am. J. Nursing, pp. 1221–1223, October, 1953.

————: Themes in Nursing Situations (Safety), Am. J. Nursing, pp. 1343–1344, November, 1953.

————: Utilizing Themes in Nursing Situations, Am. J. Nursing, pp. 325–328, March, 1954.

————: Loneliness, Am. J. Nursing, pp. 1476–1481, December, 1955.

The Surgical Addict, Am. J. Nursing, p. 1164, October, 1955, abstract from W. A. Harvey (ed.), The Surgeon and Preventive Psychiatry, Ann. Surg., vol. 142, pp. 136–137, July, 1955.

3

INFLAMMATION AND WOUND REPAIR—
FACTORS AFFECTING HEALING AND THEIR
MANAGEMENT

The surgical patient has a wound to heal. The repair of that wound is a process involved in his over-all restoration to health. Factors which affect wound healing and those which influence the general condition of the patient are interrelated. It is the whole patient who is healing —not his incision alone. *The body responds to injury or irritation by a defense mechanism known as the inflammatory reaction.* The fundamental processes involved in this reaction are similar, regardless of the nature of the insult—whether it is physical, chemical, or bacterial. The reaction of tissues to surgical *incision,* a wound made with a sterile, sharp instrument, differs only in degree from that aroused by a *laceration,* a wound made by tearing. There are always bacteria on the skin which are carried into deeper tissues, even when the wound is a surgical incision. A greater degree of contamination occurs in a laceration.

SYMPTOMS

What are the symptoms of inflammation? What are the physiologic processes responsible for these symptoms? Mr. Smith has been admitted to the hospital with the diagnosis of *cellulitis,* inflammation of the subcutaneous tissues, of the right forearm. He states that 2 days ago he cut his arm on a piece of metal and that yesterday his arm became red, warm, swollen, and painful. The nurse notices also a limitation of motion. *Inflammation is a complex cellular response to irritation.*[1] There is first a dilatation of blood vessels surrounding the area of injury. An increased amount of blood flows through the dilated vessels, causing a red flush, *erythema.* The speed of circulation is next increased, so that the blood,

[1] Adapted from W. G. MacCallum, "A Textbook of Pathology," 7th ed., W. B. Saunders Company, Philadelphia, 1942, p. 143.

19

warmed from the body's interior, courses through the area too rapidly to cool; the result is local warmth.[2] Subsequently there is a slowing of the rate of blood flow; the endothelium becomes roughened; leukocytes adhere to the vascular walls and permeate them, allowing blood cells and serum to escape into the adjacent tissues. The cells and serum compose the inflammatory *exudate*,[3] which distends the tissues, causing swelling, pain, and occasionally loss of function, especially if a joint is involved.

PURPOSE OF THE INFLAMMATORY RESPONSE

Why does the body respond in this manner to irritation or injury? Inflammation has been described as a defense mechanism. There is an initial attempt to wash out the irritant by increasing the blood flow to the area. Next the leukocytes try to counteract or destroy the irritant by *phagocytosis*, a process of engulfment and digestion. Lastly the area is prepared for healing by liquefaction of the debris left by the encounter of irritant with leukocytes and absorption of this material into the lymph stream.[4]

HEALING PROCESSES

How does healing occur? What factors influence the type of reparation which will ensue? *Healing occurs by primary or secondary intention,*[5] *depending upon the number and virulence of bacteria present, the resistance of the patient, and the size of the tissue gap to be repaired.* Healing occurs by *primary intention* when the tissue gap is minimal and very few bacteria are present, as in a sutured incision. Here the edges of the wound can be directly approximated and sealed by the serum which coagulates along the line of closure. Connective tissue cells on each side of the incision proliferate and grow across the gap, along with blood vessel sprouts; new epithelium covers the wound surface. A linear scar, *cicatrix*, results. (See Fig. 1A.) On the other hand, if injury has caused the loss of tissue, or if the wound has been held open by pus or a foreign body, healing occurs by *secondary intention*. In this type of repair the gap is slowly filled in with *granulation tissue*, new connective tissue interlaced with budding capillaries. The tissues grow in from the sides of the wound and up from the bottom; epithelium covers the

[2] *Ibid.*, pp. 145–146.
[3] *Ibid.*, pp. 148–149.
[4] *Ibid.*, pp. 150–151.
[5] *Ibid.*, pp. 212–213.

surface. Scarring is extensive because of the size of the tissue gap that must be repaired. (See Fig. 1B.)

Scar tissue is not an identical replacement for tissues which have been destroyed; therefore function is often permanently impaired. Furthermore, scar tissue contracts in time and may cause both disfigurement and disability. In some patients the granulation tissue overgrows so that it extends above the skin surface, giving rise to so-called "proud flesh," which may be removed by electric cautery. In others a keloid, composed of dense connective tissue, forms along the scar. Since this may be both unsightly and tender, it is sometimes excised; this operation is known as a *kelectomy*.

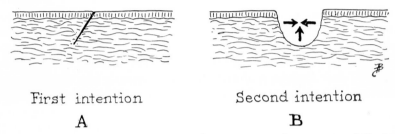

First intention   Second intention

A   B

FIG. 1. Diagram of the healing processes. Note that in first intention (A) tissues heal in direct approximation, while in second intention (B) granulation occurs in the direction of the arrows.

FACTORS INFLUENCING HEALING

What factors influence this reparative process? How does the patient's general condition affect his ability to heal a wound?

Nutrition

The patient's nutritional status is of paramount importance in repair. Especially important is protein, which is necessary for the growth of new tissues, the regulation of the osmotic pressure of blood and other body fluids, and the formation of prothrombin, enzymes, hormones, and antibodies. Chronic, severe protein deficiency, especially of albumen, leads to an increased incidence of wound infections, slower healing, and wound disruption. Patients with hypoproteinemia—lowered serum-protein level—have a lowered osmotic pressure of blood, so that fluid is allowed to escape from the vessels, causing edema and shock. A deficiency in protein and hence in prothrombin may cause hemorrhage. For these reasons the surgeon carefully evaluates his patient's protein level by using a serum test and by judging the general nutritional state from appearance, tissue turgor, and weight. When this evaluation indicates a need for protein, the surgeon will institute such replacement methods as time allows. One gram of protein per kilogram body weight is the approximate normal daily requirement, but it may be necessary to give more to a protein-deficient patient or to one whose needs are increased, as by fever or drainage. If surgery is imminent, the protein will be given intravenously in the form of whole blood, plasma, or amino acids proportionate to the need. However, such measures are costly because the kidneys rapidly excrete much of the protein. A more effective method, if time permits, is to give a high-protein diet, since more of the protein is utilized when absorbed from the gastrointestinal tract.

Also important in the healing process is an adequate supply of vitamins, especially vitamin C. Recall that healing is accomplished by connective tissue, interlaced with budding capillaries, filling in the defect. The newly formed cells lay down collagen, the main constituent of connective tissue. A deficiency of vitamin C interferes with the budding or growth of capillaries and deposition of collagen. Consequently the formation and maintenance of strong scar tissue are delayed or prevented.[6] In addition, because vitamin C influences the fragility of capillaries, a deficiency may predispose to hemorrhage. The surgeon can determine the vitamin C level by a blood test, in addition to studying the dietary history and observing symptoms such as bruises and bleeding gums. Deficiencies will be remedied by the administration of large doses of vitamin C orally or intravenously, as well as by correcting the diet to include foods rich in vitamin C.

Nutritional needs are interdependent. All the necessary amino acids and vitamins must be available to meet the needs of the body effectively. In the absence of an adequate caloric intake, body proteins and fats will be consumed for energy. One of the nurse's major responsibilities is to see that the patient actually consumes the food and water he needs. The patient is apt to have anorexia and weakness; he may need help in feeding. He will surely need encouragement and kindly persuasion. The food should be served in an appetizing manner. Frequent small feedings often help a patient consume the required amounts of nourishment.

Total Resources

Another important factor is the patient's resistance or recuperative power. *Reparation is a complex process invoking the patient's total resources, both physical and psychologic.* If the patient is weakened by infection, degenerative processes, deficiencies, neoplasm, or age, his

---

[6] Adapted from Charles C. Lund, Physiologic Principles in Wound Healing, *Therapeutic Notes*, Parke, Davis and Company, vol. 60, no. 3, p. 75, March, 1953. Dr. Lund is Assistant Professor of Surgery, Harvard University School of Medicine.

ability to recover or heal a wound is diminished. Interference with circulation is especially important. Since nutrients must reach the area of repair and waste products must be removed, it is imperative that an adequate circulation be maintained. Impaired circulation will delay or even prevent healing.[7] Also to be considered are the patient's spiritual and emotional resources, as they determine in large part how well and rapidly the patient will recover.

Infection

An essential factor related to reparation is infection, which prevents wound repair and may seriously endanger the life of the patient. Infection occurs when an overwhelming number of virulent pathogens enters the body when resistance is low, or when organisms which normally inhabit one part of the body are transferred to another where the tissues can not resist them. For example, when Mr. Smith cut his arm, the staphylococci normally present on his skin were transplanted into his subcutaneous tissue and caused an infection. Many leukocytes responded to the injury, and the battle which ensued produced a purulent discharge, pus. This discharge is composed primarily of leukocytes and bacteria in the inflammatory exudate and prevents healing by holding the wound edges apart. As long as the infection is confined to a small area, i.e., is *localized*, symptoms will be localized, too. If the bacteria overwhelm the bodily defenses, infection will spread throughout the body by way of the lymph and blood; the patient may be acutely ill with fever, prostration, and other constitutional symptoms. He will need fluids to combat dehydration resulting from fever and to aid in the elimination of wastes. Bedrest may be necessary to allow the body to conserve energy for healing. Drug therapy includes analgesics and antibiotics. Inasmuch as antibiotic drugs may cause serious reactions in sensitive patients or with prolonged administration, it is important to watch for such symptoms as gastrointestinal disturbances or dermatitis and to notify the surgeon should they occur.

WOUND CARE

Basic Principles

What local factors are important in the care of wounds? What therapeutic measures aid healing? What are the nursing responsibilities in such therapy? Recall that healing by primary intention is accomplished when the area to be healed is reduced to a minimum. This is achieved by approximating the edges of the wound as soon as possible under *aseptic conditions,* maintaining freedom from pathogenic organisms, and holding

[7] *Ibid.,* p. 74.

the closure secure with sutures or adhesive bridges. It is important to maintain the approximation until the scar tissue is as strong as the tissue it is replacing.[8] Early in the course of healing, either by primary or secondary intention, collagenous tissue being laid down is semifluid [9] and is easily disrupted unless the area is protected from motion and handling. Therefore, the body's natural tendency to put an injured part to rest by limiting joint motion or tensing muscles is reinforced through the application of dressings, slings, splints, and casts. Dressings further function to prevent exposure to pathogenic organisms and to absorb drainage.

When a wound is being dressed, it is important to avoid the abrupt removal of serum-adherent gauze; this is destructive to the delicate healing cells and is also painful. It may be necessary to moisten the dressing first with a sterile solution, such as hydrogen peroxide, normal saline, or boric acid.

The most important single factor in the care of wounds is the prevention of infection. As stated by C. W. Walter, M.D., "The primary cause of hospital wound infection is the spread of biologic organisms from infection to the environment by personnel doing routine dressings." [10] It is the responsibility of the nurse who dresses the wound under the direction of the surgeon to practice aseptic technic conscientiously. She is responsible for maintaining conditions of asepsis to assure a safe environment in which to dress wounds. She will see that the nursing unit is kept scrupulously clean and that instruments and dressings are kept sterile.

While the dressing technic will vary from one locality to another, depending upon surgeons' preferences and facilities, these fundamental principles of asepsis are basic to the care of all wounds:

1. Pathogenic organisms are present in dust which can travel on currents of air.

a. Windows and doors must be closed to prevent drafts of air.

b. Traffic must be reduced to a minimum. All persons not directly concerned with the dressing should be excluded from the room.

c. All exposed surfaces are considered contaminated.

2. Pathogenic organisms are present in salivary droplets, which can be expelled several feet into the air.

a. Talking must be reduced to a minimum.

---

[8] *Ibid.*, p. 74.

[9] Diana Clifford Kimber, Carolyn E. Gray, Caroline E. Stackpole, and Lutia C. Leavell, "Textbook of Anatomy and Physiology," 13th ed., The Macmillan Company, New York, 1955, p. 64. (Adapted with permission of The Macmillan Company.)

[10] Quoted from a personal communication from Carl W. Walter, M.D., Harvard Medical School, Cambridge, Mass.

b. Masks should be worn by all present if possible; most assuredly they must be worn for extensive wounds. Masks must be changed when moist or after being removed from the face. While masks strain out salivary droplets, they are not foolproof.

3. Bacteria are present on skin.

a. Hands must be washed thoroughly before and after each dressing and whenever contaminated.

b. Sterile gloves or instruments should be used to do the dressing.

c. Bandage scissors should be sterilized after each use.[11]

d. Soiled dressings should be wrapped in paper and burned.

e. The margins of the wounds should be cleansed with strokes moving outward from the wound with the solution ordered by the surgeon.

f. The patient must be taught to keep his hands away from the wound. Patients reacting from general anesthesia or those under sedation may handle their dressings without realizing it.

4. Bacteria can be carried through moist cloth by capillary attraction, as fluid travels through a wick.

a. Dressings wet with drainage must be changed or temporarily reinforced.

b. Sterile warm moist dressings must be dry on the outermost layer.

c. Moisture on a sterile field contaminates the entire setup.

It is important to realize that a wound already infected can be further contaminated by the introduction of more bacteria; therefore, all wounds require surgical aseptic technic. While antibiotics are extremely valuable in the prevention and treatment of infections, they in no way permit relaxation in the strict adherence to the principles of surgical asepsis. Staphlyococci, which are resistant to penicillin, streptomycin, and the tetracyline derivatives, are found in a high percentage of hospital personnel, who harbor the organisms in their nasopharynx. These carriers spread the organism to their patients by droplet and hand contact. The proper wearing of masks, use of instruments or gloves for dressings, and thorough handwashing are essential to the control of staphylococcic infections as well as of those due to other organisms which though initially sensitive to the antibiotic, later become resistant. Antibiotic therapy may only temporarily suppress bacterial growth, allowing delayed postoperative infections. A careful follow-up of discharged patients is necessary, therefore, for a true evaluation of hospital technic and morbidity rates.

Care of the Clean Wound

What is the specific care of the wound undergoing healing by primary intention? Primary repair occurs in a clean wound the edges of which

[11] Carl W. Walter, "The Aseptic Treatment of Wounds," The Macmillan Company, New York, 1948, p. 332. (Used with permission of The Macmillan Company.)

can be directly approximated as in a surgical incision. Serum coagulating along the line of closure seals the wound. Therefore, an incision usually needs only a dry, sterile dressing which is left undisturbed until changed by the surgeon approximately 5 to 7 days postoperatively.

Some surgeons omit the dressing and expose the wound to air, feeling that the serum seal is adequate protection against infection. In such cases it is essential that the bed linen coming into contact with the wound be kept meticulously clean.

How is the clean wound healing by secondary intention treated? Healing can be assisted by applying fine mesh gauze to which the fibrous strands can attach themselves; granulation is thereby stimulated. This gauze is usually kept moist to prevent drying out of the superficial cells. These dressings can be open to allow remoistening under strict aseptic conditions, but the gauze itself is usually not changed, unless necessary, to avoid tearing of the delicate granulation tissue. For the same reason the cleansing of the wound is limited to the margins. Some surgeons apply bland ointments to these wounds to aid healing and keep the area moist. This type of wound may be grafted early to cover the area.

Care of the Infected Wound

What therapeutic measures are necessary for an infected wound? While a certain amount of drainage, either serous, yellow-tinged, or serosanguineous (serum mixed with blood and therefore pink), may accompany extensive incisions and purports no danger, purulent drainage, containing dead cells and bacteria and therefore usually cream-colored, indicates that the wound is infected. There will frequently be an odor; the wound margins will be edematous and erythematous; and there will be gaps in the healing process.

A wound must be cleared of infection before it can heal. This is facilitated by the application of heat, usually moist for deeper penetration. Heat may also be applied to aid healing in an inflamed area which is not necessarily infected, and to relieve pain. Heat increases the local blood supply, which brings more leukocytes to the area and removes debris. More commonly, orders for warm moist dressings are superseding those for hot wet compresses, which tend to macerate the skin and actually delay healing. By allowing the dressings to dry intermittently the tissue turgor is maintained. The principles underlying the application of warm, moist dressings are:

1. A large area is enveloped in dressings. For example, an infected hand requires dressings to the elbow.

2. Digits are separated with gauze to prevent adherence to one another.

3. Sterile technic is used when the area is open or likely to open.

4. Ties, rather than pins, should be used to prevent transmission of the infection through accidental pricking.

5. Extremities are splinted in a position of function to permit the area a greater degree of rest and to allow maximum function in the event of *ankylosis*, stiffening, of the joint.

6. Materials used from within outward include:

a. Lubricant, if ordered, to protect margins (but lubricant tends to macerate the skin)

b. Gauze fluffed for greater absorption of moisture

c. Isotonic solution such as normal saline

d. Large absorbent pads

e. Moisture-proof material used, if ordered, to delay the drying process and to protect the bed when wet dressings are ordered

f. Flannel or towel

g. Outer wrapping

In lieu of warm moist dressings, sitz baths or foot or hand soaks are sometimes ordered. These, too, must include an extensive area to be effective. Soaks apply heat and cleanse at the same time. Dry heat may be applied with hot-water bags, electric pads, or lights.

Regardless of the type of heat applied, it is important to realize that sensitivity in an injured area may be increased or diminished. It is, therefore, essential to take precautions to avoid burning the patient.

Irrigations may be ordered to clean an infected wound and to stimulate granulation. The solution ordered may be warm, sterile saline, or an antibiotic. Sometimes a proteolytic enzyme is employed in the treatment of an infected, necrotic wound. The enzyme digests proteins such as pus and dead tissue. Several preparations are available; some are applied topically, others are given orally or parenterally. Surgical debridement, i.e., removal of foreign matter and devitalized tissues, may be necessary.

When the infected area is closed but well localized, i.e., restricted to a circumscribed area, incision and drainage may be performed in an aseptic environment. This treatment is usually followed by the application of heat to aid complete removal of material.

Nursing Responsibilities

In addition to assisting with these therapies, what further responsibilities does the nurse have? The nurse's observations of the wound are of great value in assisting the surgeon in planning the patient's treatment. Is the wound repairing evenly? Are there gaps in the healing process? Are the margins of the wound inflamed? Is the drainage increasing or decreasing in amount? What type of drainage is present?

Is there an odor to the drainage? Does the patient report a greater or lesser degree of discomfort?

The patient with a wound appreciates the tactful, empathetic nurse who provides privacy for the dressing procedure, avoids treatments at meal times, is reassuring and encouraging, and prevents unnecessary physical and emotional trauma.

It may be necessary to teach the patient or his relatives how to dress the wound at home. In this case the nurse will explain and demonstrate how to create and maintain a sterile field, how to dress the wound and dispose of soiled dressings. She will explain what equipment is necessary and where it can be obtained. She will encourage him to seek medical supervision as directed by his physician.

The therapeutic program for each patient will be designed to meet his needs. Many members of the health team will contribute to the therapy. The surgeon will depend upon the nutritionist for supplying necessary nutrients; upon the internist for treating concomitant disease; upon the clergy for spiritual encouragement; and upon the nurse for assisting with all phases of the program. The nurse must assume many roles and responsibilities. The contribution of each member of the health team is enhanced by the nurse who understands the purposes and methods of therapy, is conscientious in nursing care and teaching, and who, because of her intimate contacts and repeated opportunities, can stimulate the patient's will to recover.

SUMMARY

The inflammatory reaction is defensive in nature and is aroused by irritation. The cardinal signs of inflammation are redness, warmth, swelling, pain, and limitation of function. Wounds heal by first or secondary intention, depending upon the size of the area to be repaired and the degree of contamination present. Healing is facilitated by maintaining a high state of nutrition and by strengthening the patient's general recuperative powers. Wounds heal best when the edges can be closely approximated immediately following injury. Dressings, casts, slings, splints are protective devices preventing bacterial and mechanical trauma. Since infection prevents healing, the strict observation of the principles of surgical aseptic technic is of paramount importance in the care of wounds. A clean wound kept free from contamination needs a minimal amount of handling. An infected wound, however, must be converted into a clean area before healing can occur. This may be accomplished by the application of moist warmth, the administration of antibiotics, the enforcement of rest, and surgical drainage or debridement. Nursing responsibilities, in addition to assisting with these treatments in a tactful, reassuring manner, include observation and recording of the progress of repair, and teaching home care of the wound when necessary.

BIBLIOGRAPHY

ADAMS, R.: Prevention of Infections in Hospitals, *Am. J. Nursing*, pp. 344–348, March, 1958.

ALTEMEIR, W. A., and J. M. STEVENSON: Physiology of Wound Healing, in "Christopher's Textbook of Surgery," 6th ed., L. Davis (ed.), W. B. Saunders Company, Philadelphia, 1956, chap. 2, pp. 23–41.

——— et al.: Critical Reevaluation of Antibiotic Therapy in Surgery, *J.A.M.A.*, vol. 157, no. 4, pp. 305–309, Jan. 22, 1955.

BERRY, E. C., and M. L. KOHN: "Introduction to Operating-room Technique," McGraw-Hill Book Company, Inc., Blakiston Division, New York, 1955, pp. 22–29, 116–118.

COE, M.: "Introduction to General Pathology," Burgess Publishing Company, Minneapolis, 1954.

DOWLING, H. F., M. H. LEPPER, and G. G. JACKSON: Clinical Significance of Antibiotic-resistant Bacteria, *J.A.M.A.*, vol. 157, no. 4, pp. 327–331, Jan. 22, 1955.

LUND, C. C.: Physiologic Principles in Wound Healing, *Therapeutic Notes*, Parke, Davis and Company, Detroit, vol. 60, no. 3, pp. 74–76, March, 1953.

McCUTCHEON, M.: Inflammation, in "Pathology," 3d ed., W. A. D. Anderson (ed.), The C. V. Mosby Company, St. Louis, 1957, chap. 3, pp. 13–59.

POLLACK, H., and S. L. HALPERN: Therapeutic Nutrition, *National Academy of Sciences—National Research Council, Publication* 234, Washington, 1952.

ROBBINS, S. L.: "Textbook of Pathology," W. B. Saunders Company, Philadelphia, 1957, chap. 4, pp. 67–101.

WALTER, C.: "The Aseptic Treatment of Wounds," The Macmillan Company, New York, 1948, pp. 331–335.

4

NEOPLASMS AND SURGICAL TREATMENT

Since no tissue of the body is immune to the development of a *neoplasm* (*neo*, new + *plasm*, anything formed = new growth or tumor), surgical treatment may involve any area of the body. Therefore, this general discussion of tumor growth precedes the sections dealing with general surgery of the major areas of the body in order to serve as a basis for understanding the care required for the patient suffering from neoplastic disease of specific organs.

ETIOLOGIC FACTORS AND SYMPTOMS

A neoplasm is a more or less autonomous growth of cells performing no useful function. The exact cause is unknown, although some contributory factors, such as exposure to ionizing radiation (x-ray), radioactive elements (radium), and certain chemicals, have been identified. Awareness of the tumor occurs when it becomes palpable or visible, when it causes bleeding, or when it disturbs function by compression, obstruction, or destruction of a tissue or organ. Symptoms depend upon the organ involved. For example, a tumor of a bronchus causes a cough, while a tumor of the colon may cause bleeding or obstruction. A neoplasm of an endocrine gland may function as the involved gland but without regulation; for example, a tumor of a parathyroid gland may cause symptoms of hyperparathyroidism.

BENIGN NEOPLASM

Depending primarily upon its biologic behavior, a neoplasm may be classified as *benign* or *malignant*. A benign neoplasm is usually encapsulated and does not infiltrate or spread to other areas of the body, nor does it recur locally after its removal. It can usually be removed easily and completely. The suffix *-oma* usually indicates a benign tumor, while the prefix designates the type of tissue involved. For example, an *adenoma* (*aden,* glandular + *oma*) is defined as a benign tumor composed of cells of glandular origin.

MALIGNANT NEOPLASM

A malignant tumor, on the other hand, is composed of cells whose disorganized growth is unlimited. (See Fig. 2.) Any of the following features, or all of them, characterizes a malignant tumor:

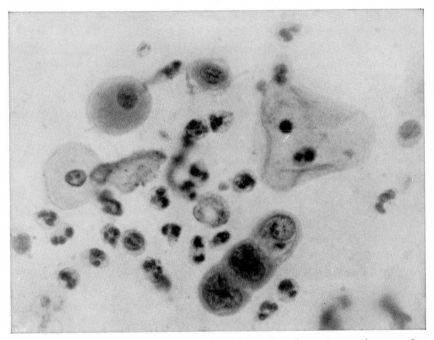

FIG. 2. The three large cells lying side by side in this photomicrograph are malignant. The larger scattered cells are normal; the smallest cells are leukocytes. (*Courtesy of the American Cancer Society, Inc.*)

1. Ability to *infiltrate* adjacent tissues by overcoming the barriers which delimit one normal tissue from its neighbors.

2. Ability to *invade* blood and lymph vascular channels—a feature probably related to the preceding point.

3. Ability of at least some of the tumor cells to survive when transplanted or after having entered the blood or lymph stream to be carried to distant points and to grow wherever they may fortuitously lodge, i.e., to *metastasize.* The point of origin of a malignant tumor is termed the *primary site,* and the area to which metastasis has occurred is known

as the *secondary site*. Metastases via the lymphatic vessels usually localize first in the proximal lymph nodes, which, as a result, become hard. Therefore, a palpable lymph node found in the region of a tumor strongly suggests that the tumor is malignant.

In addition to these features, a malignant tumor may undergo *ischemic necrosis,* i.e., death of tissues due to inadequate blood supply. It may breech a blood vessel, resulting in hemorrhage, or it may become infected, causing septicemia and bacteremia. *Carcinoma* is the term applied to a malignant tumor composed of epithelial cells, while *sarcoma* designates a malignant tumor of nonepithelial cells, usually of connective tissue. The eradication of malignant tumors is made difficult by reason of their ability to be transplanted, which permits local recurrence as well as distant metastasis from but few cells left behind or displaced locally during surgery.

DIAGNOSTIC METHODS

True early detection of tumors is possible in those sites accessible to visual examination: skin, nares, mouth, pharynx; larynx by laryngoscopy; bronchi by bronchoscopy; esophagus by esophagoscopy; certain areas of the stomach by gastroscopy; sigmoid and rectum by sigmoidoscopy or proctoscopy. In like manner also, the retina, bladder, vagina, peritoneum, and colon can be examined. As a general rule, palpation and roentgen examination, i.e., x-ray and fluoroscopy, result in somewhat later detection.

In order to determine whether a neoplasm is malignant or benign a microscopic examination of a sample of the involved tissue or cells is required. This tissue is obtained by excising the tumor en masse, in one piece, or by *biopsy,* which means the removal of a piece of the tissue during life by excision or by aspiration of fluid containing cells which have been shed by the tumor mass. The most rapid method of cytologic diagnosis is by *frozen section,* in which a portion of the tumor is removed at surgery, rapidly processed, and studied immediately. The report can be given to the surgeon, within a matter of minutes, while the patient is still on the operating-room table prepared for extensive resection, should a malignant neoplasm be detected. More effective processing takes a day or more. Excision and needle biopsy must be performed with caution to avoid spreading tumor cells. Local anesthesia for biopsy carries some hazard of seeding the tumor or distorting the specimen. The *Papanicolaou technic* of exfoliative cytology is based on the principle that desquamated cells from a malignant neoplasm retain their identifying characteristics. These specimens are obtained by aspiration of body fluids or by direct smear from a body cavity. (See Fig. 4.) This technic has proved valuable in detecting some asymptomatic, early, malignant neo-

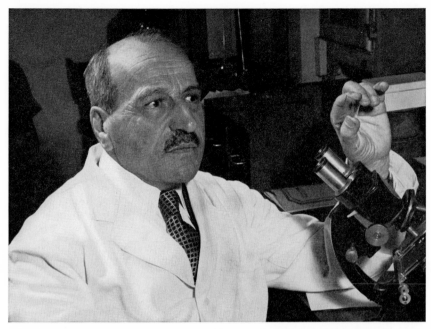

FIG. 3. Dr. George N. Papanicolaou, of the Cornell University Medical School, who developed a special cytologic technic for the detection of early carcinoma. (*Courtesy of the American Cancer Society, Inc.*)

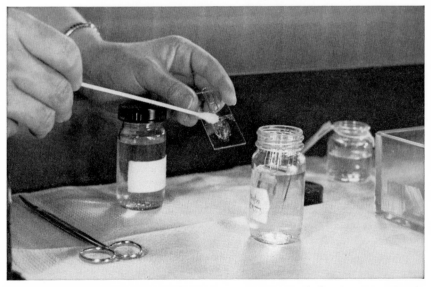

FIG. 4. Preparation of a Papanicolaou smear. (*Courtesy of the American Cancer Society, Inc.*)

plasms. Positive findings on cytologic study are meaningful. Negative findings may indicate only that the tumor was missed in obtaining the specimen.

TREATMENT

Extensive resection of the involved tissue, usually accompanied by removal of the regional lymph nodes, offers the best prognosis. Sometimes surgery is performed solely for palliation to relieve pain, obstruc-

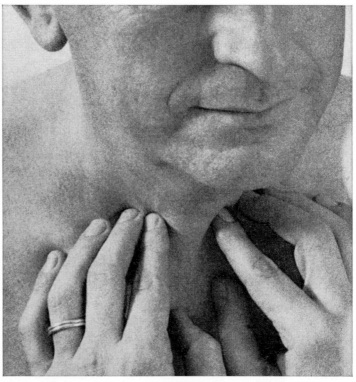

Fig. 5. The American Cancer Society emphasizes that early detection of cancer by means of periodic examinations increases the possibility of cure. Lymph nodes and glands are carefully examined as part of the annual checkup advocated by the American Cancer Society. (*Courtesy of the American Cancer Society, Inc.*)

tion, and compression. Radiation therapy may be employed as an adjunct measure postoperatively, either when it is felt that all neoplastic cells may not have been removed, or in the treatment of metastatic lesions. To this end, x-ray or radioactive isotopes may be used. Hormones may stimulate or suppress malignant growths, especially metastatic neoplasms from the prostate, mammary, or thyroid glands. Therefore, the hormonal supply may be reduced by surgery or increased by oral or parenteral administration, depending upon the particular situation. Operations performed for this purpose are *hypophysectomy*, removal of the pituitary gland; adrenalectomy; *oophorectomy*, removal of the ovaries; or *orchiectomy*, removal of the testes. The hormones administered are corticotropin, cortisone, stilbestrol, testosterone, or thyroxin.

NURSING RESPONSIBILITIES

The preoperative nursing care of a patient with a neoplasm often involves preparation for extensive and prolonged surgery. Therefore, the patient should be prepared so that he is in his optimal condition; this requires attention to his nutritional, fluid, and electrolytic balance. He should have excellent skin care and oral hygiene and should be active preoperatively if possible. Specific nursing measures in the preoperative and postoperative care required for the surgical treatment of neoplastic disease will be elaborated upon in following chapters.

The nurse shares the responsibility with other members of the medical profession for teaching the public the early symptoms of malignant neoplasm, for emphasizing the need for seeking medical attention early without arousing undue fear, and for encouraging submission to those examinations designed to permit detection of asymptomatic tumors and precancerous lesions. (See Fig. 5.) The American Cancer Society, Inc., publishes many pamphlets and excellent films designed to present the problem of cancer to the public in a realistic and helpful way. This society has listed the following seven danger signals of cancer: [1]

1. Unusual bleeding or discharge
2. A lump or thickening in the breast or elsewhere
3. A sore that does not heal
4. Persistent change in bowel or bladder habits
5. Persistent hoarseness or cough
6. Persistent indigestion or difficulty in swallowing
7. Change in a wart or mole

In conclusion, malignant neoplasms are 100 per cent fatal without early and adequate treatment. Cancer ranks second only to heart disease as a leading cause of death in the United States.[2] Many patients treated for cancer are symptom-free for 5 years and longer after surgery, and true cures have been reported. For the others, surgery usually allows greater comfort and usefulness during the remainder of their lives. Much re-

---

[1] Reprinted with permission from American Cancer Society, Inc., New York.

[2] "Cancer and the Nursing Profession," American Cancer Society, Inc., New York, 1957, p. 2.

search is being conducted to determine the cause of cancer and more effective methods of diagnosis and treatment. With the solution to these problems science will have made a remarkable contribution to the welfare of mankind.

SUMMARY

Neoplasms, which may be benign or malignant, can affect any part of the body. The primary cause is unknown although several contributory factors have been identified.

A benign tumor is usually encapsulated and neither spreads nor recurs after removal. Symptoms are due to compression primarily. A malignant tumor, on the other hand, is able to infiltrate, invade, and metastasize, setting up secondary growths. The only hope of cure for carcinoma or sarcoma is early diagnosis, employing biopsy or frozen section, and extensive surgical *extirpation,* or eradication.

The nurse shares the responsibility for encouraging the public to undergo physical examinations at regular intervals and to seek medical attention promptly should any of the symptoms suggestive of cancer develop.

BIBLIOGRAPHY

"Cancer Nursing," A joint project of the National Cancer Institute, U.S. Public Health Service, Federal Security Agency, and the New York State Department of Health, New York State Department of Health, Albany, 1950, pp. 48–51.

"A Cancer Source Book for Nurses," American Cancer Society, Inc., New York, 1950.

MOYER, C. A., and J. E. RHOADS: Neoplastic Disease—General Considerations, in "Surgery," J. G. Allen, H. N. Harkins, C. A. Moyer, and J. E. Rhoads (eds.), J. B. Lippincott Company, Philadelphia, 1957, chap. 10, pp. 163–174.

ROBBINS, S. L.: Neoplasia, in "Textbook of Pathology," W. B. Saunders Company, Philadelphia, 1957, chap. 3, pp. 30–66.

SOUTHWICK, H. W., and D. P. SLAUGHTER: Oncological Surgery, in "The Recovery Room," M. S. Sadove and J. H. Cross (eds.), W. B. Saunders Company, Philadelphia, 1956, chap. 16, pp. 404–412.

STANDARD, S., and H. NATHAN (eds.): "Should the Patient Know the Truth?" Springer Publishing Company, New York, 1955.

5

REQUIREMENTS FOR WATER, ELECTROLYTES, AND CALORIES, WITH SPECIAL REFERENCE TO PARENTERAL FLUID THERAPY

The normal daily requirements for water, electrolytes, and calories are increased by surgical conditions, general anesthesia, and operations. These experiences necessitate dietary restrictions and may be associated with abnormal losses.

REQUIREMENTS FOR WATER

How much water does a healthy adult need daily? Why is a liberal fluid intake important? Water, a basic component of all tissues, constitutes more than 50 per cent of the body by weight. Water is essential for all metabolic processes and functions in forming hormones and enzymes, transporting nutrients, excreting wastes, maintaining blood volume, regulating temperature, and bathing cells.

The greater volume of water is contained within the *intracellular compartment,* i.e., within the cells. The balance is contained within the *extracellular compartment,* i.e., outside the cells in the interstitial fluid and plasma. This compartment has direct access to the external environment through the excretory organs. (See Fig. 6.) The healthy adult daily excretes approximately 1,200 ml. water through the skin and lungs, 1,200 ml. through the kidneys, and 100 ml. through the intestines.[1] Water intake must balance output to maintain health. Therefore, a minimum of 2,500 ml. fluid intake in food and drink is required daily.

Dehydration

What special needs for fluids does the surgical patient have? When water loss exceeds intake, the person becomes dehydrated. This is a serious

[1] Adapted from Walter G. Maddock, Some Fundamentals in Water and Electrolyte Balance, *Ohio M.J.,* vol. 45, no. 5, p. 462, May, 1949.

condition which markedly interferes with recovery and may even terminate fatally. The surgical patient is especially prone to dehydration because oral intake is restricted before and after surgery; fluid is lost at surgery; there may be vomiting, drainage, fever, and excessive perspiration. The dehydrated patient is prone to surgical shock, thrombosis, and poor wound healing.

In dehydration the extracellular fluid is depleted first; in the absence of adequate treatment, loss of intracellular fluid then follows. The kidneys conserve much fluid by concentrating urine; therefore, in dehydration, oliguria occurs and the specific gravity of urine rises. The dehydrated patient will report weakness and thirst, his mucous membranes will be dry, skin turgor will be lost, and nitrogenous products will accumulate

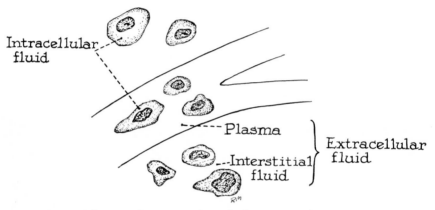

Intracellular fluid

Plasma

Interstitial fluid

Extracellular fluid

Fig. 6. Schematic drawing to show fluid compartments of the body.

in the blood.[2] Without treatment, shock ensues and is followed by coma and death. Treatment of dehydration is replacement—orally if possible, parenterally if necessary, in the form of physiologic solutions. The surgical patient usually needs 3,500 ml. or more of water daily.[3]

REQUIREMENTS FOR ELECTROLYTES

Dehydration is serious not only because of the water loss but also because of the loss of electrolytes, which govern the activity of the body, help maintain osmotic pressure of fluids, and assist in acid-base balance. An *electrolyte* is an electrically charged particle, or ion, which is released when acids, bases, and salts are put into solution.

Which electrolytes are needed most by the body? What are the conse-

[2] *Ibid.*, p. 465.
[3] *Ibid.*

quences of imbalances, and how are they treated? The major electrolyte of extracellular fluid is sodium; 6 Gm. is the normal daily requirement for a 70-Kg. male.[4] Sodium is lost in perspiration, vomiting, and diarrhea. Severe depletion causes collapse and may terminate fatally. Replacement is made with infusions of sodium chloride 0.9 per cent or with sodium lactate if the chloride ion is adequate. An excess of sodium can cause edema and loss of protein and potassium. Since the kidneys excrete excess electrolytes, it is important that replacement be made with caution in the presence of diminished renal function, which may occur early postoperatively.

Potassium is the principal electrolyte of intracellular fluid. In health adequate amounts are supplied in fruits and meats. When starvation is present, or where there has been tissue loss, as in burns and crush injuries, potassium deficiency may occur late. Severe depletion causes lassitude, muscular weakness, and paralysis, since potassium plays a role in the transmission of electrical impulses for muscular activity. Replacement is made with potassium chloride 0.2 per cent or with potassium acetate. An excess of potassium can cause death from heart block due to myocardial hyperirritability.

Electrolytes function interdependently, and replacement is often made in multiple deficiencies with physiologic solutions which contain several electrolytes in concentrations similar to those in body fluids. Three such solutions are those of Ringer, Darrow, and Hartmann.

ACID–BASE BALANCE

What is meant by acid-base balance? What are the consequences of an imbalance, and how are they treated? Closely associated with dehydration and electrolyte deficiencies is a disturbance in acid-base balance.[5] This balance is maintained by three mechanisms: carbonic acid, sodium bicarbonate, and sodium acid phosphate in the blood and tissues; by plasma protein and hemoglobin buffers; and by respiratory and renal functions. Alkalosis, i.e., plasma pH over 7.4, may result from continuous gastric drainage or excessive vomiting with attendant loss of the chloride ion. It may also occur with hyperventilation induced by severe pain or fear, in which instances the patient exhales an excess amount of carbon dioxide. The patient will have tetany, increased carbon dioxide–combining power, and slow respirations. The treatment is chloride replacement with sodium chloride. Severe cases warrant the use of ammonium chloride

[4] H. Pollack and S. Halpern, Therapeutic Nutrition, *National Academy of Sciences—National Research Council, Publication* 234, Washington, 1952, p. 41.

[5] Adapted with permission from Raymond W. McNealy and Jacob A. Glassman, "Surgical Care," Graduate Press, Inc., Maywood, Ill., 1951, pp. 8–13.

orally or potassium chloride 0.2 per cent intravenously. Acidosis, i.e., pH below 7.4, may result from the loss of alkaline secretions through diarrhea and fistulas, or from the formation of acid metabolites in dehydration, shock, starvation, or diabetes. The patient will have rapid, deep respirations and decreased carbon dioxide-combining power. Treatment is replacement of the sodium ion with sodium lactate, sodium bicarbonate, or sodium chloride.

NURSING RESPONSIBILITIES IN FLUID BALANCE

What responsibilities does the nurse have regarding the patient's fluid balance? It is important to keep an accurate record of intake and output in the surgical patient to determine whether he is balancing his output with adequate intake and whether his kidney function is normal. All intake of fluid and semifluid foods, such as ice cream and gelatin, must be recorded. Urine, drainage, and vomitus are measured and recorded. Sometimes an estimation of fluid loss in perspiration and stool is requested. Fluid intake must be adequate to balance losses and to promote a urine output of 1,000 to 1,500 ml. daily with a specific gravity of 1.030.[6]

Keeping the intake-output record is an important nursing responsibility because the physician uses these data in evaluating the patient's need for fluids. More important than keeping records, however, is the nurse's role in providing the patient with a variety of fluids and encouraging him to consume an adequate amount daily. She must also stress the value of an optimal fluid intake in health as well as in illness.

REQUIREMENTS FOR CALORIES

How is the caloric requirement affected by a surgical experience? What solutions can be given parenterally to meet the caloric need? In addition to fluids and electrolytes, the body needs calories to supply energy, heat, and reserves. When oral intake is inadequate or prohibited, calories must be supplied parenterally. It is far easier to supply fluids and electrolytes than it is to maintain an adequate caloric intake parenterally. In health a 70-Kg. male needs 2000 to 3000 calories plus 100 to 150 Gm. protein daily, depending upon his activities. In illness or under the stress of a surgical experience his requirement may be 3000 to 5000 calories daily. These may be supplied with infusions of protein, such as amino acids, or of blood in selected cases. Glucose 5 or 10 per cent is a common source of calories. Alcohol 5 per cent may be given to certain patients but may cause inebriation and phlebitis. At best, these furnish fewer calories than required. Intravenous administration of fat emulsions to furnish more

[6] W. G. Maddock, *op. cit.,* p. 463.

calories is in the experimental stage; it is especially valuable for selected surgical patients who are restricted in oral intake for prolonged periods and for those who have difficulty in the assimilation of foods. Vitamins are important nutritive adjuncts; all can be administered parenterally as well as orally.

NURSING RESPONSIBILITIES IN PARENTERAL FLUID THERAPY

What are the nursing responsibilities in the parenteral administration of water, nutrients, and electrolytes?

Care of the Patient

When bodily requirements must be met parenterally, the nurse will prepare the patient by explaining what is to happen and by assuring him that the treatment is not necessarily an indication of the severity of his condition. The physician may order that the patient be weighed or ambulated prior to the infusion. The patient should be made as comfortable as possible and a site chosen to allow maximum freedom of motion. During the infusion the nurse must anticipate and meet the patient's needs, especially if his activity is restricted. Frequent position change is necessary to his well-being and comfort.

If possible, infusions should be started early in the day to allow undisturbed rest at night. When a continuous infusion is necessary, the nurse must ensure a constant reservoir of solution and prevent air embolism by adding the next flask while the tubing is still full of fluid. Sometimes when intravenous fluid therapy is necessary for a prolonged period of time, the infusion is made through an indwelling cannula or catheter. When such a method is used for intermittent infusions, heparin is used at the site to prevent coagulation in the catheter or cannula between infusions.

Preparation of the Infusion

Fluids given parenterally for hydration and nutrition should be *isotonic*, or *isosmotic*, i.e., having the same osmotic pressure as blood. All fluids must be clear and opened immediately prior to use. Strict aseptic technic is necessary in the administration of an infusion.

Management of Reactions

One of several types of reaction may occasionally occur with intravenous infusions. The nurse must be vigilant to detect symptoms early. In general the major reactions can be classified as bacterial, biochemical, or mechanical.

Contamination of the fluid by live bacteria or by *pyrogens*, bacterial debris sometimes found in water after sterilization, may cause chills and fever, rapid pulse and respirations, nausea, and headache. The infusion should be discontinued and the physician notified immediately.

Biochemical reactions include those due to allergy or to hemolysis of red blood cells. Urticaria, dyspnea, wheezing, cyanosis, edema, and chills are manifestations of an allergic reaction. The physician may order that the infusion be discontinued or continued after or with antihistamine therapy. A hemolytic reaction will occur when a blood transfusion is incompatible with the recipient's blood. The most common symptoms include lumbar pain, hematuria, oliguria, abdominal cramps, nausea and vomiting, and chills. The transfusion must be discontinued immediately and the physician notified.

Mechanical reactions include those due to air or blood embolism, too rapid infusion, or infiltration of tissues around the vein. An embolic reaction is most commonly due to a delay in adding the next flask until all the solution has run through allowing the tubing to fill with air and the blood to clot in the needle. When this has occurred, it is best to select another site and restart the infusion with new equipment. It is also important to expel all air from the tubing initially before the infusion is started. Symptoms of an embolic reaction include sudden pain in a part and circulatory and neurologic disturbances. The physician must be notified immediately. Fluids infused too rapidly will overload the circulatory system, causing cardiac and pulmonary embarrassment. Elderly patients are especially prone to this reaction and should, therefore, be given infusions at a slower rate of speed. A speed reaction usually requires only that the rate of infusion be reduced. Infiltration indicates that the needle is out of the vein and requires that another site be selected to restart the fluids. Since infiltration with some solutions may cause the area to slough, the nurse must be vigilant for very early signs indicating that the solution is not running intravenously. Symptoms manifested during an infusion do not necessarily indicate a reaction but may rather be due to the patient's condition. Therefore, the student in nursing should consult with the supervisor or physician before discontinuing an infusion, unless symptoms are severe.

GENERAL INSTRUCTIONS FOR THE ADMINISTRATION OF SPECIFIC FLUIDS [7]

Protein. This substance is an excellent culture medium; therefore, add nothing to the solution. Infuse intravenously or subcutaneously as directed. Run slowly at 40 gtts. per minute to prevent flushing, cyanosis, and nausea. Watch for an embolic or pyrogenic reaction.

[7] Adapted with permission from a paper entitled "Commonly Used Intravenous Fluids," by Gerschen L. Schaefer, M.D., formerly of Mt. Sinai Hospital, Chicago.

Plasma. This fluid is transfused slowly with nothing added. Because plasma protein precipitates and may cause an embolic reaction, a filter is necessary.[8] Watch for an allergic, hemolytic, or pyrogenic reaction.

Blood. Blood must be typed and cross-matched so that the recipient's blood and that of the donor are compatible. Serious reactions, sometimes fatal, occur when transfused blood is incompatible with that of the recipient. Therefore, it is extremely important to verify the patient's name and blood type with the label on the flask. Blood is started only with physiologic saline solution. Add nothing to blood. Watch for hemolytic or allergic reactions and hyperpotassemia. Run slowly unless otherwise directed. Stop immediately with any reaction. The surgeon may continue the transfusion with antihistamine therapy if the reaction is mild and allergic in nature.

Glucose (dextrose). This solution may serve as a vehicle for vitamins or drugs. A 5 or 10 per cent solution of glucose in saline solution or distilled water may be given intravenously, but the 10 per cent solution may cause phlebitis. For subcutaneous administration only the 5 per cent solution is used. Infuse intravenously at 50 to 60 gtts. per minute unless otherwise ordered.

Saline. This solution may have vitamins or drugs added. A 0.9 per cent solution is given intravenously at 50 to 60 gtts. per minute unless otherwise directed. Saline solution may also be administered subcutaneously. Watch for pulmonary edema by observing the color, pulse, and respirations. Record the urine output; report if it is insufficient in amount.

Potassium. A 0.2 per cent solution of this electrolyte in saline solution is administered intravenously at 40 gtts. per minute. Symptoms to watch for are those of excess potassium, such as a slow and irregular pulse, irregular respirations, fall in blood pressure, paresthesias, and confusion. Record the urine output, and report if it is insufficient in amount.

Vitamin B. This solution is infused slowly intravenously or subcutaneously as directed. Watch for a thiamine reaction manifested by dyspnea, stridor, and shock.

SUMMARY

Water comprises more than 50 per cent of the body by weight and is contained within the intracellular and extracellular compartments. The major electrolyte of intracellular fluid is potassium; of extracellular, sodium. Dehydration and electrolyte imbalance result in profound physiologic and biochemical changes.

In a surgical experience the normal daily requirements for water, electrolytes, and calories may be increased. The surgical patient is com-

---

[8] L. Unger, Human Blood Plasma and Plasma Substitutes, *Am. J. Nursing,* p. 51, January, 1954.

monly maintained on parenteral fluid therapy until oral intake can be resumed. An accurate intake-and-output record is invaluable in helping the surgeon to determine the patient's needs for fluids.

The parenteral maintenance of an adult who has restricted oral intake, as in a surgical experience, usually includes the following:

1. Approximately 2,500 ml. water daily minimum to meet losses, prevent dehydration, and maintain renal function

2. 3000 to 5000 calories met by 5 or 10 per cent glucose solutions, fat emulsion, and protein solutions

3. Sodium, potassium and chloride replacement as needed following the immediate postoperative period when urine output is satisfactory

4. Vitamins A, B complex, C, and possibly D

Fluids used parenterally for hydration and nutrition must be isotonic, sterile, and pyrogen-free. Glucose and saline solutions may serve as vehicles for the administration of drugs and vitamins, but protein solutions, blood, and plasma should have nothing added.

It is the nurse's responsibility to prepare the patient for the infusion and to promote his comfort and well-being during this treatment. She will watch for a reaction of a bacterial, biochemical, or mechanical nature and notify the physician immediately should symptoms occur.

BIBLIOGRAPHY

ELMAN, R.: Fluid Balance from the Nurse's Point of View, *Am. J. Nursing,* pp. 222–225, April, 1949.

FARR, H. W.: Fluid and Electrolyte Balance with Special Reference to the Gastrointestinal Tract, *Am. J. Nursing,* pp. 826–831, July, 1954.

GAMBLE, J. L.: "Chemical Anatomy, Physiology, and Pathology of Extracellular Fluid," 6th ed., Harvard University Press, Cambridge, 1954.

LOWE, C. N.: Principles of Parenteral Fluid Therapy, *Am. J. Nursing,* pp. 963–965, August, 1953.

MACBRYDE, C. M.: Dehydration, in "Signs and Symptoms," 3d ed., J. B. Lippincott Company, Philadelphia, 1957, chap. 29, pp. 703–745.

MADDOCK, W. G.: Some Fundamentals in Water and Electrolyte Balance, *Ohio M.J.,* vol. 45, no. 5, pp. 462–474, May, 1949.

ZIMMERMAN, B., Management of Fluid and Electrolytes in Surgical Practice, in "Christopher's Textbook of Surgery," 6th ed., L. Davis (ed.), W. B. Saunders Company, Philadelphia, 1956, chap. 5, pp. 132–142.

6

MAJOR POSTOPERATIVE COMPLICATIONS

Postoperative complications are best prevented. Sometimes, how-ever, because of the nature of the patient's condition, anesthesia, and surgery, complications may occur. In addition to causing pain and suf-fering, they prolong the period of hospitalization and disability and raise the cost of medical care. Postoperative complications can often be pre-vented or minimized by skilled effort and constant vigilance on the part of the health team. This chapter deals with conditions which may com-plicate any surgery; it precedes the chapters on preoperative and post-operative care because an understanding of these complications is basic to rendering effective care throughout the surgical experience. In each of these postoperative complications the nurse will give first aid to the patient while the surgeon is being called and then prepare the equip-ment for anticipated therapeutic measures. All care must be given deftly and calmly to reduce the patient's apprehension.

SHOCK

Probably the most common and one of the most serious complications encountered postoperatively or with trauma is *shock*. This term is used to describe a syndrome, the essential feature of which is a diminished volume of circulating blood with resultant tissue *anoxia*, i.e., oxygen lack in the tissues. This reduction in blood volume, *hypovolemia*, can be an actual loss, as when blood leaves a vessel through a cut or when plasma leaves the body through a burn. Sometimes the loss is relative, as when, in response to stress, massive vasodilatation enlarges the vascular bed out of proportion to the amount of fluid circulating. Many factors, such as the following, play a role in causing shock: fear; prolonged anesthesia; extensive surgery, especially when much visceral manipula-tion has been necessary; and severe trauma. (See Table 1.)

TABLE 1   FACTORS CONTRIBUTING TO SHOCK *

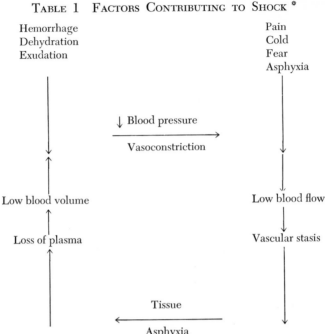

Hemorrhage
Dehydration
Exudation

Pain
Cold
Fear
Asphyxia

↓ Blood pressure

Vasoconstriction

Low blood volume

Low blood flow

Loss of plasma

Vascular stasis

Tissue

Asphyxia

* Diagrammatic representation of chain of events contributing to the production of inadequate circulation following which irreversible shock can occur. (*Reprinted with permission from I. S. Ravdin and J. E. Eckenhoff, Shock, in "Christopher's Textbook of Surgery," 6th ed., L. Davis (ed.), W. B. Saunders Company, Philadelphia, 1956, chap. 4, p. 101.*)

Symptoms

The symptoms of shock are directly related to a decreased circulating blood volume. The systolic blood pressure drops below 100 mm. mercury; the heart beats faster and harder to compensate for the reduced blood volume, and therefore the pulse rate rises while force and volume progressively grow weaker. Tissue anoxia develops, causing the formation of acid metabolites; [1] respirations become deeper and faster as these metabolites affect the respiratory center in the medulla; cyanosis occurs. As cellular metabolism fails, body temperature falls below 97°F. (36.1°C.); the skin becomes cool and moist. Simultaneously, the adrenal glands are reacting to shock as to other stress situations, causing constriction of the peripheral blood vessels in an effort to service the viscera with available blood. Kidney failure occurs, evidenced by oliguria

[1] C. Fox and S. Lasker, Fluid Therapy in Surgical Emergencies, S. *Clin. North America*, vol. 35, no. 2, p. 340, April, 1955.

progressing to anuria. The patient grows increasingly restless but usually retains consciousness until the terminal stage.

Prevention

Preventive measures include adequate preoperative explanation and reassurance to minimize fear. The surgeon prepares the patient for the impending surgical procedure; the nurse supports and reassures the patient in his decision to undergo surgery. Adequate preoperative build-up, especially of protein levels, helps prevent shock. Blood or plasma administered before, during, and after surgery, as necessary, is effective in the prevention as well as the treatment of shock. Sometimes elastic bandages are applied to both legs from ankle to groin to help move the blood from the large veins into the arteries to keep the blood moving in the vital areas.

Treatment

Postoperative shock usually occurs early. When the several symptoms of shock are recognized, the nurse should place the patient in bed with head low and feet raised, if not contraindicated, to encourage circulation of blood to the vital centers of the brain. Body temperature should be maintained at normal levels; external heat applied in excess of need serves only to increase fluid loss through perspiration and to deepen the state of shock. If a hot-water bag is ordered, it should be well covered to avoid burning the patient, who during shock is more susceptible to burns.

The major aim of treatment in shock is to increase the blood volume. This is best achieved by the administration of plasma, or of blood if there has been hemorrhage, but 5 per cent glucose in distilled water may be used initially if plasma or blood is not readily available. A plasma expander, such as dextran, may also be used satisfactorily in the treatment of shock.[2] The fluids are allowed to run rapidly, unless this is contraindicated by the patient's condition.

Pain, which enhances the state of shock, must be relieved, but the liberal use of narcotics is prohibited because of their general depressing action. Stimulants, such as adrenal cortical extract, or vasoconstrictors, such as levarterenol (Levophed), may be used. Narcotics and stimulants must be administered subcutaneously with caution because circulation is so impaired that the drug will not be absorbed readily; as circulation improves, there is danger of the drug being absorbed suddenly with overwhelming effects. Levarterenol is administered intravenously in a 5 per cent glucose solution. Because a severe hypertension may suddenly be

[2] Use of Dextran in the Civilian Hospital, *What's New*, Abbott Laboratories, no. 195, pp. 1–2, Summer, 1956.

produced by the administration of levarterenol, the blood pressure should be taken at least every 2 to 5 minutes, and the patient should be under the constant supervision of a physician or nurse.

HEMORRHAGE

Another serious complication is *hemorrhage,* loss of blood from the vascular system. This may be due to trauma, as when a blood vessel is lacerated; to the slipping of a ligature in surgery; or to faulty coagulation, most commonly caused by insufficient prothrombin formation, as in liver disease. (See Table 2.) Visible blood loss is described as *overt.* Sometimes bleeding is into a body cavity, where only skilled observation of symptoms can aid in its detection; this bleeding is called *occult.*

TABLE 2   CHEMISTRY OF BLOOD COAGULATION *

Prothrombin
- Calcium ions
- Thromboplastin
- Ac-globulin
- Platelet derivatives
- Antihemophilic factor
- PTC
- Other activators

- Heparin
- Antithromboplastin
- Other inhibitors

Thrombin

Fibrinogen $\longrightarrow$ Fibrin + Fibrinopeptide
+
Antithrombin
↓
Inactive thrombin

* Conversion of prothrombin (which is present in plasma and synthesized in the liver in the presence of vitamin K) to thrombin requires catalytic activators such as calcium ions and thromboplastin. Heparin and other inhibitors check the reaction to keep blood normally in a fluid state. Thrombin reaction with fibrinogen produces a fibrin clot which soon retracts with the aid of platelets. Thrombin has a short survival time because it is inactivated by plasma antithrombin. This formula is important from the viewpoint of hemorrhage and thrombosis. Factors such as excess heparin or want of prothrombin prevent coagulation and can cause hemorrhage; failure of prothrombin inhibition or inactivation of thrombin can increase the possibility of thrombosis. (*Reproduced with permission from Walter H. Seegers, The Blood Clotting Mechanism, Theraupeutic Notes,* PARKE, DAVIS AND COMPANY, *vol. 61, no. 2, p. 44, February, 1954. Dr. Seegers is Professor of Physiology, Wayne University College of Medicine.*)

Symptoms

The symptoms are due to decreased blood volume and anoxia, as in shock. Indeed, shock accompanies any prolonged or massive hemorrhage. The patient is rapidly dehydrated and will have extreme thirst and vertigo. He will be pale, restless, and apprehensive. He may see spots before his eyes and/or experience *tinnitus,* ringing in his ears. Respirations, of a sighing nature, are described as "air hunger." Early the red blood cell count and hematocrit will be normal; hemoconcentration occurs with dehydration so that the count will be elevated, but as the body compensates for blood loss by pouring interstitial fluid into the vascular system, anemia will be evident.

If bleeding is into the chest cavity, there will be signs of heart and lung compression; if into tissues, swelling and pain will be noted. Bleeding from an artery, evidenced by bright red blood issuing in spurts, is usually more serious than venous bleeding, marked by darker blood flowing in a steady stream, or than capillary oozing. When bleeding is massive and prolonged, the patient is in danger of death from exsanguination.

Prevention

Preventive measures include ensuring adequate protein and vitamin C levels preoperatively. Vitamin K, which supplies the precursor to prothrombin, is given the patient with a bleeding tendency, which is due to a deficiency of prothrombin, as in the presence of jaundice. Careful, adequate hemostasis in surgery, gentle operative technics, and packing when indicated help prevent hemorrhage.

Treatment

Early recognition of hemorrhage is a lifesaving responsibility shared by surgeon and nurse. Therapy must be instituted promptly. The nurse will be especially alert to the possibility of hemorrhage early postoperatively or late in the first week after operation when sutures are being absorbed. If bleeding is overt and pressure can be applied safely, it is important to realize that arterial flow is interrupted between the bleeding site and the heart; venous flow is interrupted distad to the area. If bleeding is incisional, a pressure dressing can be applied. The patient should be positioned in dorsal recumbency with head lowered unless bleeding is from the head, in which case it should be elevated. If the hemorrhage is from an extremity, elevation of that part is necessary. An ice bag and pressure dressing can be applied to the area. It is essential to reassure the patient and to promote quiet, since apprehension may increase bleeding. Blood-stained linen and dressings should be saved for the surgeon to see to help him approximate blood loss. Transfusion of whole blood is the treatment of choice in hemorrhage. Narcotics may be ordered to allay apprehension and quiet the patient. Sometimes the local application of coagulants such as Gelfoam and thromboplastin is feasible. The patient may need to return to surgery for resuturing.

THROMBOEMBOLIC PHENOMENA

Another serious postoperative complication is clotting within the blood vessels. When circulation is slowed, as it is following general anesthesia and postoperative inactivity, a clot, *thrombus,* may form on the wall of the blood vessel. *Phlebothrombosis* (*phleps,* vein + *thrombosis,* a becoming curdled = formation of a blood clot within a vein) is usually not attended by symptoms, but there may be calf pain and a palpable vein. Should part of this thrombus dislodge and be carried in the blood stream as an *embolus,* occlusion of the blood supply to a vital area could cause sudden death. (See Fig. 7.)

One dramatic type of embolism is pulmonary embolism with infarction. The embolus occludes the pulmonary artery, causing necrosis of that part of the lung beyond the obstruction and right heart failure. This type of embolism usually occurs in a patient who has been progressing satisfactorily and is walking for the first time after the operation. The patient will experience sudden severe chest pain, hemoptysis, and dyspnea; he will be cyanotic. If he survives this experience initially, oxygen and anticoagulant drugs will be used in his treatment.

Sometimes inflammation of the vascular wall is associated with the clot, a condition called *thrombophlebitis.* This patient is in less jeopardy than the one with silent phlebothrombosis, since the tendency toward embolism is less marked and symptoms aid early detection. Symptoms include a palpable vein, swelling, pain in the calf when the foot is dorsiflexed (positive Homan's sign), increased clotting time, and sometimes constitutional symptoms of infection, such as fever and increased pulse rate.

Prevention

Preventive measures against all three types of thromboembolic phenomena are the same. Phlebothrombosis is prevented by avoiding venous stasis, i.e., stagnation. A better return of venous blood to the heart can be aided by encouraging activity, especially walking, and by foot and leg exercises, such as alternate flexion and extension. Prolonged flexion of pelvis and knees is to be avoided, since circulation is impeded at the sites of flexion. Therefore, the postoperative patient should be fully extended several times daily while in bed; knee rests should not be provided. It should be noted that "dangling" encourages venous stasis and that sitting in a chair still allows flexion. Abdominal distention or constriction with tight binders also hinders circulation and should be avoided. Elastic bandages applied to the legs help prevent venous stasis. Another helpful measure is adequate hydration to keep the blood thin enough to flow readily.

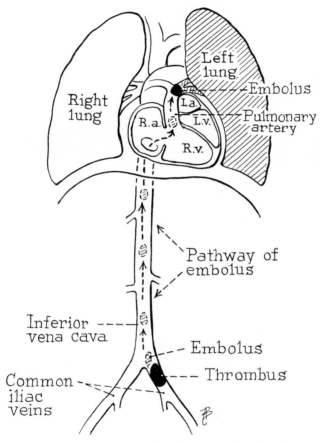

FIG. 7. Pulmonary embolism. Note the thrombus situated in the left iliac vein and the pathway taken by the embolus to reach and occlude the left branch of the pulmonary artery.

It may be necessary to administer anticoagulant drugs, such as heparin or dicoumarin, to retard or prevent the extension of a thrombus. Heparin is given intravenously or intramuscularly and apparently prevents the formation of thrombin from prothrombin. It has an immediate but short-lived action when administered intravenously. The dosage is determined for each patient on the basis of clotting-time determinations prior to each dose. Bishydroxycoumarin (Dicumarol) is given orally and prevents the formation of prothrombin. It has a slower, more prolonged action. Daily studies of prothrombin levels are made to determine dosage. Heparin and dicoumarin may be used together. When either drug is given prophylactically or therapeutically, the patient must be watched for evidences of hemorrhage, such as hematuria or bleeding from the wound. The patient must be protected from trauma. Vitamin K must be readily available for the patient on dicoumarin therapy to counteract possible serious hemorrhage.

Treatment

Once a thrombus is suspected the patient should be kept in bed until the surgeon has evaluated his condition. Treatment varies considerably. Anticoagulants are commonly used, as described above. Elastic bandages are applied from ankle to groin. Fluid intake is encouraged. Bed rest is usually ordered, especially if the thrombus is in the femoral vein. Warm, moist dressings are applied to the legs, which are elevated to encourage venous return. A cradle may be used to relieve the patient of the weight of the bedding. Every effort is made to prevent embolism. Therefore, the legs are *never massaged*. Deep-breathing and coughing exercises are forfeited, as such activity could dislodge an embolus into the chest. Sometimes the vein is ligated above the thrombus to prevent embolism, or the thrombus may be excised. Occasionally a sympathetic nerve block is performed to reduce vasospasm and improve circulation.

ATELECTASIS

One of the most common surgical complications is *atelectasis*, a condition in which a lung collapses in part or whole. It is caused by aspiration of mucus or vomitus which plugs the bronchial passages. The air in the lung beyond the obstruction is slowly absorbed, with the result that the affected part of the lung collapses. (See Fig. 8.) This may occur in any patient who has been unconscious or whose pharyngeal reflexes are diminished; therefore, it is found in patients who have had general anesthesia. Since the anesthetist is in constant supervision of the patient's respiratory functioning during surgery, atelectasis is more likely to occur in the recovery period unless the patient is very closely attended.

Symptoms

When atelectasis is impending, the patient's pulse will be rapid; respirations will be rapid and shallow; apprehension or restlessness may be present. With actual atelectasis, respirations may be unilateral, i.e., the

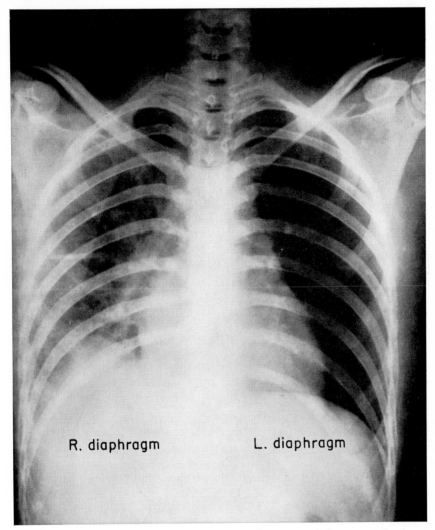

R. diaphragm   L. diaphragm

Fɪɢ. 8. Atelectasis. Note in this roentgenogram the increased density in the lower right lung field, indicating collapse of the right lower lobe. The space created by collapse is partially filled by elevation of the right diaphragm; in time a mediastinal shift to the right will occur.

chest fails to rise on the affected side with inspiration. Cyanosis will occur if the atelectasis involves a large enough area to interfere markedly with oxygen and carbon dioxide exchange. The patient may have chest pain.

Prevention

It is regrettable that atelectasis occurs as often as it does since it is almost wholly preventable. Preventive measures include emptying the stomach before surgery, by withholding fluids and food for several hours preoperatively. It is necessary to aspirate the stomach before emergency surgery if the patient has eaten recently and must have a general anesthetic. In addition, care is taken when the patient vomits to turn his head to one side to allow the vomitus to drain out. The use of anti-secretory drugs, such as atropine and hyoscine, prior to a general anes-thetic helps prevent the aspiration of mucus. Adequate hydration helps to prevent atelectasis by keeping mucus thin so that it can be coughed up.

Postoperatively it is essential to enforce activation of the patient, i.e., he should be turned every 1 to 2 hours and encouraged to cough and breathe deeply at more frequent intervals to raise sputum, aerate the lungs, and hasten removal of the anesthetic. If the patient's secretions are copious, suctioning may be required, or he may be positioned with head lowered to facilitate drainage of tracheobronchial secretions. Overseda-tion is to be avoided, since it depresses both respirations and the cough reflex.

Treatment

Once atelectasis has occurred, immediate treatment is necessary to prevent the formation of a lung abscess and necrosis. The patient should be turned on his unaffected side with head low and encouraged to cough. To reduce pain and strain on the incision the nurse should press gently against the dressings while the patient coughs. Carbon dioxide inhala-tions may be necessary to stimulate respirations. Expectorants and steam inhalations may be used to thin mucus. It may be necessary to remove the obstruction through a bronchoscope.

PNEUMONIA

Pneumonia can also complicate the surgical patient's condition. This secondary infection occurs in a patient with lowered lung resistance following atelectasis or general anesthesia, or in one who fails to be active enough to prevent secretions from collecting in the lungs. This latter condition has been called *hypostatic pneumonia*. Pneumonia is marked by fever and chills, rales and dyspnea, chest pain, rapid pulse, and the production of sputum.

Prevention

Preventive measures include the avoidance of general anesthesia and surgery, when possible, if resistance is low or if a respiratory infection is present. If surgery is emergent, a spinal anesthetic may be used. It is essential to enforce turning, coughing, and deep-breathing exercises post-operatively. Oversedation must be guarded against to prevent depression of respirations and the cough reflex. Abdominal distention hinders adequate respirations, as do tight binders; both must be avoided. Frequent oral hygiene is helpful in reducing the number of oral bacteria. Chilling must be avoided postoperatively, especially since many patients are diaphoretic and resistance is low immediately after surgery.

Treatment

Pneumonia usually occurs, if at all, rather late in the postoperative period. Bed rest with head elevated, if feasible, is ordered during the acute stage. A liberal fluid intake is encouraged. Activation is essential. Antibiotic drugs, oxygen, and steam inhalations may be used.

WOUND DISRUPTION (DEHISCENCE)

In a small percentage of postoperative patients wound disruption, *dehiscence*, occurs because of faulty healing or occasionally because of inadequate closure of the wound. During the first few days of repair the wound is held together solely by sutures and the initial cohesiveness of the healing tissues. Following this so-called "latent period" the wound becomes increasingly stronger as the tissues regenerate until maximum strength is reached in approximately 14 days.[3] Sutures are usually removed 1 week after surgery so that the period of greatest danger of dehiscence lies within the first two postoperative weeks, although disruption can occur several weeks later.

The factors contributing to dehiscence have been discussed in Chapter 3. Wound infection is a major cause of dehiscence. Therefore, every effort is made to prevent infection by scrupulous adherence to the principles of surgical asepsis. (See pages 23 to 25.) If infection does occur, antibiotic therapy is usually instituted promptly. Other factors contributing to dehiscence are dehydration, malnutrition, especially protein lack; obesity; age; debility; and concurrent disease such as diabetes and carcinoma. Postoperative conditions causing increased intra-abdominal pressure, such as distention, vomiting, hiccoughing, and excessive coughing, place a strain on the incision and may disrupt the closure. Hemorrhage into the wound may also cause dehiscence.

Prevention

Prevention of this complication lies in improving the general condition of the patient preoperatively and in remedying the above factors known to result in dehiscence.

[3] W. Mersheimer and J. Winfield, Abdominal Wound Disruption, A Review of the Etiology, Recognition and Treatment, *S. Clin. North America*, vol. 35, no. 2, p. 472, April, 1955.

Symptoms and Treatment

Usually wound disruption is superficial, but unless detected and treated early, the condition may progress to evisceration and consequent bowel obstruction. Detection should not be difficult with careful observation. The patient will usually experience sudden, sharp incisional pain and report that "something gave way"; there will be copious serosanguineous drainage. The wound should be inspected immediately and a tight binder applied, with the patient in the dorsal recumbent position with knees flexed to encourage abdominal relaxation. Should evisceration occur, the protruding loops of intestine should be covered with sterile moist packs and compression avoided. Shock if present demands immediate attention. The patient will usually need to return to surgery for secondary closure. If the patient is a poor risk for immediate re-suturing, a gauze tamponade and firm dressing may be applied by the surgeon until the patient's condition improves enough to allow surgical repair.[4]

GASTRIC DILATATION

In gastric dilatation the stomach dilates markedly, rupturing capillaries within its walls. The patient has projectile vomiting of blood which has been curdled by hydrochloric acid and is therefore described as "coffee ground." Abdominal distention is usually marked. Preventive measures include activation of the patient preoperatively and post-operatively, and the administration of potassium to increase gastric tonus when indicated. In addition gastric decompression through a naso-gastric tube which is connected to gentle suction is necessary to relieve the vomiting and distention.

PARALYTIC ILEUS

Paralysis of the intestine, called *paralytic ileus,* is common, especially following abdominal surgery when there has been much visceral manipulation or prolonged exposure of the abdominal contents to air. The major symptom is distention due to the cessation of peristalsis. There may be vomiting if oral intake is not restricted. This condition is usually self-limited. Peristalsis returning 2 to 3 days postoperatively is the indication for the resumption of oral intake. If the condition does not relieve itself, the patient is treated as for intestinal obstruction with decompression through a nasogastric tube, and intravenous infusions to maintain nutrition and hydration.

[4] *Ibid.,* p. 479.

SUMMARY

Postoperative complications are more easily prevented than treated. Since early detection and treatment are often lifesaving, the nurse must be familiar with the symptoms of complications and report their occurrence immediately to the surgeon. She should conscientiously practice preventive measures in nursing care, such as the activation of the patient to prevent pulmonary and circulatory stasis. She must be able to employ emergency measures and anticipate further specific types of therapy so that valuable time will not be lost.

The major postoperative complications affecting the vascular system are shock, hemorrhage, and thromboembolic phenomena (phlebothrombosis, thrombophlebitis, and embolism). Atelectasis and pneumonia are the major respiratory complications. The integrity of wound closure may be threatened by infection and/or dehiscence and evisceration. Gastric dilatation and paralytic ileus are usually less serious complications since they usually respond to treatment rather promptly.

BIBLIOGRAPHY

Shock and Hemorrhage

ELMAN, R.: "Surgical Care," Appleton-Century-Crofts, Inc., New York, 1951, pp. 442–477.

Fox, C., and S. LASKER: Fluid Therapy in Surgical Emergencies, S. Clin. North America, vol. 35, no. 2, pp. 335–352, April, 1955.

HAYES, M. A.: Shock and the Adrenal Cortex, Surgery, vol. 35, no. 2, pp. 174–190, February, 1954.

NELSON, R. M.: Current Concepts in the Pathophysiology of Shock, Am. J. Surg., vol. 93, no. 4, pp. 644–646, April, 1957.

QUICK, A. J.: Problem of Defective Hemostasis in Surgery, Am. J. Surg., vol. 84, no. 5, pp. 614–616, November, 1952.

RAVDIN, I. S., and J. E. ECKENHOFF: Shock, in "Christopher's Textbook of Surgery," 6th ed., L. Davis (ed.), W. B. Saunders Company, Philadelphia, 1956, chap. 4, pp. 100–108.

ROBBINS, S. L.: Disturbances of Body Fluids, in "Textbook of Pathology," W. B. Saunders Company, Philadelphia, 1957, chap. 7, pp. 160–170.

Thromboembolic Phenomena

COHEN, M. B.: Treatment of Thrombophlebitis, Am. J. Surg., vol. 8, no. 1, pp. 44–51, July, 1950.

PATERSON, J. C., and T. McLACHIN: Precipitating Factors in Venous Thrombosis, Surg., Gynec. & Obst., vol. 98, no. 1, pp. 96–102, January, 1954.

PRATT, G. H.: The Surgical Significance and Management of Pathologic Blood Clotting, Surg., Gynec. & Obst., vol. 97, no. 5, pp. 589–596, November, 1953.

ROBBINS, S. L.: Thrombosis, Embolism, and Infarction, in "Textbook of Pathology,"
    W. B. Saunders Company, Philadelphia, 1957, chap. 8, pp. 171–196.
STANTON, J. R.: Venous Thrombosis and Pulmonary Embolism, Am. J. Nursing, pp.
    709–711, June, 1955.

Atelectasis

MOYER, C. A.: Nonoperative Surgical Care, in "Surgery," J. G. Allen, H. N. Harkins,
    C. A. Moyer, and J. E. Rhoads (eds.), J. B. Lippincott Company, Philadelphia,
    1957, chap. 14, pp. 220–223.
ROBBINS, S. L.: The Respiratory System, in "Textbook of Pathology," W. B. Saunders
    Company, Philadelphia, 1957, chap. 19, pp. 629–632.

Dehiscence

JORGENSON, E. J., and E. T. SMITH: Postoperative Abdominal Wound Separation
    and Evisceration, Am. J. Surg., vol. 79, no. 2, pp. 282–287, February, 1950.
MERSHEIMER, W., and J. WINFIELD: Abdominal Wound Disruption, Review of the
    Etiology, Recognition and Treatment, S. Clin. North America, vol. 35, no. 2, pp.
    471–485, April, 1955.
TWEEDIE, F., and R. LONG: Abdominal Wound Disruption, Surg., Gynec. & Obst.,
    vol. 99, no. 1, pp. 41–47, July, 1954.

7

ANESTHESIA AND NURSING CARE

Progress made by anesthesiologists in inducing safe, pain-free relaxation of the patient has allowed surgeons to operate with less haste and greater skill, making surgery possible on areas heretofore inaccessible for surgical intervention. *Anesthesia* means literally without feeling (*an,* without + *esthesia,* feeling). Loss of sensation affecting the entire body and accompanied by unconsciousness is called *general anesthesia;* loss of feeling restricted to a limited area without loss of consciousness is termed *local anesthesia.*

GENERAL ANESTHESIA

How is the state of general anesthesia accomplished? General anesthesia is induced by anesthetics, or drugs, administered to the patient intravenously, rectally, or by inhalation. (See Table 3.) The selection of the anesthetic and method of administration depends upon the surgeon's and anesthetist's preferences; the area to be operated upon; the degree of relaxation required; the extent of surgery to be performed; the patient's age, condition, preparation, and emotional state.

Routes of Administration

Anesthetics may be administered by inhalation in one of several ways. In the open-drop method the liquid anesthetic is dripped onto a gauze mask and subsequently vaporized. This method requires the least amount of equipment; carbon dioxide is exhaled into the atmosphere and room oxygen is used with the anesthetic. If necessary, additional oxygen can be administered through a catheter placed under the mask. The anesthetist must be concerned with the oxygen and carbon dioxide exchange to maintain proper acid-base balance. Closed or semiclosed methods of administration require a series of cylinders from which the anesthetic gas and oxygen are fed to a mask. If the system is closed, provision must be

59

TABLE 3   MAJOR GENERAL ANESTHETICS

Anesthetic	Route of administration	Advantages	Disadvantages	Postoperative complications
Chloroform	Inhalation Open-drop	Noninflammable; little excitement; excellent relaxation	Toxic to such a degree that it is rarely used	Nausea, vomiting, respiratory depression, profound circulatory depression, cardiac arrhythmias, heart failure, hypotension, liver necrosis
Cyclopropane	Inhalation Closed Endotracheal	Pleasant induction	Inflammable, explosive	Shock, respiratory depression, cardiac damage, laryngospasm
Diethyl ether (ether)	Inhalation Open-drop Closed Endotracheal Rectal	Good abdominal relaxation; fairly safe since large amounts are necessary to produce toxicity	Inflammable, explosive if used with oxygen	Vomiting, acidosis, respiratory complications
Divinyl ether (Vinethene)	Inhalation Open-drop Semiclosed	Rapid, pleasant induction; short action; rapid recovery; fair muscular relaxation; useful for ether induction, for children, and for minor surgery for very short periods	Explosive; stages passed very rapidly	Liver damage if used for prolonged periods; respiratory depression if used in high concentrations
Ethylene	Inhalation Closed Endotracheal	Good for elderly patients and poor risks	Explosive, inflammable	Increased clotting time, therefore hemorrhage
Nitrous oxide	Inhalation Closed	Pleasant, safe for short operations	Poor relaxation of muscles; supports combustion	Cyanosis if used with less than 20% oxygen
Thiopental sodium (Pentothal sodium)	Intravenous Rectal	Potent, short action; well tolerated by aged; no excitement stage; nonexplosive	Somnolence, delayed reaction with large amounts, poor relaxation of muscles	Respiratory depression if prolonged; laryngospasm

TABLE 3   MAJOR GENERAL ANESTHETICS (*Continued*)

Anesthetic	Route of administration	Advantages	Disadvantages	Postoperative complications
Tribromo-ethanol (Avertin)	Rectal	Pleasant induction; amnesia for operating room; good for children; noninflammable; nonexplosive		

made for absorbing carbon dioxide with soda lime; if semiclosed, carbon dioxide is exhaled into the atmosphere. Endotracheal intubation, the insertion of a soft catheter into the trachea, is used for the administration of anesthesia for surgery in the facial area where a mask would be in the way of the surgeon, or when it would be difficult to use, as with the patient prone for surgery on the back or cranium. It may also be used when general anesthesia is necessary soon after the patient has eaten; a collar on the catheter can be inflated at the neck of the trachea, acting as a plug to prevent the aspiration of food and mucus.

Intravenous anesthesia is promptly and pleasantly induced but affords poor relaxation of muscles. It is, therefore, frequently used for induction, especially for apprehensive patients, and is followed by inhalation anesthesia. Rectal administration of an anesthetic is usually reserved for children and extremely apprehensive adults who find undergoing anesthesia too frightening. The drug is administered as a retention enema. The patient is unaware that the solution contains an anesthetic, loses consciousness in bed, and is thereby saved the emotional strain of a conscious trip to the operating suite. Intravenous anesthesia can be used with the same intent, but is usually not used for children. The state of light anesthesia is referred to as "basal"; in the operating room other methods and more potent anesthetics will be used.

Anesthetic Adjuncts

All anesthetics are toxic. In order to minimize the toxic effects and enhance the advantages of anesthetics, combinations of drugs and methods of administration are often used. Every effort is made to reach the stage of surgical anesthesia quickly and smoothly with as little excitement as possible and to use a minimal amount of drug throughout.

Curare and similar drugs are used to relax muscles. These drugs have no anesthetic properties but are useful adjuncts in anesthesia. By relaxing muscles, they permit milder anesthetics and smaller doses to be used.

Their action is at the myoneural junction, where they prevent the transmission of impulses; therefore, it can be seen that overdosage can paralyze the patient. Respiratory paralysis is the chief danger, and equipment for resuscitation must be readily available. (3-hydroxyphenyl) dimethylethylammonium bromide (Tensilon) is an antidote.

Stages of General Anesthesia

What are the stages of general anesthesia? The patient goes through three stages as the drug's effect is deepened. First is the induction or analgesic stage, in which sense of pain and consciousness are progessively lost. Second is the stage of delirium or excitement, in which a loss of consciousness and often violent activity occur. The third stage, that of surgical relaxation, permits operation. The toxic stage is reached if the anesthetic is given in increasing doses beyond the third stage; respiratory paralysis, cardiac failure, and death may ensue. Each of the stages requires definite nursing measures from the operating-room personnel and from the nurses caring for the patient postoperatively, because recovery from general anesthesia proceeds in orderly fashion from the third stage back to the first.

Nursing Care during Recovery from General Anesthesia

What are the principles of care for a patient recovering from general anesthesia? *Foremost in importance is the maintenance of a clear airway.* Muscular relaxation allows the jaw to drop and the tongue root to fall backward, occluding the pharyngeal orifice. Thus the patient is deprived of oxygen with prompt and serious consequences, for prolonged anoxia can cause brain damage; unrelieved anoxia is incompatible with life. A mechanical airway may be inserted by the anesthetist and should be left in place until the patient has regained his muscle tone and protective reflexes of swallowing and coughing. (See Figs. 9 and 10.) In the absence of a mechanical airway, gentle mandibular traction will bring the jaw and tongue forward and clear the airway. Positioning the patient with his head turned to one side is also effective.

The patient must be protected from injury. Protection from injury is necessary both for the immobile patient and for the hyperactive one. The nurse must watch for areas of pressure in the unconscious patient who is not moving. The patient must be aligned comfortably, especially so that his limbs are not under his body or exerting pressure on each other. If the patient must be moved while his muscles are relaxed, he must be moved gently in one plane to prevent strain, especially of the large dorsal muscles. He can be positioned on his side usually, well supported, to ensure comfort and a clear airway. An unconscious patient must never be left unattended.

When the patient becomes active during the excitement stage, he must be guarded from injuring himself or his wound. Restraints may be necessary, temporarily, but should always be used as a last resort; they may serve only to heighten the patient's excitement. Side rails should be used to prevent falls. Since the ability to move returns before judgment, the patient may attempt to get out of bed.[1] Fatal leaps from hospital windows have been known to occur in this stage.

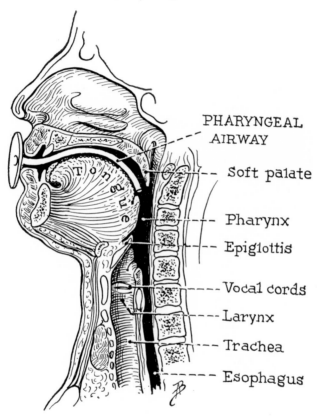

PHARYNGEAL
AIRWAY

Soft palate

Pharynx

Epiglottis

Vocal cords

Larynx

Trachea

Esophagus

FIG. 9. Pharyngeal airway. Note in this diagram of the upper respiratory tract in sagittal section that the mechanical airway reaches only to the pharynx.

Care must be exercised in transporting the patient to his bed on the clinical division. Drainage and intravenous tubes must be kept from dislodging. Medical supervision should be provided in transit. Since motion can deepen shock, the patient must be moved gently and easily. The nurse who receives the patient from surgery must know the type of anesthetic

[1] E. M. Greisheimer, The Physiological Effects of Anesthesia, *Am. J. Nursing*, p. 338, June, 1949.

used, the site of incision, and whether there are tubes or clamps present which might be dislodged, in order to assist with the safe transportation of the patient to the bed. Relaxed muscles must be protected from strain. There must be enough personnel on hand to lift the patient in one plane. This is best accomplished by the use of a lifting sheet or roller device.

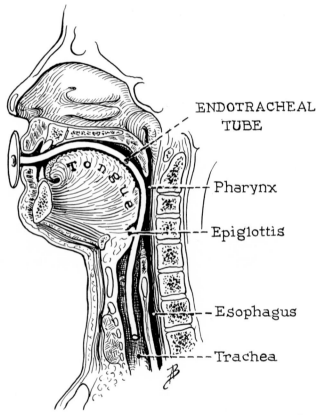

ENDOTRACHEAL
TUBE

Pharynx

Epiglottis

Esophagus

Trachea

FIG. 10. Endotracheal airway. Note that the tube extends into the trachea.

Psychic trauma is to be avoided. Conversation must be guarded, because hearing is the last sense to be lost in experiencing general anesthesia (or unconsciousness from any cause) and the first to be regained in recovery.[2] The patient must be reassured in a normal tone of voice repeatedly during recovery. He should be called by name, assured that surgery is over, and told that he is back in bed being cared for.

Postoperative complications are to be avoided.[3] The previous chapter

[2] *Ibid.,* p. 337.
[3] See Chapter 6.

has described the major complications of general anesthesia and surgery. With an understanding of what may occur, together with a knowledge of preventive and therapeutic measures necessary, the alert nurse can do much to make the recovery period far less crucial.

Pulse, respiration, and blood pressure should be taken and recorded at least every 15 minutes until stable, i.e., approximately the same for four consecutive readings, thereafter every ½ hour for 2 hours, then every 4 hours. Surgeons may order a different schedule for these observations, but the nurse can not take these cardinal signs too often during the immediate postoperative period. A fall in blood pressure, *hypotension*, may indicate surgical shock or hemorrhage. A rapid pulse is one of the first signs of respiratory distress. The patient's type of respirations may indicate hemorrhage, shock, or atelectasis. His color should be noted: cyanosis can indicate respiratory obstruction or severe shock; pallor may be indicative of hemorrhage. The temperature should be taken every 4 hours. A drop in temperature may indicate shock; an elevation, infection. The nurse will note the patient's state of consciousness and will record when full recovery occurs. Consciousness is determined by the patient's ability to respond to his name and by the return of the swallowing, gag, and eye reflexes.

The nurse will watch the dressings for seepage, reinforce wet dressings, and notify the surgeon of excess drainage or bright red blood. She will connect drainage tubes as directed and will ensure the administration of infusions. The nurse will prevent atelectasis, guarding against the aspiration of mucus or vomitus by positioning or suctioning as necessary. The patient who is vomiting should be placed in a side-lying position, if possible, to prevent aspiration. Frequent oral hygiene is appreciated and frequently is successful in allaying nausea. No oral intake is allowed while vomiting occurs.

In the recovery period the patient's diaphoresis and the depression of his heat-regulating center combine to render him highly susceptible to chilling. The nurse will guard against drafts, therefore, and will keep the patient dry. It is essential to avoid excess heat, which causes perspiration and further dilates blood vessels, increasing the loss of fluids and heat, and producing a risk of shock. The patient is especially susceptible to burns; if heating devices are ordered, they must be used with extreme caution.

Recognizing her responsibility for preventing pulmonary and vascular stasis, the nurse will institute the *activation regime* early in the recovery period. This includes turning the patient from side to side every 1 to 2 hours, and encouraging deep-breathing and coughing exercises and leg motion. Respirations and coughing can be stimulated with inhalations of carbon dioxide. If 90 to 100 per cent carbon dioxide is used, it is administered through a catheter held 6 to 8 in. above the patient's nose; the gas, being heavier than air, settles over the patient's nose and mouth. Lesser concentrations are administered with oxygen through a mask. Carbon dioxide is irritating to the eyes, so the patient should close them during this treatment. Sometimes the patient's own carbon dioxide is used by having him breathe into a paper bag. Usually it is sufficient to encourage the patient to take from six to eight deep breaths every hour. The nurse must realize that deep breathing and coughing are painful to the patient; for this reason his respirations are often guarded, especially when incisions infringe upon the costal margin. Demonstration, encouragement, and gentle pressure against the dressing during deep-breathing and coughing exercises help to achieve activation. Turning is also painful and is often better accomplished by allowing the patient to turn at his own rate of speed, but his reluctance to turn must be overcome by kindly persuasion and assistance when needed.

Lastly, the nurse will allow the patient to recover fully from the anesthetic before further depressing him with narcotics. This permits the nurse to activate the patient and observe him for signs of complications. Excessive pain is to be alleviated, but the nurse who meets a patient's restlessness with the prompt administration of a narcotic without adequate observation may be masking this early symptom of internal hemorrhage, shock, or pulmonary distress, and consequently may cause treatment to be delayed too long.

LOCAL ANESTHESIA

When is local anesthesia used? How is it accomplished? A local anesthetic may be used instead of a general one for minor surgery, or for the poor-risk patient, such as one with a severe cardiac condition, who could not tolerate a general anesthetic. Sometimes the surgeon's or patient's preference dictates its use. (See Table 4.)

Routes of Administration

The local anesthetic can be applied topically by spray, as in the pharynx, or by instillation, as in the eye. It can be administered by infiltration i.e., injection into tissues such as the skin, mucous membrane, and joints. Conduction, or regional, anesthesia refers to the injection of the drug into the cerebrospinal fluid, as in spinal anesthesia, or into nervous tissue to interrupt the condition of sensory impulses.

Nursing Care Following Local Anesthesia

What is the nursing care for a patient who has had a local anesthetic? The nurse must realize that the patient has no feeling in the anesthetized part and must, therefore, be protected from injury, such as that from pressure, friction, burns, and falls. She should reassure the patient that sensation will return gradually. She should record the time of motion and/or sensory return. It is important to observe and record the cardinal signs as carefully as for patients who have had general anesthesia, as well as to watch drainage tubes, dressings, and the patient's general condition. The patient who has had local anesthesia needs the activation regime, but if he has had a spinal anesthetic he is kept flat in dorsal recumbency for several hours; then he is turned from side to side

TABLE 4   MAJOR LOCAL ANESTHETICS

Anesthetic	Route of administration	Advantages	Disadvantages	Complications
Benzoylmethyl-ecgonine hy-drochloride (cocaine)	Topical Infiltration		Rapid, toxic reaction	Nausea, vomiting, cardiac depression, respiratory failure
Dibucaine hy-drochloride (Nupercaine hydrochloride)	Topical Spinal Regional	Potent	Toxic	Vasomotor dilatation
Procaine hydro-chloride (Novocain hydrochloride)	Topical Infiltration Regional-block Spinal	Relatively prompt and powerful		Hypotension, sensitivity reaction
Tetracaine hy-drochloride (Pontocaine hydrochloride)	Spinal Eye	Potent	Toxic	

every hour. If the patient is permitted to sit up too early, the anesthetic agent may rise to dangerous levels in the subarachnoid space, where the cerebrospinal fluid circulates. Headache is common following spinal anesthesia; the patient should be kept quiet and given analgesics as ordered. Urinary retention is not uncommon; catheterization may be necessary.

THE RECOVERY UNIT

This immediate postoperative care is best rendered in a recovery unit located close to the operating suite, staffed by skilled personnel, and equipped to meet postoperative emergencies. (See Fig. 11.) Such intensive therapy units designed for postanesthetic and postoperative care provide the patient with the benefits of constant, skilled observation and care during the most crucial hours of a surgical experience. The period of time during which this service is provided varies. The patient may be transported to the clinical division as soon as he has fully recovered from the anesthesia and has regained his protective reflexes. He may be kept in the recovery unit for a longer period of time, depending upon the facilities of the hospital and/or upon his condition.

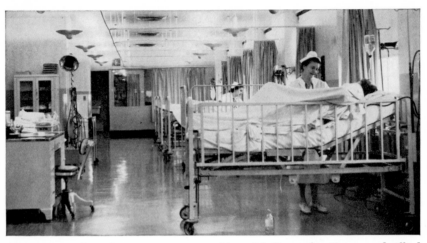

Fig. 11. Scene from the recovery room at Memorial Center for Cancer and Allied Diseases, New York. Note the bed sides used to prevent falls. Sphygmomanometers are attached to the wall beside the suction and oxygen inlets. Professional personnel give continuous attention to these patients. (*Courtesy of Memorial Center for Cancer and Allied Diseases.*)

Visitors are usually excluded from this unit and must, therefore, be made to understand the patient's delay in reaching the clinical division. They should be notified of the patient's condition at regular intervals to allay their apprehension during the waiting period. In units where patients are kept for several hours or days, visitors may be allowed.

SUMMARY

General anesthesia involves total loss of bodily sensation and unconsciousness. This state can be induced by drugs administered intravenously, rectally, or by inhalation. Each anesthetic bears risks which must be recognized in the nursing care given during the recovery period. The nurse must protect the patient from asphyxia, falls, psychic trauma, and postoperative complications during the crucial period of recovery from anesthesia and surgery. The cardinal signs, which include blood pressure, must be observed frequently until fully stabilized, and the general condition of the patient must be carefully scrutinized.

Local anesthesia causes regional loss of sensation only and is accomplished by injection, instillation, or spray. This patient also needs protection from trauma and postoperative complications. His condition must be closely observed. He needs reassurance that sensation will return in the affected area. If he has had a spinal anesthetic, he must be kept in the horizontal position.

The activation regime is initiated early in the recovery period: the patient is turned and positioned hourly; deep breathing and coughing can be stimulated by carbon dioxide inhalations after the patient has regained his reflexes. After consciousness has returned, the patient must be encouraged to turn voluntarily, cough, and breathe deeply at frequent intervals.

BIBLIOGRAPHY

ADRIANI, J.: "The Pharmacology of Anesthetic Drugs," 3d ed., Charles C Thomas, Publisher, Springfield, Ill., 1952.

ARROWHEAD, J. G.: Current Practice in Anesthesiology, Am. J. Nursing, pp. 1098–1100, September, 1954.

CULLEN, S. C.: "Anesthesia in General Practice," 4th ed., Year Book Publishers, Inc., Chicago, 1954.

DRIPPS, R. D.: Anesthesia, in "Surgery," J. G. Allen, H. N. Harkins, C. A. Moyer, and J. E. Rhoads (eds.), J. B. Lippincott Company, Philadelphia, 1957, chap. 12, pp. 184–202.

GREISHEIMER, E. M.: The Physiological Effects of Anesthesia, Am. J. Nursing, pp. 337–343, June, 1949.

JORDON, E. P. (ed.): "Modern Drugs Encyclopedia and Therapeutic Index," 7th ed., Drug Publications, Inc., New York, 1958.

WEYL, R.: Determination of the Anesthetic Procedure of Choice, J. Internat. Coll. Surgeons, vol. 13, no. 1, pp. 78–84, January, 1950.

8

PREOPERATIVE AND POSTOPERATIVE CARE
AND TEACHING—BETTY MARROW—
LAPAROTOMY

This chapter presents the general principles of preoperative and postoperative care and teaching which are applicable to the majority of patients undergoing general anesthesia and major, soft-tissue surgery. Because the plan for the care of every patient must evolve from that patient's needs, this material is adapted to the fictitious person Betty Marrow, who represents a composite of many patients undergoing a surgical experience.

THE PREOPERATIVE EVALUATION OF NEEDS

The preoperative evaluation of a patient's needs is basic to planning her care throughout the entire surgical experience. This evaluation is a continuous process and results in frequent revisions of the plan for nursing care. The more that is learned about the patient's background and personality, the more she is appreciated as an individual, the better her needs can be met. The nurse can plan to meet as many needs as possible in such a way that the patient is helped to achieve not only physical health but also a better understanding of her problems and a more objective view of them. This is important since health implies a harmonious interrelationship of mind, body, and soul.

Socioeconomic Status

The evaluation begins with a consideration of the socioeconomic status, which serves to point out concerns the patient may bring to the hospital. For example, Betty Marrow is a 33-year-old housewife and mother of two children, ages 4 and 6 years. She lives in a middle-class neighborhood. The family carries hospitalization insurance through the department store where Mr. Marrow is employed as a salesman. The nurse will realize that the care of the children and the separation caused by hospitalization will be uppermost in Betty's thoughts. Some patients might need the assistance of a social agency in finding someone to care for the children; however, Mrs. Marrow can rest assured that her children are in the capable care of her mother. The fact that this patient has medical insurance means she will be financially able to meet the major burden of the cost of hospitalization and surgery. Since the patient is not the wage earner, the family income will not be interrupted as it would have been had Mr. Marrow been the patient.

Psychologic Characteristics and Needs

Next in the evaluation of Betty Marrow is an understanding of her psychologic characteristics. She is worried about undergoing surgery because she knows that her grandmother died of carcinoma of the uterus and she fears that she may have the same disease. She states that she has little patience with illness. She asks many questions, such as:

Will I be sick afterward from the ether?
Will they wait until I'm asleep to cut?
Will I have gas pains like my neighbor had after her operation?
What if I do have cancer?

What needs are indicated by Mrs. Marrow's behavior and questions? How does the nurse respond to these questions? Betty Marrow's questions reveal concerns common to surgical patients. However, some people are less direct. They may hint or ask these same questions in a disguised manner. For example, "I know I don't have to worry about cancer anyway," may mean, "What will happen to me if I do have cancer?" It is important to allow a person to express herself. Feelings are thus brought out into the open, where they can be faced in the light of reality. Allowing a patient expression is not a mere passive permission: it is conveying a feeling of genuine acceptance of that person as she is so that she will not hesitate to disclose attitudes and feelings. Every effort should be made to answer a patient's questions and allay anxiety, especially in the preoperative period. Fear has a decided effect upon the way a patient undergoes anesthesia and surgery; then too, the postoperative period can be prolonged and complicated for a fearful patient. The nurse is reminded that she is part of a skilled team and that deep anxieties are best referred to the physician for treatment. It is, however, the alert nurse who often detects morbid fears.

Fear of the anesthetic rivals fear of surgery itself. Many patients are secretly convinced that they will talk and disclose guarded personal information while under the anesthetic. Some fear that they may not recover from anesthesia at all. But the greater dread of ridicule makes patients hesitate to express these feelings openly. Betty questions whether the anesthesia will be complete before the operation is begun. The nurse can assure the patient that the anesthetist, who is skilled in the use of anesthesia, will evaluate her condition and give her the benefit of individualized attention. The nurse may also comment that methods of anesthesia have been greatly improved. Betty's fear of ether can be dispelled by saying that ether is seldom used as the only agent: that ether, if used at all, is usually added after the patient is no longer awake. Postoperative recovery is more comfortable than previously, and nausea is minimized with the newer anesthetics. The nurse can honestly assure the patient that talking under the influence of an anesthetic is a fear not based upon fact: patients very seldom utter complete or meaningful statements.

The nurse, knowing that Betty's dread of cancer is due to inadequate understanding, will be able to help Betty realize that her condition is not necessarily cancer just because her grandmother had cancer. She can further assure her that early and adequate treatment effects a large percentage of cures. This learning will come about for the most part as the nurse listens and rephrases what has been said and supplies facts for hearsay when indicated.

This is an opportune time for the nurse to teach postoperative activation. To ensure postoperative cooperation, teaching must be started in the preoperative period when the patient is alert and interested. If properly instructed before surgery, a patient who is recovering from anesthesia, or who is in pain or discomfort, will nevertheless cooperate in turning, coughing, and taking fluids. It is not wise to suggest dreaded complications to patients in order to gain their cooperation in preventive measures. However, since gas pains seem to be expected by the majority of patients, and because postoperative activation helps reduce the severity of these pains, Betty can be assured that if she should have gas pains they will be minimized if she turns frequently after surgery. She should be told that should she have severe pain it will be alleviated by drugs if necessary.

The nurse will reassure Betty throughout all nursing contacts by realizing that she fears the unknown in this experience; by encouraging Betty's belief in her doctors, nurses, and other members of the health team; and by reinforcing her decision to undergo surgery and subsequent treatments. The nurse will thus reinforce Betty's desire to effect a speedy recovery by preoperative instruction and understanding.

What further teaching and orientation does Mrs. Marrow need? The orientation to the hospital will depend in large measure upon the patient's previous contacts. Because it has been 4 years since Betty was in the hospital she may need an explanation of changed concepts of care and what is expected of her in a surgical experience. She should be introduced to all personnel caring for her and to the patient who shares the two-bed room. She should have an idea of what is to happen to her before any treatment is carried out so that she can cooperate and be relieved of fear. Nurses are sometimes not aware of the anxiety which may accompany any treatment which is unfamiliar to the patient and which may be painful or uncomfortable. Because of the very strangeness of a hospital experience and the patient's condition on admission, she is more likely to react to all situations in a heightened manner and may need a great deal of reassurance. It is important that explanations of procedures be honest without being frightening; confidence is weakened whenever patients are deceived. Betty will also need to have an understanding of the general hospital rules and regulations, as well as specific directions relating to signal lights, bathroom facilities, and personal activities, e.g., she should be informed that to be up walking before the operation helps maintain visceral function in an optimal condition. It helps make a patient feel more comfortable also to know the hospital schedule for meals, visiting hours, and the usual hour for her physician's rounds. Many hospitals have much of this information written in attractive, easily read booklets for their patients.

Betty Marrow's need for some diversion is to be considered in this plan for care and teaching. She likes to knit and should be encouraged to do so while in the hospital. She can also be interested in radio or television programs and the newspaper. Patients seem to recover more rapidly if their interest in events outside the hospital can be maintained.

Spiritual Needs

The preoperative evaluation continues with a consideration of the patient's spiritual needs. What responsibility does the nurse have for helping the patient meet her spiritual needs? What activities would provide a suitable means of reinforcing Betty's religious convictions and preparing her for surgery?

Spiritual preparation for surgery immeasurably influences a patient's recovery. An undergirding faith helps the patient attain a tranquility not possible through drugs alone. Betty is Protestant and will appreciate a visit from her minister, Reverend Johns. In addition, Bible reading will comfort and strengthen her. She may wish to have Communion before the operation; this can be arranged through her minister or the hospital chaplain.

Physical Needs and Medical Status

The evaluation next centers on the patient's physical condition, medical history, and diagnostic impression. What responsibility does the nurse have for observing the physical condition of the patient? How are these observations applied to the plan for care and teaching? There is growing recognition among nurses of their responsibility in assisting with the evaluation of the physical condition of the patient. Although the physical examination is a medical responsibility, the nurse can observe the patient and assist in formulating a plan for care and teaching. Such observations as those of the condition of the patient's hair, nails, and skin, as well as of habits of oral hygiene, elimination, oral intake, posture, and sleep, should be made. Significant deviations from health should be recorded, and plans for corrective teaching instituted.

Betty's skin is noted to be dry and chapped; her hair lusterless. The nurse can substitute a lotion for daily back rubs in place of alcohol, which is drying. She can teach Betty to use lotion freely, especially after exposure to extremes in temperature, wind, and moisture. She can teach Betty how to brush and shampoo her hair to stimulate more luster. These hygienic habits are personal and unless discussed with a great deal of tact can offend a patient who has probably felt her habits were satisfactory. The nurse can also teach much in matters of hygiene by her own general appearance, care of skin and nails, and by the proper use of cosmetics and deodorants. Teaching is oriented toward rehabilitation of the patient for living outside the hospital environment.

What is the purpose of the medical history and physical examination? What is meant by diagnostic impression? Since concurrent infection or systemic disease increases the surgical risk, the surgeon will make every effort to detect and treat such conditions preoperatively. The surgeon elicits in the medical history of Betty Marrow that there has been no serious illness or previous surgery and that both deliveries were normal. He notes that the patient is a well-developed, fairly well-nourished but pale female in no acute distress. Mrs. Marrow complains of a sensation of pressure which has persisted for 2 years in the lower right side of her abdomen. Her vital signs are 98.6°F. (37°C.)–84–20; blood pressure 124/84 mm. mercury. An inventory by systems reveals no abnormalities. Her chest is clear and resonant. The pelvic examination reveals a palpable, fluctuant, freely movable, slightly tender mass approximately 20 cm. (or the size of a fist) in the right lower quadrant (R.L.Q.) of the abdomen; the uterus is normal. There is slight tenderness upon abdominal palpation, only in the R.L.Q. These findings are essentially negative, except for the pelvic symptoms, which suggests that Betty is in good condition for surgery.

Mrs. Marrow's physical condition is further studied and evaluated by the use of certain laboratory tests. First, a complete blood count (C.B.C.), which indicates the total number of erythrocytes (R.B.C.) and leukocytes (W.B.C.), is usually done for all patients undergoing general anesthesia and major surgery. Normally there are 4,600,000 to 4,800,000 R.B.C. per cubic millimeter blood for women and 5,400,000 to 5,800,000 for men, with a hemoglobin concentration of 12 to 15 Gm. A decrease may indicate anemia—either primary, due to hemorrhage, or secondary, due to faulty metabolism. An anemic patient may heal more slowly and poorly, with risk of wound disruption; be more prone to shock and thrombosis; and have a longer recovery period. The normal leukocyte count is 6,000 to 10,000 per centimeter; an increase may indicate infection, which increases the operative risk.

In addition a plasma protein is often taken to determine whether the patient has sufficient protein to promote healing and avoid postoperative complications. Normally the plasma contains 6.3 to 8 Gm. protein per 100 ml., with the ratio of albumen to globulin being 2:1.

A serologic test is performed to determine the presence of syphilis, a venereal disease. Such tests are the Kahn, Wassermann, and Kline. If the test result is positive, treatment will precede surgery to render the patient noninfectious and to make her a better surgical risk. It should be noted that a positive test result can be obtained with diseases other than syphilis, e.g., malaria and infectious mononucleosis.

Blood is typed, cross-matched, and made available when the surgeon anticipates prolonged surgery, hemorrhage, or shock. A transfusion, then, can be prophylactic as well as therapeutic.

The chest is x-rayed to determine the presence of lung diseases, such as tuberculosis, and also the size of the heart. This again is an effort to rule out or diagnose for treatment systemic conditions which increase the surgical risk.

A urinalysis is done to determine the condition of the urinary tract. The specific gravity of urine, which normally is 1.010 to 1.030, gives an indication of kidney function. An elevated specific gravity may indicate dehydration, as there is then not enough fluid to dilute the solid constituents of urine. Blood, casts, bacteria, and leukocytes, if found, necessitate further investigation to rule out urinary tract disease.

These tests then are performed to detect systemic conditions which increase the surgical risk and invite postoperative complications. Betty Marrow's test results are all within normal limits, which confirms the surgeon's impression that she is a good surgical risk.

Of what value to the nurse is an understanding of the purpose of laboratory procedures and their results? The nurse should know why a test is being done so that she can understand the interpretations of results and assist in planning for the patient's care. It is necessary for the nurse to know the procedure so that she can prepare the patient properly. It is not necessary to withhold oral intake before a blood count, but this is necessary before a blood chemistry test, such as a plasma protein determination. Since dehydration distorts the laboratory findings, a sufficient amount of water to ensure adequate hydration is usually permitted. It is also important that the nurse be accurate in making out requisitions and appointments for these tests to avoid delay and the expense of repeated or delayed tests. She must be accurate in getting the reports of the tests included on the patient's record.

Having evaluated the patient's condition, the surgeon forms a diagnostic impression. Betty Marrow's diagnostic impression is "Right ovarian cyst—rule out carcinoma." The diagnostic impression usually contains, in order of likelihood, the conditions the surgeon suspects to be present. The differential diagnoses are listed to be "ruled out," i.e., to be proved erroneous. Therefore, in interpreting the diagnostic impressions for Mrs. Marrow, it can be said that a cyst will probably be found on her right ovary. Through further examinations and surgery itself, the possibility of carcinoma can be ruled out—or may be proved to be correct.

There are times when the surgeon can not say with certainty what the true diagnosis is until he can see, feel, biopsy, or take a smear of the involved tissue. It is in such a situation that a laparotomy may be scheduled, as it is with Betty Marrow. *Laparotomy* (*laparo,* loin + *otomy,* cut) has come to mean an incision made into the abdomen. (See Fig. 15.) *Celiotomy* is a synonymous term. Upon examination of the surgical field the diagnosis can be confirmed, and usually the diseased tissue can be removed. Therefore, Betty Marrow's preoperative diagnosis is "possible ovarian cyst," but after the laparotomy the diagnosis may be "ovarian cyst—right oophorectomy." Lest this discussion convey the impression that surgical diagnosis is neither scientific nor certain, it is pointed out that surgery is itself a scientific diagnostic tool as well as a therapeutic method.

IMMEDIATE PREOPERATIVE PREPARATION

The immediate preoperative preparation is designed to assist the patient safely through anesthesia, surgery, and the postoperative period. The medical orders for the immediate preoperative preparation are concerned chiefly with activity allowed, skin preparation, oral intake, emptying the gastrointestinal tract, and medication. They may be written by the surgeon or anesthesiologist. What are the purposes of each of the orders? What are the nurse's responsibilities in fulfilling them?

Activity

Ambulation, which is usually encouraged preoperatively when possible, serves several purposes. A patient allowed out of bed can usually occupy herself more easily and so is happier. Elimination is more normal, appetite is stimulated, skin and muscle tonus is maintained, circulation is kept active, and respirations are more adequate. Knowing that sitting in a chair is a poor substitute for ambulation, the nurse will encourage the patient to walk and be active.

Skin Preparation

The order for the skin preparation involves an extensive area and includes a margin of safety around the proposed site of incision. (See Fig. 12.) The skin is made as clean as possible but can never be con-

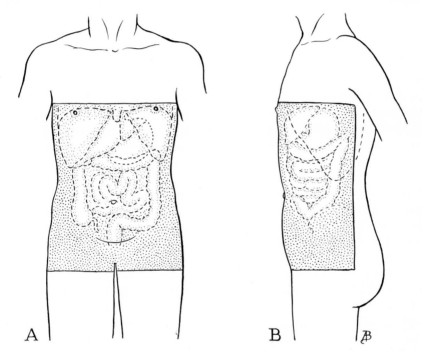

A   B

FIG. 12. Area of skin preparation for laparotomy. Note that the area prepared extends from just above the nipple line to and including the pubic area, and from bed line to bed line.

sidered sterile. There are always bacteria present on the skin, and these organisms, while harmless on the surface of the intact skin, may become pathogenic if introduced below the skin surface, as through an incision. It is, therefore, essential that the skin be prepared meticulously. The entire area is shaved to remove hair, which holds grease and bacteria. Care must be taken to avoid nicking the skin. In some hospitals the shave is done on dry skin, in others on skin moistened with soapy solution. In either case the area is scrubbed and rinsed well, with due caution to avoid skin irritation. The skin preparation may be done by professional or nonprofessional personnel from the operating rooms or from the nursing division. Usually this procedure is performed the night before surgery, but in some hospitals it is done in the operating room immediately prior to surgery.

Oral Intake

The orders regarding Betty Marrow's oral intake are as follows: (1) serve a regular diet for supper, (2) encourage fluid intake until the hour of sleep, and (3) withhold all oral intake after midnight. These are representative of the orders usually given prior to general anesthesia and surgery, although there will be variations depending upon the policies of individual hospitals, the preferences of the surgeon and anesthesiologist, and the time and type of surgery scheduled.

The basic principles underlying these orders are that the patient must have optimal nutrition and hydration for as long as possible preoperatively and yet must have an empty gastrointestinal tract to prevent aspiration of gastric contents or distention of the intestine. Fluids are encouraged when feasible until the hour of sleep to combat dehydration and acidosis, which may occur with preoperative and postoperative restriction of oral intake, fluid loss at surgery, and postoperative vomiting. Oral intake after midnight is usually restricted when surgery is scheduled for the morning. In view of the fact that the stomach normally empties itself in 3 to 4½ hours,[1] some surgeons allow oral intake of fluids until 4 to 6 hours preoperatively in the interest of more adequate hydration. Each surgeon considers his patient's individual needs. The nurse is responsible for instructing the patient about the need to abstain from eating or drinking after the time set by the surgeon. The order to withhold intake must be shared by all personnel in order to spare the patient the necessity of having surgery delayed because intake was allowed. If a patient must undergo emergency surgery sooner than 3 to 4 hours following his last oral intake, he may require gastric aspiration preoperatively.

Elimination

An enema is often ordered to clear the colon: (1) to prevent contamination of the surgical area with relaxation of the sphincters during general anesthesia; (2) to remove feces and flatus which could distend the sigmoid and rectum, thereby obscuring the surgeon's view and working area and risking surgical trauma to a loop of distended intestine; and (3) to help prevent postoperative distention. The order for the enema varies with each surgeon's preference as well as with the patient's condition. Nurses will see the order varying from several

[1] D. C. Kimber, C. E. Gray, C. E. Stackpole, and L. C. Leavell, "Textbook of Anatomy and Physiology," 13th ed., The Macmillan Company, New York, 1955, p. 582. (Used with permission of The Macmillan Company.)

enemas, to one, to none. Repeated enemas seem to weaken a patient and are usually more a part of preparation for intestinal surgery.

Preoperative Medication

The preoperative medications given have a twofold purpose: to promote relaxation and to diminish mucus secretion. Betty Marrow has an order for a barbiturate to help her sleep. It is important that she rest well the night before surgery. The nurse should check at frequent intervals to note the effectiveness of the hypnotic; if the patient is not sleeping by midnight, at the latest, the surgeon should be notified. He will probably order another dose or drug. In addition to the preoperative hypnotic, generally but not always given the night before surgery, a narcotic, tranquilizer, or potent antihistamine with sedative qualities, such as promethazine hydrochloride (Phenergan), is given the morning of surgery. Betty has an order for morphine sulfate grain ¼, which is used to quiet the patient and allow her to go to surgery with minimal apprehension. Such a relaxed patient goes through the induction period more easily and requires less anesthetic. Morphine, however, depresses respirations and causes nausea in sensitive patients. Therefore, meperidine (Demerol) is widely used in place of morphine. In addition to these drugs, a belladonna derivative such as atropine or scopolamine (hyoscine) is used to stimulate respirations and to lessen bronchial secretions, which are increased in general anesthesia and may be aspirated during unconsciousness. The preoperative medication should be given on time as ordered. If given too late, i.e., if the patient is called for ahead of schedule, notify the anesthetist, who will regulate the anesthesia accordingly. Otherwise the medication will take effect during surgery and not only will deprive the patient of the benefit when needed but may dangerously intensify the stage of anesthesia during surgery. Furthermore, the patient may react from the anesthetic and then be sedated by delayed action, thereby jeopardizing the recovery period. If the preoperative medication is given too early, i.e., if surgery is delayed, notify the surgeon, who may order another dose. If the patient is "on call," medication is given when the nursing division is notified. Mrs. Marrow is to be transported to surgery 1 hour after her medication is given. This time interval will vary, but it is generally felt that the medication, given parenterally, reaches its full effect in approximately 1 to 1½ hours. When the medication is given, the patient should be told that she may feel drowsy and should stay in bed. The unit should be arranged so that it is conducive to rest, and all preparation for surgery should be completed before the medication is given. Visitors should be restricted to two at one time and should be instructed to refrain from conversation so that the patient can rest. The nurse must observe the patient who is under the influence of a narcotic to prevent accidents, such as a fall from bed.

Further Nursing Responsibilities

In addition to carrying out these medical orders, what further nursing responsibilities must be attended to preoperatively? Several hours prior to surgery the nurse should check the patient's chart to be sure the

---

Name .... Ward .... Patient's No ....

Operation No ....

Consent to Operation and Treatment, and
Release of Claims to Medical and Surgical Staff of
Cook County Hospital

For and in consideration of the medical treatment, including any and all surgical operations or procedures, which I may receive while a patient in Cook County Hospital, Chicago, from or through the duly appointed members of the medical and surgical staff of the said hospital, either severally or collectively, consent is hereby given, voluntarily and knowingly, by me, if of age and competent, or for me, if a minor or incompetent, by my parents, guardian or best friend, as the case may be, to the said members of the said medical and surgical staff, or any of them, severally or collectively, to prescribe and carry out, or cause to be carried out, such medical treatment, including any and all surgical operations or procedures, which they, or any of them, in their best judgment, may deem proper for my best interest; and furthermore, the said members or any of them, are hereby released from any and all liability, of whatsoever kind or nature, for any damage which may result from anything done, suffered to be done or omitted, by reason of such treatment, operation or procedure, or any or all of them.

Dated at Chicago, Illinois, this .... day of .... A. D. 19....

.... (SEAL)

Witness:

....

By .... (SEAL)
His or her (as the case may be) parent, guardian or best friend.

NOTE: If an adult, sign personally on first line. For a minor or incompetent, the parent, guardian or best friend as the case may be, must sign the name of the minor or incompetent on the first line, and the name of such parent, guardian or best friend on the second line.

		Date	Hour	
1. Operation Scheduled. Relatives Notified By _____		_____	_____	M.
2. Operation Scheduled. Relatives Notified By _____		_____	_____	M.
3. Operation Scheduled. Relatives Notified By _____		_____	_____	M.

63 20M 8-56 (FORM 39)

Fig. 13. A surgical permit. (*Used with permission from the Cook County Hospital, Chicago.*)

laboratory reports for blood and urine are present. She must also be sure that the surgical permit is signed and witnessed. (See Fig. 13.) Students in nursing are usually not permitted to witness legal records; this is usually a function of the medical staff. It is important that the patient understand the full significance of this consent for surgical treatment. If the patient is under age (twenty-one years for a male, eighteen years for a female), the parent or guardian signs the permit. Whoever signs the permit should realize that it gives the surgeon full legal permission to carry out any surgical treatment necessary for the patient's welfare.

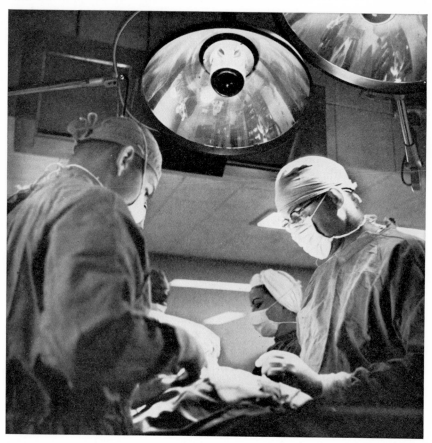

Fig. 14. General scene in the operating room of the M. D. Anderson Hospital, Houston, Tex. (*Courtesy of the American Cancer Society, Inc.*)

Next the nurse takes the temperature, pulse, and respirations, and records them; abnormalities are reported to the surgeon. A pulse over 100 is especially important to report. A preoperative blood pressure reading is not always ordered, but since it serves as a standard for comparison to detect postoperative shock, the nurse would do well to take and record the blood pressure. At this time the nurse observes the patient and reports such contraindications for surgery as excessive fear, rash, or signs of an upper respiratory infection.

The patient is then assisted with her personal care. Oral hygiene should be thorough. A tub bath, if permitted, helps ensure cleanliness. A clean hospital gown is provided. Laparotomy stockings may be applied at this time or later in the operating room. Hair is combed and pins are removed. As with the stockings, the hair covering may be applied at this time or later, depending upon the hospital's policy. Nail polish and lipstick should be removed to allow the anesthetist to observe for cyanosis. In the interest of minimizing negative feelings preoperatively, some hospitals allow cosmetics in moderation when the patient goes to the operating room; some allow the patient to wear her own gown; and some let the patient go to surgery in a wheelchair. All jewelry, dentures, and other prostheses are removed and placed in safekeeping. It is generally felt that dentures should be removed to facilitate the administration of anesthesia, to ensure a clear airway, and to prevent their loss. However, some anesthetists prefer to leave the dentures in place to preserve the facial contour, thereby helping to ensure a clear airway. If the wedding band is to stay on the patient, it should be secured to the finger with bandage slipped through the ring and brought to encircle the wrist loosely; constriction is to be avoided.

Immediately prior to administering the medication, the nurse should encourage the patient to void. An empty bladder prevents involuntary micturition during anesthesia, avoids trauma to a full bladder, and helps ensure a clear operative field. This is especially important in pelvic surgery, and for this reason a catheter is often introduced in surgery.

The final charting is done, usually including information on observations, treatments and medications, and voiding, and a note indicating that the patient is prepared for surgery. The time the patient goes to surgery is usually the last notation. The chart is sent to the operating suite along with the patient.

Transportation to the Operating Suite

Lastly the nurse assists the patient to the cart, taking precautions to avoid straining the back muscles, which are relaxed because of the preoperative medication.

Throughout the preoperative period, Betty Marrow and her nurse have worked cooperatively toward the goal of health. Now at the crucial moment of transportation to the operating room, this relationship can no longer be shared. The patient realizes that, in spite of her reliance upon surgeon and nurse, she must go through surgery alone. An operation has unique meaning for each individual. However, the nurse can extend the relationship already established and give the patient supportive reassurance to take with her by expressing a feeling of genuine interest through gestures, attitudes, and speech. Such a comment as, "I will be here when you wake up," reassures the patient that (1) she will wake up, (2) she will be cared for, and (3) the relationship already established will continue. It is therefore highly desirable that the nurse accompany the patient to the operating suite. This will make the transition from bed to operating table more gradual and less of a threat to the patient's sense of security.

POSTOPERATIVE NURSING CARE

Nursing care and teaching in the postoperative period are designed to prevent complications and to hasten full recuperation. Postoperatively Betty Marrow's care centers on her recovery from anesthesia and surgery, her convalescence, and her preparation for discharge. Measures necessary to prevent complications and promote comfort in the initial period of recovery have been described in the two preceding chapters. This discussion will, therefore, emphasize the care and teaching required in convalescence.

Transition from Recovery Unit to Clinical Division

Betty Marrow's convalescence may be considered as beginning with her transfer from the recovery unit to the clinical division. How is a smooth transition from recovery unit to the clinical division effected? What information must be exchanged by the personnel of these departments to ensure continuity of nursing care?

First to be considered is the length of time the patient is in the care of recovery-unit personnel. This varies with the facilities of the hospital. In some, the recovery-unit personnel care for the patient only until she has reacted fully from the anesthetic and her cardinal signs have stabilized. In others, the patient remains in this unit for 12 to 24 hours, or longer, depending upon her condition. If the hospital lacks such a unit, or if it is closed, the patient will be received on the nursing division directly from surgery. The plan for continuity of nursing care must then begin with the degree of recovery the patient has reached. In addition the personnel on the nursing division must know the type of anesthetic used, the exact nature of the surgery performed, the postoperative diagnosis, and the course of progress during surgery and recovery in order to anticipate possible complications and nursing needs in convalescence.

To illustrate, the nurse who receives Betty Marrow from the recovery unit will want to know that the exploratory laparotomy revealed an ovarian cyst, so that a right oophorectomy was performed. This will relieve Mrs. Marrow's symptoms, as well as the fear that she had cancer, and will interfere in no way with her normal physiologic functioning. Cyclo-propane, the anesthetic used, tends to cause cardiac arrhythmia, so the nurse will be especially careful to note the quality of the pulse frequently. Since no complications occurred during surgery, and since her progress in the recovery unit, where she remained for 5 hours, was uneventful, it is probable that she will have a smooth convalescence.

Care in Convalescence

What special needs does the patient have in the convalescent period? How does the nurse meet these needs? Some nursing problems originate in the recovery period but may extend beyond it. They are, therefore, described here with the care necessary in early convalescence.

Intake-Output. Thirst is a common postoperative problem and can be allayed by frequent oral hygiene and lubrication of lips. Adequate fluid intake parenterally, or orally when tolerated, helps combat thirst and promotes renal function. An accurate record of intake and output is necessary for the first two to three postoperative days, to determine needs for fluids and adequacy of urine output. Urinary retention is common following general anesthesia and surgery. Its exact cause can not always be clearly determined. It may be due to manipulation and exposure of pelvic viscera, to packing, to the anesthetic, to interruption of nervous impulses, or to fear. Spontaneous voiding is to be encouraged by fluid intake, privacy, suggestion, and sitting if possible. Bathroom privileges frequently are allowed the day of surgery. Catheterization every 8 to 12 hours may be necessary but should be considered as a last resort because the risk of cystitis and of catheter dependence increases with each treatment. Once spontaneous voiding has been initiated, the surgeon not uncommonly orders catheterization for residual urine to determine the adequacy of bladder function.

Prevention of Distention. Abdominal distention, another distressing problem, is best met by prevention. Frequent turning and early ambulation encourage peristalsis. Once peristalsis has returned, the patient should be encouraged to eat a full diet as ordered and to push fluids. A rectal tube, enema, and/or gastrointestinal decompression may be necessary to treat distention.

Analgesia. Excessive pain must be relieved by the administration of the narcotic or analgesic ordered by the surgeon. The nurse bears a major responsibility for preventing narcotic addiction in her patient by giving the drug only when absolutely necessary and for the reason ordered, and by substituting nursing measures to promote comfort and diversion of attention. Narcotics should not be necessary for the majority of patients after the third to fourth postoperative day. The nurse must also observe the patient carefully to determine the cause of pain: is it incisional soreness? is it due to abdominal or bladder distention? is it sharp and shooting? where is the pain in relation to the surgical area? are other symptoms present?

Wound Care. The incision must be protected from injury and infection; the nurse must be watchful for signs of either. Usually the dressings are left undisturbed until sutures are removed in approximately 3 or 4 days postoperatively. The first dressing is done by the surgeon. Wound healing has been described in Chapter 3 and should be reviewed at this point.

Medical Orders. Usually all preoperative orders are discontinued with surgery. The surgeon writes new orders postoperatively regarding intake, activity, and medication. Not infrequently dietary supplements and antibiotics are ordered to hasten full recuperation and to prevent complications.

Ambulation. Early ambulation, an extension of the activation regime, is introduced early in the convalescent period, sometimes even on the day of surgery. Activity counteracts the hazards of bed rest, stimulating circulation and respirations, improving visceral function and muscle tone, and raising the patient's morale. The patient needs a great deal of reassurance and support as she first attempts to walk because she is weak and such activity is painful. She should be allowed to sit up for a few minutes until she has regained her equilibrium. She should have a substantial pair of shoes or slippers for adequate foot support. She may also need support such as is furnished by a handrail or by pushing a light chair ahead of her. Because she will favor her incision she must be encouraged to assume an erect position to prevent permanent postural deformities. Ambulation is always achieved more readily when the patient has a purpose, such as walking to the solarium to meet her visitors. Ambulatory patients require supervision of their activities to prevent falls; they must be discouraged from prolonged rest periods sitting in a chair, being encouraged rather to return to bed where they can rest fully extended. As convalescence nears the date of discharge the patient should be up most of the day.

Preparation for Discharge

How does the nurse assist in preparing the patient for discharge from the hospital?

The Patient Who Is Cured. Throughout Betty Marrow's postoperative course the nurse makes every effort to prevent an excessive dependency attitude and to promote a desire to regain an active independent status as soon as is clinically sound. The patient's activities are progressively increased in keeping with her regaining strength and she is encouraged to help herself in her care as much as is wise. Her attention is directed toward her return home and she is helped to anticipate problems in rehabilitation which may arise there. She should know how soon to return to her surgeon for medical supervision, what restrictions in activity will be made and for how long, and how to adapt her routine to meet these restrictions. With the rapid turnover in hospital population it is likely that the patient will go home with a dressing in place; therefore, she must know how to change the dressing if necessary, that it must be kept dry, and that the wound must be protected from irritation. She must also understand dietary restrictions, if they are necessary, and changes in hygiene necessitated by her condition, such as whether intercourse is permissible and whether a tub bath is allowed. The surgeon will give the patient instructions regarding her home care. The nurse must be prepared to support and clarify these orders. She must ascertain whether they are clear to the patient and whether she understands how to follow them at home.

The Patient Who Is Not Cured. If surgery has not been able to effect a cure, the health team must anticipate the type of problem the patient will meet at home and plan with relatives or an agency, such as the Visiting Nurses' Association, for the care of the patient. The patient may require injections, frequent changes of dressings, or even bedside care. The patient may or may not realize her prognosis, as in the case of a patient with inoperable carcinoma. If she does, she will need much support and encouragement, best given her by her clergy but offered also by the entire health team. The relatives who assume her care will also require understanding, guidance, and reassurance.

SUMMARY

The preoperative evaluation of a patient's needs is basic to planning her care throughout the entire surgical experience. This evaluation centers upon the following areas of need: socioeconomic status, spiritual-psychologic characteristics, physical findings and history, diagnosis, and treatment.

The immediate preoperative preparation is designed to assist the patient safely through anesthesia, surgery, and the postoperative period. This preparation includes attention to activity, skin preparation, oral intake, elimination, medication, personal care, and reassurance.

Postoperative nursing care is designed to prevent complications and to hasten full recuperation. Continuity of nursing care and observations, from the recovery unit to the nursing division, is facilitated by a full report to the nursing personnel regarding the surgery, anesthesia, and recovery progress. The first 12 to 24 hours postoperatively are crucial. Careful, frequent observations of the patient's condition are essential.

Methods of inducing comfort and preventing complications throughout the postoperative period include attention to intake, output, oral hygiene, activation, analgesia, and wound care.

Preparation for discharge requires that the patient understand how to take care of herself to promote full physical, emotional, and social rehabilitation. When recovery is not possible, arrangements must be made for the care of the patient, and much encouragement must be given to sustain the patient and her relatives.

STUDY GUIDE FOR PART ONE

1. How can the nurse best assist the minister in meeting Betty Marrow's spiritual needs throughout her surgical experience?
2. How much of the financial burden of care is borne by the usual type of hospitalization insurance? (Consult literature from leading insurance companies.)
3. What are some of the attitudes and feelings revealed by Betty Marrow's questions preoperatively which might help her nurses understand how she is viewing her problems?
4. What responsibility does the nurse have for meeting the psychologic needs of surgical patients?
5. Pain in the right lower quadrant of the abdomen could arise from what organs located there?
6. What drugs other than morphine and atropine are used preoperatively?
7. What serious complication is avoided by the preoperative use of an antisecretory drug such as atropine?
8. Complete in detail the plan for *preoperative* care which you would use for Mrs. Marrow from the afternoon before until the day of surgery.
9. If Mrs. Marrow were going for elective surgery early in the afternoon, how would this plan have to be altered?
10. What orders would you expect the surgeon to give regarding oral intake, elimination, medications, activity, and wound care during the first 12 to 24 hours postoperatively? The next 3 to 5 days? What is the reason for each of these orders?
11. Assuming that Mrs. Marrow's oral fluid intake was only 700 ml. the first 24 hours postoperatively, list the types and amounts of fluids she would probably have as an intravenous supplement.
12. What factors are important in promoting primary repair of Mrs. Marrow's incision?
13. What observations should be made of the patient the first 12 to 24 hours? The next 3 to 4 days?

14. How would these observations be affected if the patient had had a spinal anesthetic instead of general anesthesia?

15. What responsibility does the nurse have for preventing narcotic addiction in the surgical patient? What nursing measures help relieve the patient in pain?

16. What is the reason for each measure in the activation regime? How can the nurse help the patient cooperate in this program?

17. If you found postoperatively that Mrs. Marrow's blood pressure was 80/40 mm. mercury, pulse 120, respirations 32, and that she was pale and extremely restless, what would you do first? Next? What is the reason for each of these actions?

18. In terms of possible specific postoperative complications, what is the significance of the fact that Betty Marrow has a low intake of protein and vitamin C owing to a poor appetite? Outline a teaching program which the health team can institute to correct this habit. Apply principles of teaching and cite appropriate methods which could be used.

19. What are the teaching needs of Mrs. Marrow preparatory for discharge?

20. Suppose that one day, shortly after her uncle's death due to carcinoma, your neighbor asks you, "How could I know if I have cancer?" What would you say to furnish adequate information in answer to this question? What must this person know in order to safeguard her health?

21. How does a benign tumor differ from one that is malignant on the basis of pathology, symptomatology, prognosis, and treatment? What diagnostic methods are used to differentiate these two types of neoplasms?

Part Two

CARE OF THE PATIENT UNDERGOING ABDOMINAL SURGERY

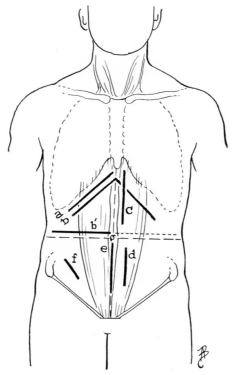

FIG. 15. Abdominal incisions: (*a*) subcostal, (*b*) and (*b'*) transverse, (*c*) paramedian, (*d*) transrectus, (*e*) midline or median, and (*f*) McBurney.

9

SURGERY OF THE STOMACH AND DUODENUM

Surgery of the stomach and duodenum is performed primarily in the treatment of carcinoma and of peptic ulcer and its complications.

GASTROSTOMY

When the esophagus is obstructed, some means of feeding other than oral must be instituted. Recall that prolonged parenteral fluid therapy is not feasible; the patient benefits most from food taken directly into the gastrointestinal tract. Therefore, a *gastrostomy* (*gastro,* stomach + *ostomy,* making an opening into = the creation of an opening from the stomach to the outside) is performed to permit nutrition and hydration in a patient with esophageal obstruction. (See Fig. 16.) The obstruction may be due to carcinoma or stricture formation, which occurs most commonly after the accidental or intentional swallowing of a caustic, such as lye. The patient with a stricture is usually in a good state of nutrition because the operation is performed promptly. The gastrostomy is usually temporary, sustaining the patient until esophageal repair can be made. If the esophagus is obstructed with carcinoma, which is a slow-growing process gradually reducing alimentation over a period of time, the patient will probably be severely malnourished. The procedure may then be performed as a permanent palliative measure, although a *jejunostomy,* making an opening into the jejunum, may be preferable.

Regardless of the circumstances requiring a gastrostomy, the patient must be helped to accept the idea of taking food and water directly into his stomach rather than orally. Preparation for a gastrostomy is the same as for laparotomy. A tubular gastrostomy may be performed which permits the insertion and removal of a catheter for feeding, or a retention catheter may be left in place.

The plan for postoperative nursing care centers upon gastrostomy feedings, skin care, oral hygiene, and teaching self-care. The patient with a permanent gastrostomy, or his relative, must be taught how to insert, remove, and clean the catheter; how to prepare and administer the formula; and how to keep the skin margins free from excoriation. Approximately 200 ml. high-protein, high-vitamin formula alternating with water is introduced into the gastrostomy tube every 2 to 4 hours and the tube is clamped to prevent reflux. Air must not be introduced with the formula for then the patient will be unable to take the full feeding. The feeding should be given at room temperature. The patient should be in a sitting position to facilitate the passage of the fluid into the stomach

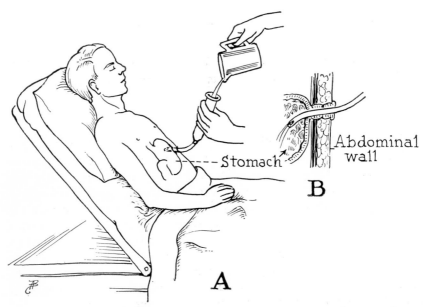

Fig. 16. Gastrostomy. (A) Patient receiving the feeding. Initially, the nurse clamps the catheter with her fourth finger to prevent entrance of air. (B) Catheter inserted through the stoma.

and hence into the duodenum. Privacy should be provided. When a patient is unable to take food orally, he is deprived of the pleasure of tasting food and the consequent stimulation of gastric secretion which aids digestion and appetite. Such a patient may be allowed to chew some food and expectorate the material without swallowing. This also helps, along with frequent oral hygiene, to prevent *parotitis*, inflammation of the parotid glands, which may ensue when the salivary glands are not exercised.

When the catheter is left in place, it is likely to cause irritation, leakage of gastric juices around the tube, and the sour odor of curdled milk. Water flushed through the catheter after each feeding helps prevent odor by removing traces of formula. The catheter may need to be irrigated before each feeding, especially if gastric retention is present. If the catheter is removed after each feeding, some leakage of gastric juices and formula may occur through the *stoma,* or opening. The skin around the gastrostomy opening must be kept scrupulously clean and dry, protected as necessary by a water-repellent ointment or aluminum powder. Dressings must be changed as often as necessary to reduce odor and moisture. The patient should be encouraged to develop interests outside of himself to prevent undue concentration upon his feeding handicap.

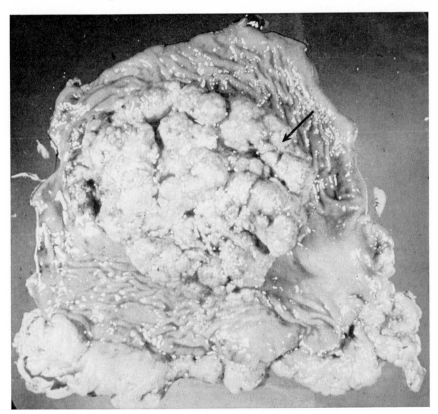

Fig. 17. A specimen showing a proliferating type of gastric carcinoma. Arrow points to the neoplasm. (*Courtesy of the American Cancer Society, Inc.*)

GASTRIC CARCINOMA

Carcinoma of the stomach can occur as a proliferating neoplasm (Fig. 17) or as an ulcerating lesion which is difficult to differentiate from a benign peptic ulcer. Differentiation is essential because the only chance for cure in gastric carcinoma depends upon early and extensive gastric resection. Carcinoma of the stomach has an insidious onset and a rapid rate of invasion. There is mounting evidence that the high degree of malignancy in gastric carcinoma is biologically predetermined [1] and that the patient who presents the usual symptoms of anorexia, especially for meat, persistent indigestion, and weight loss is often inoperable. Nevertheless, extensive gastric resection, together with removal of all adjacent, involved structures, offers the patient the best prognosis for life and/or comfort.

Statistics ranking the most common sites for cancer causing death list the stomach as second in males and fourth in females in the United States in 1954.[2]

Diagnostic Methods

X-ray or fluoroscopy following a barium meal will reveal a proliferating neoplasm but will not adequately differentiate the malignant ulcer from a benign peptic ulcer, since both show a filling defect. The only conclusive method of diagnosis is by histologic studies. *Gastroscopy*, examination of the interior of the stomach with a gastroscope, with biopsy is conclusively diagnostic if positive, but a negative report may only indicate that the neoplasm was missed in obtaining the specimen. Papanicolaou smears obtained by direct erosion of the surface of the gastric mucous membranes using a lavage technic are also significant only if positive. The specimen must be examined immediately before the cells are digested by gastric juices.[3]

The location of the lesion may suggest the presence of a malignancy. A gastric ulcer is more likely to be malignant if it is located on the greater curvature, high on the lesser curvature, in the prepylorus, or in the fundus. An ulcer located in the duodenum is almost always benign. A malignant gastric ulcer is commonly associated with an absence of free hydrochloric acid or *achlorhydria*, pernicious anemia, and atrophic gastritis. A duodenal ulcer is usually associated with *hyperchlorhydria*, an excess of free hydrochloric acid.

Surgical Technics

One treatment commonly employed is total gastric resection, or gastrectomy, with an *esophagoenterostomy* (*esophago* + *enteron*, intestine + *ostomy* = anastomosis of esophagus and intestine). It may be

---

[1] I. Macdonald and P. Kotpin, Biologic Predeterminism in Gastric Carcinoma as the Limiting Factor of Curability, *Surg., Gynec. & Obst.*, vol. 98, no. 2, p. 152, February, 1954.

[2] "Cancer and the Nursing Profession," The American Cancer Society, Inc., New York, 1957, pp. 8–9.

[3] R. W. McNealy and J. A. Glassman, "Surgical Care," Graduate Press, Maywood, Ill., 1951, p. 85.

possible to resect only two-thirds to three-fourths of the stomach, a *subtotal resection,* and reestablish continuity with a *gastroenterostomy,* anastomosis between the stomach and intestine. (See Fig. 18.) With either procedure, the regional lymph nodes must be resected. It is sometimes necessary to remove, in addition, the spleen, tail of the pancreas, and the omentum. If the carcinoma is too far advanced to warrant resection, palliative bypassing procedures will be used. Usually the abdominal approach is used, but sometimes a combined thoracoabdominal route may be used for total gastrectomy. The nurse then needs to know the principles of care for gastric surgery as well as those for thoracic surgery, which are described in Part Three.

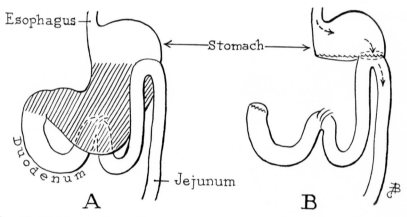

Fig. 18. Gastric resection with gastroenterostomy. (*A*) The shaded portion represents the amount of stomach and duodenum to be resected. (*B*) The completed resection and anastomosis, with arrows indicating the direction of the food and fluids postoperatively.

PEPTIC ULCER

A benign peptic ulcer is usually located in the pylorus or duodenum. (See Fig. 19.) This lesion causes an eroding process and may extend into a blood vessel, causing hemorrhage, perforate through a free wall, or penetrate into the pancreas. Repeated activity in an ulcer results in edema and scarring, which may cause gastric obstruction. An ulcer may be *intractable,* i.e., symptomatic despite adequate medical management.

The major symptom of a peptic ulcer is that of boring epigastric pain between meals when the stomach is empty. Medical management aims to coat the ulcer, neutralize the gastric juices, and put the stomach at rest. To these ends the patient is given antacids, antispasmodics, sedatives, and a soft, bland diet with milk and cream supplements between meals. He is taught that he must minimize worrying and abstain from rough, spicy foods, alcohol, coffee, and smoking—all of which aggravate the ulcer. Failure to follow this regime may lead to any of the serious complications listed previously.

The Role of Surgery in the Treatment of Peptic Ulcer

An ulcer becomes operable when it is complicated. However, some surgeons feels that gastric resection should be performed for all patients with peptic ulcer to avoid serious complications and the possibility of malignant neoplasm. The ulcer-producing mechanism is not yet completely understood. However, it is known that adequate excision of the gastric antrum removes the source of gastrin, a hormone which stimulates

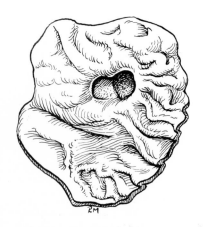

FIG. 19. Diagrammatic representation of a duodenal peptic ulcer.

the parietal cells of the corpus and fundus to secrete hydrochloric acid. Pepsin, secreted by the chief cells, is activated in an acid medium and digests the gastric lining, resulting in ulcer formation. Therefore, a subtotal gastric resection is usually the procedure of choice for benign peptic ulcer of the stomach or duodenum. Gastrointestinal continuity is reestablished by an anastomosis of the gastric remnant to the duodenum, a procedure termed *Billroth I*, or to the jejunum, *Billroth II*. With either procedure, the ulcer may or may not be resected, depending upon the feasibility of resection. If the ulcer is left in place, it will usually heal.

All the complications previously listed can be treated by gastric resection.

Hemorrhage. An initial hemorrhage from a peptic ulcer may require an emergency gastrectomy if conservative measures fail to control bleeding. This is most likely to occur when a large blood vessel has been eroded, and when the body's ability to combat bleeding by retraction of the blood vessel and coagulation fails. Such a hemorrhage is usually manifested by hematemesis and symptoms of shock. However, the majority of patients come to surgery after having had several episodes of bleeding, when it seems evident that a future recurrence may cause exsanguination. When hemorrhage is repeated or occurs in a patient with arteriosclerosis it is much more difficult to control by conservative measures.

Perforation. When an ulcer perforates through a free wall, the gastric contents (air, acid, food, and fluids) escape into the peritoneal cavity, causing pain, shock, peritonitis, and *paralytic ileus,* i.e., paralysis of the small intestine. The operation performed for an acute perforated ulcer may be simple closure of the opening with *peritonealization,* i.e., sealing the area by covering with omentum, and aspiration of the peritoneal cavity. This may be followed in 3 to 6 weeks by subtotal gastrectomy, or the gastric resection may be performed as the initial procedure, providing the patient's condition will tolerate this amount of surgery.

Penetration. If the ulcer erodes through a wall adjacent to another viscus, most commonly the pancreas, gastric resection must be performed.

Gastric Obstruction. Obstruction to gastric outflow sometimes requires gastric resection. This may occur with repeated episodes of activity and healing of a peptic ulcer in the pyloric or duodenal area. The treatment is conservative, at first, to determine whether the obstruction is due to edema and spasm, or to scarring. Nausea, vomiting, and gastric dilatation are usually relieved by aspiration. However, if symptoms persist more than a few days, surgery is necessary. Procedures, other than gastrectomy, which may be used include *pylorectomy,* removal of the pylorus, followed by gastroenterostomy, or *gastrojejunostomy,* anastomosing a loop of jejunum to the stomach to bypass the obstructed area.

Intractability. An ulcer may be truly intractable, the patient may be discouraged with the discipline of medical management and may request surgery, or he may make no consistent effort to adhere to the physician's orders. Gastric resection may be performed in such cases. Sometimes the vagus nerve is interrupted by *vagus neurectomy* or *vagotomy* to reduce the cephalic stimuli for gastric secretion and motility, thereby promoting healing of the ulcer. This procedure is almost always combined with a gastroenterostomy. Sometimes it is combined with a subtotal gastric resection. Unfortunately, a vagus neurectomy may produce undesirable sequelae, such as alternating diarrhea and constipation, or immobility of the stomach with subsequent gastric retention. Drainage procedures, such as pylorectomy, or a gastroenterostomy may be necessary to relieve gastric retention. Vagus neurectomy is reserved largely for the treatment of patients with true intractability, often associated with penetration into the pancreas, or for those with a chronic, recurring ulcer.

In the following discussion two patients are presented to illustrate the care and teaching required when a gastric resection is necessary. Mr. Olger represents a patient undergoing elective gastric resection because of a duodenal ulcer which has bled profusely on several occasions. Mr. Malcolm represents a patient undergoing emergency surgery because of a perforated peptic ulcer. The underlying principles of care for a patient undergoing gastric surgery are basically the same regardless of the condition which necessitated that surgery.

NURSING CARE AND TEACHING OF A PATIENT UNDERGOING ELECTIVE GASTRIC RESECTION

Preoperative Care of Mr. Olger

The preoperative plan for nursing care and teaching of Mr. Olger is that of preparing a 67-year-old man for a rather drastic change in his life habits. He is a retired foreman living on a modest pension; his hospitalization will seriously strain his economic status. His wife is living and well; she will be able to help her husband in his dietary regime and in his total adjustment.

His previous hospitalizations, required because of recurrent hemorrhage, have prepared him somewhat for what he should expect in this experience. He has been on ulcer management for 20 years and has been able to accept this discipline fairly well. Therefore, his nurse must concentrate on the change in living to be necessitated by a gastrectomy and emphasize the need to remain on ulcer management, realizing that this patient will probably be able to make the adjustment satisfactorily.

The principles of geriatric nursing must be employed in Mr. Olger's care. His skin is thin and dry; therefore the nurse will use soap sparingly, rinse thoroughly, and apply a lubricant. Vigorous measures to prevent the hazards of bed rest must be employed, since these patients develop complications readily. Protective measures to prevent falls must be used when the patient is ambulatory or after the administration of sedatives. Nursing care must be given skillfully, without haste, because these patients may become confused when rushed. The nurse must help the patient maintain an interest in activities outside himself to prevent depression and withdrawal. To this end she must take time to engage the patient in conversation. If the patient is hard of hearing, the nurse must speak slowly and enunciate clearly in full view of the patient; shouting is unnecessary and is resented by the patient.

Diagnostic Methods. Preoperative diagnostic procedures aim to detect active bleeding, to rule out malignancy, and to determine the presence of conditions requiring correction before surgery. A stool specimen is tested for occult blood several days after a meat-free diet has been instituted. The blood is typed and cross-matched for transfusion to correct the anemia resulting from chronic blood loss. A full blood count, hematocrit reading, and measurements of prothrombin time and serum-protein level are usually made. Gastrointestinal roentgen studies with barium are made to rule out a malignant neoplasm as the cause of bleeding. The patient is prepared for these studies by abstaining from oral intake and by taking enemas or cathartics. The lower intestinal tract is studied prior to the barium meal. Complete evacuation of the barium is necessary to prevent intestinal obstruction.

Patient Teaching. The nurse will have ample time to reassure Mr. Olger throughout these preoperative procedures and to teach him what he must know about his postgastrectomy care. She must emphasize the need for activation, decompression, and intravenous fluid therapy. She must explain that oral intake will be resumed gradually and that the medical management for ulcer, previously followed, will still be necessary to Mr. Olger's comfort and welfare.

Decompression Therapy. Gastrointestinal decompression is a procedure commonly employed before and after surgery on the gastrointestinal tract to keep the suture line clean, to prevent or relieve distention, and to prevent excessive vomiting. This procedure may be used in a variety of conditions, not necessarily surgical, e.g., paralytic ileus, when it is necessary to prevent an accumulation of fluids and gases in the gastrointestinal tract. The principles of care in decompression therapy are described here in detail, because this procedure is almost universally used in gastric surgery.

The principle underlying effective gastrointestinal decompression is the maintenance of a partial vacuum which creates gentle suction to remove fluids and gas from the stomach and intestines. This can be accomplished by several methods. (See Figs. 20, 21, 22.) All require the intubation of the patient with a catheter, usually passed through the nose, into the stomach or small intestine. The most commonly used tubes are the single-lumen Levin, which reaches only into the stomach, or a double-lumen tube, such as that of Miller-Abbott or Harris. Double-lumen tubes contain a balloon which can be distended with air, water, or mercury to facilitate passage of the tube past the pyloric sphincter; the balloon acting as a bolus of food is aided in passage by peristalsis. The care required when these intestinal decompression tubes are used will be described in Chapter 11.

The patient must be helped to accept this procedure by realizing that it will prevent vomiting and will be discontinued as soon as his condition allows. If the water-displacement apparatus is used, he may think the procedure is similar to intravenous therapy and may therefore be concerned if there is not a steady dripping of water. He should be told that the water does not enter his system but is only a method of creating suction to relieve him of nausea and distention.

The patient with gastrointestinal decompression requires a definite plan for nursing care to achieve the full therapeutic effectiveness of the procedure, to prevent complications, and to promote comfort. The nurse must ensure the functioning of the system by checking frequently to be sure that there are no kinks in the tubing, by maintaining the apparatus

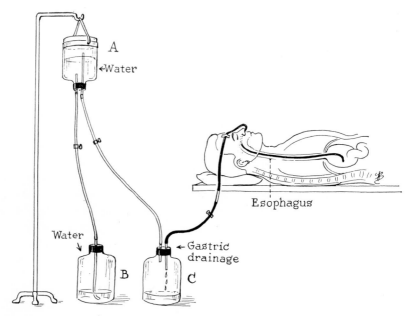

Fig. 20. Gastric decompression using the Wangensteen three-bottle method. Water falling from bottle *A* to *B* creates a partial vacuum in *A* which is transmitted to *C*. (While bottle *C* can be omitted, its use is recommended, because it allows an accurate measurement and observation of drainage. It also facilitates the handling of bottles *A* and *B* by eliminating the need for washing these containers each time they are reversed.) *Caution:* The end of the tubing leading from the patient must never contact fluid.

creating the suction in working order, and by irrigating the nasal gastroduodenal catheter as ordered. The Levin tube, the type most commonly used in gastric surgery, is irrigated at regular intervals of 2 to 4 hours, or only as necessary, with 10 to 30 ml. air or solution as ordered by the surgeon; positive pressure should not be exerted in the irrigation. Sterile solutions are used after surgery on the stomach and upper small intestine. The amount and character of the returns must be noted. The amount of irrigating solution used and not aspirated by syringe must be deducted from the total returns to give a true index of the amount of gastric drainage. Distention and vomiting indicate that the system is not functioning properly, usually because the outflow is obstructed or the tube is not in the correct position.

Complications which may ensue are due to mechanical irritation of the pharynx or larynx and to lack of stimulation of the salivary and parotid glands. Pharyngitis can be minimized and parotitis prevented by giving oral hygiene every 4 hours. Chewing gum or sucking fruit drops, if permitted by the surgeon, helps moisten the mouth and activates the

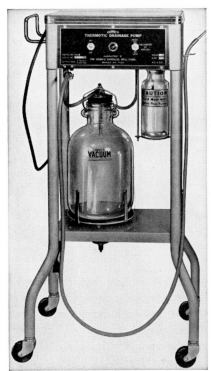

FIG. 21. Gomco thermotic drainage pump. This commercial electrical apparatus creates suction by alternately heating and cooling air. (*Gomco Surgical Manufacturing Corp., New York.*)

salivary glands. Parotitis is evidenced by fever, prostration, and tenderness of the parotid gland; this type of parotitis is noninfectious. Pharyngitis may be relieved by allowing the patient sips of water, at the discretion of the surgeon. The water returning with the apparatus serves as an effective irrigation but invites electrolytic imbalance by acting as a gastric wash. If local anesthetic troches are ordered to relieve pharyngeal discomfort, the nurse must realize that the patient may aspirate fluid into his lungs because his throat is anesthetized. Irritation of the larynx, causing laryngeal edema, is evidenced by hoarseness and dyspnea. This is a serious complication which demands removal of the nasal gastroduodenal tube to prevent permanent damage or asphyxia. Frequent position change and ambulation help prevent tissue necrosis due to constant pressure of the tube. Some surgeons obviate these complications by establishing a temporary gastrostomy, which can be used to decompress the stomach.

The patient is maintained in nutritional-fluid-electrolytic balance by parenteral fluid therapy. He will need to have his chlorides, sodium, and potassium, which are removed by suction, replaced by the intravenous route. An accurate intake-output record and frequent urinalyses are necessary to help determine renal function and guide parenteral fluid therapy.

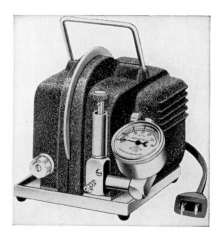

Fig. 22. Stedman continuous suction pump. This commercial pump is activated by electromagnetic coils. A vacuum collecting bottle is interposed between the patient and the pump. (*American Cystoscope Makers, Inc., New York.*)

When a patient has intranasal intubation and is not permitted oral intake, a rectal temperature must be taken to obtain an accurate reading. The temperature should be taken every 4 hours.

Decompression will be discontinued when peristalsis has resumed and the operative area is ready for oral intake. The surgeon may order the prompt removal of the nasal gastroduodenal tube. He may prefer to have the tube clamped for a period of time and to have the patient resume oral intake so that his tolerance may be noted. In this case the nurse will watch for nausea and distention, and gastric retention, which is evidenced by the amount of drainage obtained when the tube is unclamped. The tube is withdrawn with suction applied to prevent aspiration of material in the end of the tube as it passes the trachea.

Immediate Preparation for Surgery. In preparation for gastric surgery, frequent aspirations and lavage may be employed to empty the stomach. The patient may be given a liquid diet or nothing orally for a day or more preoperatively. A Levin tube is commonly inserted and left in place the morning of surgery. Laparotomy orders are carried out in addition to the measures described. Oral hygiene is particularly important before gastric surgery.

Surgical Technic

The operation performed for Mr. Olger included resection of three-fourths of his stomach, including the duodenal area containing the ulcer, closure of the duodenal stump, and gastrojejunostomy. (See Fig. 18.)

Postoperative Care

The postoperative care for a patient who has had such an operation, whether for carcinoma or peptic ulcer, follows closely the care outlined for a laparotomy. The major additional considerations include the use of decompression and intravenous fluids, the gradual resumption of oral intake, and watching for the complications which are the most likely to occur following gastric surgery. Leakage due to blowout of the duodenal stump is evidenced by symptoms of shock and peritonitis. Because the stomach has an excellent blood supply, healing usually occurs rapidly, but hemostasis may be difficult. Therefore, the nurse will be alert to symptoms of postoperative hemorrhage and shock.

A small percentage of patients may have nutritional problems following gastric resection with gastroenterostomy. Although the gastric remnant dilates in time to assume more of the stomach's natural reservoir function, it never completely reaches normal capacity. Therefore the patient feels satiated early in the course of eating and may fail to take adequate nourishment. Weakness and weight loss follow. In addition, food is projected into the intestines at a more rapid rate than normal without the adequate churning effect of an intact stomach and without being mixed with gastric juices. The food reaching the small intestine is hypertonic so that fluid is poured into the intestine from the extracellular compartment, and hypovolemic shock may ensue. The resultant sudden overdistention of the intestine coupled with hypovolemia may result in diarrhea and/or the "dumping syndrome." This latter phenomenon is an experience of faintness, weakness, cardiac palpitation, nausea, and diaphoresis which occurs shortly after eating in a small percentage of patients. Symptoms are relieved when the patient abstains from liquids with his meals and lies down for 20 to 30 minutes after eating. Many patients experience a transitory dumping syndrome for 2 to 3 days after oral intake is initiated. It is important to allay apprehension when these symptoms first appear in order to minimize their severity and to prevent a pattern formation, especially in patients who have many emotional problems. "Dumping" may occur with either a gastroduodenostomy or gastrojejunostomy but is more common with the latter.

Another factor which may contribute to postgastrectomy malnutrition in a patient who has had a gastrojejunostomy is the absence of food in the duodenum to stimulate the flow of bile and pancreatic secretions which aid digestion. It is sometimes helpful in intractable nutritional invalidism to convert a gastrojejunostomy into a gastroduodenostomy, which is the more normal route.

Another condition which may interfere with nutrition is gastric retention owing to a stoma which is too small. If this is due to edema, relief is usually obtained by gastric decompression, lavage, liquid feedings, and correction of electrolytic imbalance. If the line of anastomosis is too tight, reoperation for revision of the stoma is necessary.

Many of these complications are minimized when oral intake is initiated gradually, postoperatively, and a positive attitude toward eating is developed in the patient. The incidence of nutritional invalidism, when it does occur, is usually in direct proportion to the extent of gastric resection; however, the cure rate also rises as more of the stomach is removed. When a total gastrectomy with an esophagoenterostomy is performed, a reflux esophagitis may be added to the nutritional problem. Sometimes a pouch can be formed from a double loop of jejunum, or part of the colon can be transplanted, to serve as a gastric reservoir.

The patient who has had a gastrectomy should be taught to eat frequent, small amounts of food, gradually increasing the amount and lengthening the intervals between meals. He must eat slowly, chew his food thoroughly, and stop when he feels full. Usually he is started on clear-to-full liquids, then progresses to a bland, soft diet, then to a full diet which is high-caloric, high-protein, high-fat, low-carbohydrate. If his gastrectomy was performed for peptic ulcer, he must remain on ulcer management to prevent a recurrence.

NURSING CARE AND TEACHING OF A PATIENT UNDERGOING EMERGENCY GASTRIC SURGERY

Preoperative Care of Mr. Malcolm

Mr. Malcolm typifies a patient who is to undergo emergency surgery for another complication of peptic ulcer, namely, perforation. On his way to work this morning he collapsed with an acute, knifelike pain in his upper abdomen accompanied by faintness, nausea, and diaphoresis. He was brought to the hospital by ambulance.

The physician notes that Mr. Malcolm is in shock, has grunting respirations, and appears to be more comfortable lying on his left side with knees and thighs flexed. The physical examination further reveals boardlike rigidity of the abdomen; bowel sounds are absent; tympany is elicited over the liver area. An upright and left lateral x-ray of the abdomen reveals free air under the diaphragm and over the liver.

As has been stated, when an ulcer perforates, gastric contents escape into the peritoneal cavity. Leakage is minimized with the patient lying on his left side when the site of perforation is through the anterior duodenal surface. With the rupture of any hollow viscus, air escapes and rises to press against the diaphragm, causing tympany and grunting respirations. Peritoneal response to acid is due to chemical peritonitis which is evidenced by rigidity. Paralytic ileus, detected by absence of bowel sounds, eventually causes more distention.

Emergency Care. It is necessary that the nurse form a general concept of the medical management of conditions which may become surgical emergencies in order to anticipate equipment which will probably be needed. Having equipment immediately available saves valuable time in the treatment of the patient and may be lifesaving. For example, in ulcer perforation the patient's prognosis is considerably improved if he can be readied for surgery and operated upon within 3 to 6 hours, before bacterial peritonitis ensues. Therefore, the nurse receiving Mr. Malcolm would have ready equipment for intravenous fluids and gastrointestinal decompression. She will also anticipate the administration of an antibiotic, narcotic, and antisecretory drug. It is pointed out that anticipation of equipment needed is the nurse's responsibility but that she must await specific orders from the surgeon.

Preparation for Surgery. Because Mr. Malcolm is to undergo emergency surgery, the plan for nursing care will be limited to the immediate preparation for laparotomy and to assisting with measures to correct fluid-electrolyte imbalance, control pain, counteract infection, combat shock, and decompress the stomach and intestine. The nurse must reassure the patient throughout these many procedures that he will be well cared for. She must make frequent determinations of the patient's cardinal signs in this early period of perforation. The temperature should be taken rectally because the patient is in shock and pain and has difficult respirations.

Laboratory Procedures. Laboratory procedures in emergency surgery are usually limited. A complete blood count and urinalysis are performed immediately, and blood is drawn for serologic testing. It may be necessary to catheterize the patient to obtain a urine specimen. The blood is typed and cross-matched preparatory to transfusion, which helps combat shock and possible hemorrhage. If the patient is vomiting, the vomitus may be tested for blood.

Postoperative Care

Mr. Malcolm's surgeon closed the perforation with the intention of performing a gastric resection after convalescence.

In the postoperative period the nurse has a better opportunity to plan for care and teaching to meet Mr. Malcolm's personal needs, as well as those imposed upon him by his medical condition and surgical intervention. It is important for the nurse to learn that Mr. Malcolm is a tense, impatient, overly conscientious person who tends to neglect his health in the interest of his responsibilities as president of a large business corporation. He has been in the habit of eating irregularly, smoking excessively, and worrying habitually. While the patient with a peptic ulcer need not necessarily have this type of personality, these traits are not uncommonly a part of the "ulcer personality." Irregular eating, excessive smoking, and repressed emotions all tend to aggravate an ulcer.

His postoperative care is essentially the same as that described for Mr. Olger except that his resumption of oral intake need not be so gradual. He must be watched for symptoms of gastric retention.

In preparation for assuming responsibility for self-care following his discharge from the hospital, Mr. Malcolm must be helped to understand and accept the need for adequate physical rest and recreation, for moderation in all areas of living including his emotional responses, for abstinence from smoking and from alcohol, and for strict adherence to the prescribed intake of antispasmodics, antacids, sedatives, and bland diet. He must remain under medical supervision and be helped to accept the need for further surgery following convalescence to prevent a recurrence of peptic ulcer complications.

SUMMARY

Gastrostomy may be necessary to provide for the intake of water and nutrients in a patient who has an obstructed esophagus. The patient requires a plan for care and teaching designed to prevent complications, maintain adequate intake, and promote comfort.

Gastric surgery is more commonly performed in the treatment of carcinoma and of peptic ulcer and its complications. Carcinoma requires a total gastric resection, whereas a partial resection usually suffices in the treatment of peptic ulcer and/or its complications. The complications of peptic ulcer include hemorrhage, perforation, penetration, obstruction, and intractability. A peptic ulcer must be differentiated from one that is malignant on the basis of histologic studies.

The patient is prepared for gastric surgery as for laparotomy. In addition, decompression therapy is commonly instituted to remove all gastric contents. Decompression therapy automatically implies a need for giving nothing by mouth, administering intravenous fluids, frequent oral hygiene, frequent position change, and the taking of rectal temperatures. In addition, it is important to ensure the functioning of whatever equipment is used to decompress the stomach.

In the postoperative period, the plan for care includes the measures just described. In addition, a program of gradually increased oral intake is initiated after decompression therapy is no longer needed. If surgery was performed in the treatment of a peptic ulcer, the patient must be helped to understand the need to continue with medical management to prevent a recurrence. The patient with carcinoma must also remain under medical surveillance to detect recurrence.

BIBLIOGRAPHY

ALTHAUSEN, T. L., and I. S. RAVDIN: Treatment of Gastric Ulcer, *Spectrum Forum,* Chas. Pfizer and Company, Inc., vol. 5, no. 6, pp. 170, 171, 173, 1957.

BARBORKA, C. J., and E. C. TEXTER, JR.: Peptic Ulcer and Benign Gastric Lesions, in "Christopher's Textbook of Surgery," 6th ed., L. Davis (ed.), W. B. Saunders Company, Philadelphia, 1956, chap. 20, pp. 589–606.

"A Cancer Source Book for Nurses," American Cancer Society, Inc., New York, 1950, pp. 76–78.

COLE, W. H.: Surgical Considerations in Peptic Ulcer, *S. Clin. North America,* vol. 35, no. 1, pp. 81–91, February, 1955.

DONHAUSER, J. L.: Peptic Ulcer Perforations, *A.M.A. Arch. Surg.,* vol. 68, no. 5, pp. 605–607, May, 1954.

GROVE, W. J.: Surgery of the Abdomen, in "The Recovery Room," M. S. Sadove and J. H. Cross (eds.), W. B. Saunders Company, Philadelphia, 1956, chap. 9, pp. 259–294.

HARKINS, H. N.: Stomach and Duodenum, in "Surgery," J. G. Allen, H. N. Harkins, C. A. Moyer, and J. E. Rhoads (eds.), J. B. Lippincott Company, Philadelphia, 1957, chap. 29, pp. 627–678.

HARVEY, H. D.: Acute Massive Hemorrhage and Acute Perforation in Peptic Ulcer, *S. Clin. North America,* vol. 35, no. 2, pp. 369–380, April, 1955.

HEGER, C.: Surgical Nursing Care of Patients with Duodenal Ulcer, *Am. J. Nursing,* pp. 861–862, July, 1952.

KELLY, W. D., L. D. MACLEAN, J. F. PERRY, and O. H. WANGENSTEEN: A Study of Patients Following Total and Near-total Gastrectomy, *Surgery,* vol. 35, no. 6, pp. 964–980, June, 1954.

MACLEAN, L. D., J. F. PERRY, W. D. KELLY, D. G. MOSSER, A. MANNICK, and O. H. WANGENSTEEN: Nutrition Following Subtotal Gastrectomy of Four Types, *Surgery,* vol. 35, no. 5, pp. 705–718, May, 1954.

MCNEALY, R. W., and J. A. GLASSMAN: "Surgical Care," The Graduate Press, Maywood, Ill., 1951, pp. 80–99.

MARSHALL, S. F., and H. W. REINSTEIN, JR.: The Role of the Pyloric Antrum in the Production of Gastrojejunal Ulcer Following Gastrectomy, *S. Clin. North America,* vol. 35, no. 3, pp. 711–717, June, 1955.

MATHEWSON, JR., C.: Conversion of Billroth II to Billroth I for the Relief of Postgastrectomy Symptoms, *Surgery,* vol. 90, no. 2, pp. 317–324, August, 1955.

MEDWID, A., J. WEISSMAN, H. T. RANDALL, H. N. BANE, P. VANAMEE, K. E. ROBERTS: Physiologic Alterations Resulting from Carbohydrate, Protein, and Fat Meals in Patients Following Gastrectomy: the Relationship of These Changes to the Dumping Syndrome, *Ann. Surg.,* vol. 144, no. 6, pp. 953–959, December, 1956.

PALUMBO, L. T.: Surgical Treatment of Duodenal Ulcer, *Am. J. Nursing,* pp. 857–861, July, 1952.

————, T. T. MAZUR, and B. J. DOYLE: Partial Gastrectomy with or without Vagus Resection for Duodenal or Marginal Ulcer, *Surgery,* vol. 36, no. 6, pp. 1043–1050, December, 1954.

ROSS, J. R.: Dumping Syndrome and Other Postoperative Symptoms Following Partial and Total Gastrectomy, *S. Clin. North America,* vol. 35, no. 3, pp. 703–710, June, 1955.

SCHELL, R. F., M. B. DOCKERTY, and M. W. COMFORT: Carcinoma of the Stomach Associated with Pernicious Anemia, *Surg., Gynec. & Obst.,* vol. 98, no. 6, p. 719, June, 1954.

STRODE, J. E.: In Support of Surgical Removal of Small Ulcerating Lesions of the Stomach without Benefit of Medical Treatment, *Surg., Gynec. & Obst.,* vol. 98, no. 5, pp. 607–618, May, 1954.

WALLENSTEN, S., and L. GOTHMAN: An Evaluation of the Billroth I Operation for Peptic Ulcer, *Surgery,* vol 33, no. 1, pp. 1–19, January, 1953.

WEINBERG, J. A., S. J. STEMPIEN, H. J. MOVIUS, and A. E. DAGRADI: Vagotomy and Pyloroplasty in the Treatment of Duodenal Ulcer, *Am. J. Surg.,* vol. 92, no. 2, pp. 202–207, August, 1956.

WILKINSON, S. A.: Indications for Surgical Intervention in Peptic Ulcer, *S. Clin. North America,* vol. 35, no. 3, pp. 679–682, June, 1955.

10

SURGERY OF THE GALLBLADDER AND BILE DUCTS, LIVER, SPLEEN, PANCREAS, AND ADRENAL GLANDS

Abdominal surgery performed for the treatment of conditions affecting the gallbladder and bile ducts, liver, spleen, pancreas, and adrenal glands can be described collectively inasmuch as these structures share a common anatomic region and are subject to similar types of disease, and operations on them require essentially the same nursing measures. The close cooperation of the medical- and surgical-care teams is necessary, since many of the conditions affecting these structures become surgical only after a prolonged period of medical management or for palliation only. In order to understand better the role of surgery in the treatment of these diseases, it is imperative that the student first develop an understanding of the basic pathologic processes and medical aspects of care. Therefore, the student is urged to refer to a medical textbook prior to or concurrent with the study of this chapter and to refer freely to Figure 23.

SURGICAL CONDITIONS OF THE GALLBLADDER AND BILE DUCTS

Cholecystitis with Cholelithiasis

Jean Thorenson is a 42-year-old mother of three children, ranging in age from 14 to 22 years. She and her husband own their large dairy farm and are active members of the Lutheran Church. Mrs. Thorenson is fair-complexioned and rather obese, with a pleasant, outgoing personality.

One night, following a banquet, she awoke with severe colicky pain which started in the epigastrium and radiated to the right upper quadrant and scapula. This pain was accompanied by nausea and vomiting and was relieved only by an injection of meperidine and atropine administered by her physician. Since this was the third such attack within a year, she was told that she could no longer delay surgery and that arrangements for hospitalization would be made the following morning.

This description is typical of biliary colic and of the person who has such attacks, although it by no means follows that all patients conform to this pattern. Biliary colic is due to *cholecystitis* (*chole*, gall or bile + *cyst*, bladder or sac + *itis* = inflammation of the gallbladder) with

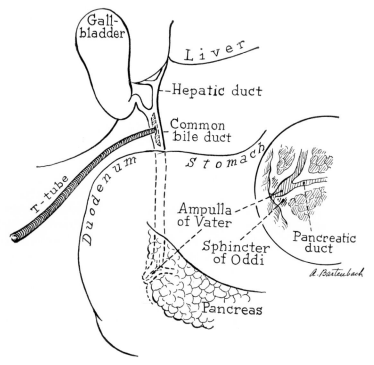

Fig. 23. Diagram of the anatomy of the extrahepatic biliary system. Note the T-tube in place. The insert shows the anatomic relationships of the common bile duct passing through pancreatic tissue to enter the duodenum.

cholelithiasis (*chole* + *lith*, stone or calculus + *iasis*, being with = condition of having gallstones). These disease entities almost always occur together and affect women more commonly than men. The incidence of the disease increases with age.

Etiology and Pathology. Etiologic factors associated with biliary calculi include an increased serum-cholesterol level, such as may occur in obesity with the eating of rich, fatty foods, and in pregnancy. Disturbances in bile metabolism and excretion are important factors. Stasis of bile, which may be caused by obstruction to outflow due to compression, a neoplasm, calculi, or spasm of the sphincter of Oddi, is almost always present. Inflammatory changes are also present and cause further stasis owing to edema. The edema which accompanies the inflammation causes further obstruction and stasis. Whether stasis of bile precedes or follows inflammation initially has yet to be determined. At any rate, once initiated, the pathologic process tends to be cyclic. With stasis of bile there is precipitation of bile salts to form calculi which irritate the mucous membranes, evoking an inflammatory reaction which causes further stasis.

If a calculus becomes impacted at any point along the common bile duct, causing complete obstruction, dilatation of the duct proximal to the site occurs. Bile forced back into the liver ruptures the sinusoids, allowing bile constituents to be reabsorbed into the bloodstream to cause jaundice. If the cystic duct is obstructed by a gallstone, the gallbladder dilates and secretes a clear mucoid fluid, a condition termed *hydrops*. *Empyema* of the gallbladder supervenes when bacteria gain access by the hematogenous route or by ascending through the common bile duct from the duodenum. Both hydrops and empyema are emergency conditions requiring *cholecystostomy*, drainage of the gallbladder, to prevent gangrene and perforation of the gallbladder wall, which may cause a fatal peritonitis.

Symptomatology. Acute cholecystitis with cholelithiasis is commonly manifested by biliary colic such as Jean Thorenson experienced. These attacks typically occur several hours after eating and at night, causing such agonizing pain that the patient is reluctant to breathe or move and fears impending death. She may become profoundly depressed. The surgeon easily obtains consent for surgery during such an attack, but the following morning the patient is usually much more comfortable and, therefore, tends to put off surgical intervention until the next attack. Relief occurs with cessation of spasm following the administration of a narcotic and atropine. Narcotics, while often necessary in the height of an attack, tend to increase spasm and intrabiliary pressure; therefore, atropine or scopolamine is given concurrently to reduce spasm.

There may be a moderate elevation in temperature and a leukocytosis. The gallbladder may be palpable. Following the acute attack, there may be residual soreness and muscle spasm in the right upper quadrant. Jaundice and acholic stools may or may not occur, depending upon whether the common bile duct is obstructed. If obstruction is due to unimpacted stones, jaundice will be intermittent, subsiding when the stones move; if due to a tumor or stricture, jaundice will be more gradual in onset and unrelenting in character.

Following the acute stage the disease may become chronic, manifested by flatulence, belching, and intolerance to fatty foods. Fat in the duodenum initiates the release of cholecystokinin, a hormone responsible for stimulating the gallbladder to contract. If this organ is inflammed, these contractions cause pain.

Diagnostic Methods. Diagnosis is made on the basis of history, physical findings during an acute attack, and by x-ray studies made during a quiescent period. Visualization of the biliary tract by *cholecystography* is accomplished by the use of a radiopaque contrast medium which is administered orally or intravenously and is excreted by the liver in the

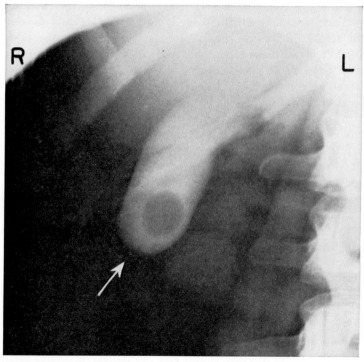

Fig. 24. Cholelithiasis. Note in this cholecystogram the large nonopaque calculus contained within the gallbladder. The calculus displaces the contrast medium and appears as a negative shadow.

bile. Provided no obstruction is present, the contrast medium fills the gallbladder and ducts. Intraluminal or extraluminal lesions are revealed by obstruction to the flow of the contrast medium. Biliary calculi are usually detectable as negative shadows. (See Fig. 24.) A series of cholecystograms taken before and after the ingestion of a high-fat meal helps to evaluate how well the gallbladder can concentrate and excrete bile and whether there is obstruction to the outflow of bile through the sphincter of Oddi. An x-ray of the abdomen is taken prior to the ingestion of contrast medium, since some stones are of the same density as the contrast medium and would be obscured by cholecystography.

In preparing the patient for cholecystography it is important that the patient understand what is to take place, both to minimize apprehension and to ensure her cooperation in taking the tablets as directed and in abstaining from oral intake. The tablets are taken with a light, fat-free supper, after which no oral intake is permitted except for sips of water until bedtime. Reactions to the contrast medium may occur and must be promptly reported. They may be of an allergic nature, manifested by urticaria, although vomiting and diarrhea are more common. It is important to notify the physician if the patient vomits the medium so that he may order the tablets to be repeated or decide to administer the medium intravenously in the morning. However, intravenous administration involves more risk. An enema is usually given in the morning to prevent a distended colon from obscuring the x-ray findings. After the first x-ray, a high-fat breakfast is given and followed by one or more films at stated intervals. It is imperative that nothing be given orally until ordered by the roentgenologist, since failure to comply with the orders may render the examination invalid and necessitate the expense of repeating the procedure.

Liver-function tests are usually ordered to determine the degree and type of hepatic involvement which may be present. The operative risk is increased in the presence of hepatic damage. When jaundice is present, hypoprothrombinemia may result and predispose the patient to hemorrhage. The administration of vitamin K usually restores the prothrombin level to normal. A serum bilirubin test is helpful in evaluating the degree of jaundice which may be present. With obstructive jaundice, bilirubin is excreted in the urine, and no urobilinogen is found in the stool.

Duodenal drainage, which entails intubating the patient and aspirating samples of bile from the duodenum, is helpful in evaluating the site of obstruction as well as the quality of bile and presence of sediment.

The nurse's observations can be of great value to the surgeon during this period of diagnostic work-up. She should observe excreta carefully and report promptly the passage of clay-colored stools and golden-brown, foamy urine. She must note the onset and character of pain in relation to food intake. The onset and intensity of jaundice must be reported; jaundice is usually noticeable in the sclera and mucous membranes before the skin becomes yellow-tinged.

Preoperative Preparation. If jaundice is present, vitamin K must be administered orally or parenterally for the associated hypoprothrombinemia to prevent hemorrhage. Vitamin K is necessary for the formation of prothrombin in the liver. Since this vitamin is fat-soluble, bile salts must be administered simultaneously when the oral route is used, to allow emulsification and absorption.

The nurse's role during the preoperative preparation of a patient like Mrs. Thorenson is largely supportive. She has had three acute attacks which she is not eager to repeat, and, therefore, having decided to undergo surgery, she needs encouragement primarily in feeling that she has made a wise decision. She is a good risk for surgery since she is relatively young, has had the disease for only a year or so, and has no complications. Her socioeconomic status is not threatened too seriously by this hospitalization. Her children are old enough to carry on satisfactorily with their father's guidance. In addition, Jean's strong religious faith lends her much support.

Although Jean is still somewhat overweight, the reducing diet she was using is not continued in the hospital because the liver needs carbohydrate to withstand surgical stress. Therefore, she is given a diet moderately high in carbohydrate, adequate in protein, and low in fat, with vitamins and minerals supplemented. A liberal fluid intake is encouraged. Mrs. Thorenson is urged to be ambulatory throughout the preoperative period.

The immediate preparation for cholecystectomy is the same as for laparotomy with two exceptions. A low-fat, light supper is usually given. Meperidine or Phenergan may be substituted for morphine in the preoperative medication. Blood for transfusion is made available, especially for a patient with jaundice.

Surgical Technic. Cholecystectomy under general anesthesia is the procedure of choice for cholecystitis with cholelithiasis. Such surgery involves far less risk if it can be performed prior to the onset of complications, such as obstructive jaundice. Since the number and size of the calculi increase with age,[1] and since surgery carries a higher morbidity and mortality in older patients, operative intervention is preferred early in the course of the disease.

Should multiple small calculi be found which could pass through the cystic duct into the common bile duct, *choledochostomy*, i.e., making an opening into the common bile duct, would be performed in addition to cholecystectomy. This procedure permits exploration and irrigation of the common bile duct and is followed by T-tube drainage of bile to the exterior. (See Fig. 23.) Choledochostomy is performed also when calculi are known to be in the duct or when, in spite of the presence of jaundice, no calculi are found in the gallbladder.

Postoperative Nursing Care and Teaching. The basic care following cholecystectomy is also the same as for laparotomy. The vital signs must be closely observed, catheterization may be necessary, the activation regime is instituted early, an intake-output record is kept, and analgesics are administered as necessary. In addition, the nursing measures necessary

[1] F. Glenn, The Liver and Biliary System, in "Christopher's Textbook of Surgery," 6th ed., L. Davis (ed.), W. B. Saunders Company, Philadelphia, 1956, chap. 21, p. 729.

with gastrointestinal decompression and intravenous fluids are employed for the first 2 days postoperatively when this therapy is used. After decompression therapy is discontinued, oral alimentation is resumed without dietary restriction. This is possible because the bile ducts dilate in time to assume some of the reservoir function of the gallbladder, and, although bile is no longer concentrated, digestion is unimpaired.

Wound care in this case differs somewhat from the usual in that bile is drained to the exterior. Bile escaping through a Penrose drain or around a T-tube is extremely irritating to the skin and requires that the area be kept scrupulously clean, dry, and protected with a moisture-repellent ointment or aluminum paste or powder. When aluminum paste is used, the surface is kept clean and reapplications are made as necessary, but the basic layer is not disturbed. A T-tube is used following choledochostomy to prevent obstruction due to edema, to splint the duct, and to allow egress of bile. When the gallbladder has been opened but not removed, catheter drainage is instituted. Both tubes require strict aseptic technic. Bile is collected in a light-weight, sterile container, such as a rubber glove, fastened in such a way that no traction is exerted on the tube. The nurse must note the color, consistency, and amount of bile drainage. The bile occasionally is returned to the patient through an indwelling nasogastric feeding tube. The exact amount collected and returned must be added to the intake-output record. If bile is not returned, bile salts may be ordered to be administered orally during the period of bile drainage.

As healing progresses, and edema subsides, the bile flows around, rather than through, the short arm of the tube into the duodenum. In approximately 2 weeks, bile no longer escapes to the outside, and the T-tube is clamped as tolerated for a trial period. During this time the nurse must be particularly observant for evidences of pain, jaundice, and fever which might indicate obstruction of the bile duct. Stools are examined for urobilinogen content. Patency of the common bile duct is confirmed by *cholangiography*, roentgenologic visualization of the bile ducts. The tube is then removed by gentle traction. The duct seals itself.

Activation and deep-breathing exercises are particularly important following cholecystectomy because the incision impinges upon the costal margin, making respiratory movements painful. These patients tend to have shallow respirations, and, therefore, respiratory stasis is a real hazard. Elevation of the head of the bed for short periods of time relaxes tension upon the incision, promoting comfort and more effective ventilation.

In addition to the complications of pulmonary and vascular stasis, shock, hemorrhage, and wound infection, there are complications peculiar to surgery on the biliary tract. Chills, fever, and jaundice may indicate surgical trauma to the bile ducts, common bile duct obstruction, or infection. Leakage of bile can cause a fatal peritonitis. Liver abscess formation can result from the introduction of bacteria at surgery or through the drainage tube. Hemorrhage may occur in a patient who has jaundice. Wound healing may be slow.

Antibiotics, vitamin K, and cholagogues are administered as necessary. The surgeon will usually order laboratory determinations of bilirubin, prothrombin time, and fecal urobilinogen.

The patient is discharged with instructions to return to her surgeon or physician for follow-up care. Her diet is not restricted, but rich, fatty foods should be avoided. A liberal fluid intake and moderate activity help promote the flow of bile. Frequent rest periods and the avoidance of physical and emotional strain are beneficial for any patient postoperatively. Convalescence will be more prolonged for the patient who had marked jaundice preoperatively, and close medical supervision will be necessary. Some patients will be discharged with the T-tube in place and will need to be instructed in its care. Such a patient can benefit by referral to a public health agency who can help her with her care at home.

Stricture of the Bile Duct

A stricture is an abnormal narrowing of a lumen by cicatrical contraction or neoplastic growth. Stricture of the hepatic and/or common bile duct is usually due to surgical trauma, inflammation, or neoplastic growth. Indigestion and jaundice with or without pain develop insidiously. The gallbladder can not be visualized by cholecystography because the dye is not excreted by the liver when jaundice is present. If the stricture is segmental rather than diffuse, and if liver damage is not too extensive, resection of the area of stricture followed by an end-to-end anastomosis is attempted.

Neoplasms of the Extrahepatic System

Patients with malignant neoplasms of the biliary tract are resistant to treatment and have a poor prognosis, with a short survival time. The majority of such neoplasms arise in the gallbladder and occur more commonly in women over fifty-five years of age.[2] Cholelithiasis is present in approximately 90 per cent of the patients with carcinoma of the gallbladder.[3] Radical cholecystectomy with resection of the gallbladder bed, with or without partial hepatectomy, is attempted, but metastasis or extension into the liver usually has occurred and results are poor.

Less frequently the extrahepatic bile ducts are the site of a primary neoplasm. A malignancy of the ampulla of Vater carries the best prognosis, with a few 5-year survivals having been achieved by radical pancreatoduodenectomy (see page 124).

[2] *Ibid.*, p. 736.
[3] *Ibid.*

Sometimes diversionary procedures are attempted for palliation when neoplasm of the common bile duct obstructs the flow of bile. An anastomosis between the gastrointestinal and biliary tracts permits bile to flow directly into the jejunum from the gallbladder or proximal common bile duct. This is accomplished by *cholecystojejunostomy* or *choledochojejunostomy,* using a defunctionalized loop of jejunum in an effort to minimize intestinal reflux. Some palliation is achieved but survival time is short.

Benign neoplasms of the extrahepatic ducts are of little significance since they are usually asymptomatic and are rarely diagnosed during life.

SURGERY OF THE LIVER

Advances in physiology, pharmacology, biochemistry, anesthesiology, and surgical technics have made surgery of the liver a feasible though formidable treatment for a limited number of conditions. Wounds may be repaired; a solitary *cyst* (a sac containing fluid or solid matter) or *abscess* (a localized collection of pus) may be drained; and occasionally a localized, primary carcinoma may be resected by lobectomy or partial *hepatectomy* (*hepar,* liver + *ectomy*).

Hepatic Trauma

Hepatic injuries are not uncommon, since the liver, being large and relatively unprotected anatomically, is easily lacerated, ruptured, or penetrated in battle, automobile collisions, and falls. Injuries to the liver and spleen comprise approximately 72 per cent of all intra-abdominal injuries.[4] Surgical intervention is warranted regardless of risk, since the mortality rate with conservative management ranges from 57.1 to 96 per cent, increasing with the length of time surgery is delayed.[5]

Pathology. On the basis of pathology, there are three major types of hepatic injuries.[6] A subcapsular rupture is probably least serious, because the hematoma which forms is tamponaded by the capsule and adjacent hepatic tissues, preventing frank hemorrhage; however, abscess or cyst formation may supervene. A transcapsular rupture results in a stellate splitting of the liver, producing persistent, profuse hemorrhage which is increased by respiratory movements. Cholerrhagia also occurs, and the bile which is spilled delays clotting and increases the risk of infection. In addition, the veins are without valves and neither contract nor retract to hasten coagulation. Bleeding from portal and hepatic vessels interferes

---

[4] Adapted with permission from H. Gans, "Introduction to Hepatic Surgery," Elsevier Publishing Company, Houston and Amsterdam, 1955, p. 144.

[5] *Ibid.,* p. 149.

[6] *Ibid.,* pp. 144–146.

with the blood supply to the liver, resulting in multiple infarctions, focal necrosis, and sequestrations. Percutaneous injuries due to penetration or perforation by a missile or fractured rib may fragment the liver; these fragments may be carried into the inferior vena cava and cause fatal embolism or may be deposited within the peritoneal cavity; they may also cause toxemia.

Symptomatology. Hepatic trauma is manifested by hemorrhage, shock, and peritonitis. If slight oozing of blood occurs, the patient may only report pain over the right hypochondrium radiating to the shoulders. As bleeding continues and shock supervenes, free fluid will be found in the peritoneal cavity. There may be distention, fever, tachycardia, pallor, weakness, and restlessness. There may or may not be biliary colic, hematemesis, and melena. There is almost always dullness over the right flank. A mass may or may not be palable. Jaundice may supervene 48 to 72 hours after the injury. The diaphragm may be elevated, and *pneumothorax*, the presence of air in the pleural cavity, may be present.

Secondarily the patient may develop a subphrenic abscess or hepatic and renal failure. The damaged liver loses its detoxifying ability, imposing an increased demand for this function upon the kidneys, which in turn fail because of tubular degeneration. The symptoms of hepatorenal failure are similar to those of uremia. Renal output diminishes, and erythrocytes, casts, and albumen appear in the urine. Acidosis, delirium, shock, and coma develop as toxemia increases. The process is fatal unless halted by early surgical intervention.

Treatment. A damaged liver is especially susceptible to infection and withstands anoxia poorly. Therefore, in preparation for surgery, antibiotics and oxygen are administered, and shock is combated with transfusions of whole blood. The patient is prepared for emergency exploratory laparotomy. Cyclopropane, being least toxic to the liver, is the anesthetic of choice, although ether or nitrous oxide and ethylene may be used if adequate amounts of oxygen are administered.

At surgery, fragmented segments are removed, lacerated areas are sutured over omentum or gelatin sponge to avoid cutting into the hepatic tissues; the area is packed or tamponaded with an absorbable, hemostatic material, such as gelatin sponge or oxidized cellulose soaked in thrombin. The peritoneal cavity is aspirated prior to closure. Drains must be left in the hepatic bed to permit egress of bile which interferes with reparation. Deep lacerations interfering with hepatic blood supply require partial hepatectomy. A missile lodged in the liver may give rise to abscess formation and should be removed if possible.

The plan for postoperative care is designed to combat hemorrhage, shock, and infection, and to support the liver during the crucial period of reparation. Glucose, blood, and antibiotics are administered parenterally.

Decompression therapy is employed to rest the gastrointestinal tract, to prevent vomiting, and to relieve the distention which accompanies peritonitis and paralytic ileus. The nurse must be especially vigilant in observing vital signs and in watching for evidence of blood or bile draining through the dressings. She must keep an accurate intake-output record and describe all drainage accurately.

Cysts and Abscesses of the Liver

Although a solitary cyst of the liver is not a common condition, surgery is sometimes performed to incise and drain an infected cyst, or to incise one that is causing compression.

Hepatic abscess formation is a serious condition carrying a mortality rate of 27 to 70 per cent. The incidence has been markedly reduced with earlier recognition and surgical treatment of intraperitoneal infections and with antibiotics. While multiple abscesses are inoperable, a large, solitary lesion, or aggregate of several which have coalesced, requires surgical drainage.

Although the etiology may be unknown, hepatic abscess is often caused by infection extending from the bile ducts or transmitted by way of the portal vein. The onset may be insidious with vague digestive disturbances and right upper quadrant discomfort. In some patients the disease is more acute, marked by toxicity, chills and fever, tenderness and severe radiating pain in the right upper quadrant. Vomiting and jaundice may be present. Moderate-to-marked leukocytosis is a consistent finding. The right half of the diaphragm may be elevated.

Antibiotic drug therapy is combined with incision and drainage. The extraperitoneal route is preferred, to minimize spread of infection. It may be necessary to use a transperitoneal or transpleural route, in which case a preliminary operation is necessary several days prior to the incision for drainage to create inflammatory adhesions between the peritoneal or pleural surfaces and so wall off these cavities. Resection of one or two ribs may be necessary with the transpleural or extraperitoneal routes. The nursing care, therefore, may entail measures necessary for either thoracic or abdominal surgery.

A subphrenic abscess, such as may develop after appendical perforation, is differentiated from a liver abscess primarily on the basis of location, being situated between the diaphragm and the liver. Symptoms and treatment are the same as for an hepatic abscess.

Hepatic Neoplasms

Carcinoma of the liver infrequently lends itself to surgical extirpation because, in the majority of cases, it is either metastatic or diffuse in growth. Primary carcinoma of the liver is comparatively rare, and only a few such carcinomas are accessible for surgery. The neoplasm is usually asymptomatic until considerable growth has been attained. Metastasis to the lung occurs early, and the survival time is short.

Some surgeons perform *metastectomy*, removal of metastatic lesions, if the secondary growths are small and limited, and if the primary lesion is resectable. Surgery is, however, more commonly reserved for resection of a primary hepatic neoplasm which is accessible. Resection is also advocated for carcinoma of the gallbladder in its initial stage of liver invasion.[7] The liver has remarkable reserve and regenerative powers, allowing a considerable amount of hepatic tissue to be removed without jeopardizing life, provided the patient survives surgery. Indeed, liver-function test results may still be normal in spite of disease or absence of a considerable amount of hepatic tissue. Surgery performed along the relatively avascular planes of the interlobar fissures allows as much as the entire left lobe, both segments of the middle lobe, or the entire right lobe to be removed.[8]

Early diagnosis of a primary hepatic neoplasm is very difficult. Symptoms, if present, are vague. A rapidly growing tumor may cause compression of adjacent tissues. The tumor may be discovered incidentally in abdominal surgery or may be detected by hepatography. Treatment consists of removal of the involved lobe.

Preoperative Preparation for Partial Hepatectomy. In order for a partial hepatectomy to be successful, it is essential that optimal liver function be attained preoperatively. The reserve and regenerative powers of the liver are enhanced by a diet high in carbohydrate, protein, and vitamins. Oral or intravenous supplements may be necessary. Intravenous glucose furnishes the liver with immediate and reserve energy. Hypoprothrombinemia, if present, is treated with vitamin K. The cardiovascular, respiratory, and renal systems must also be brought to their optimal level of functioning.

Immediate preparation for surgery includes prelaparotomy measures. The area for the skin preparation depends upon the anticipated type of incision. The right upper quadrant can be explored through a right subcostal, transverse, or right rectus incision requiring a laparotomy preparation. A left hemihepatectomy may require an incision which extends from the umbilicus to mid-chest, splitting the sternum.[9] The area to prepare for this procedure, therefore, includes the anterior thorax and abdomen from the neck to and including the pubes. A right hemihepatectomy may be performed through an incision which extends from the midaxillary line, along the eighth intercostal space, to join a right paramedian or right

[7] Gans, *op. cit.*, p. 237.
[8] *Ibid.*, p. 118, p. 235.
[9] *Ibid.*, p. 185.

rectus incision which extends to the umbilicus.[10] Therefore, the area of skin preparation must include not only the anterior thorax and abdomen, but also the right lateral aspect of the thorax including the axilla.

Postoperative Nursing Care. Basic to postoperative care is a realization of the fact that liver function has probably been impaired by operative manipulation. Anesthetics can not be detoxified readily, and recovery may be delayed. Shock, hemorrhage, and infection are likely to develop. Hepatorenal failure may occur and may be immediate or delayed.

Liver anoxia must be combated by the administration of oxygen immediately after operation and by preventing impairment in flow or oxygen content of the blood supply to the liver. Gastrointestinal decompression is used to treat the accompanying paralytic ileus and prevent distention, which hinders circulation. Dressings must not be so tight that they constrict. Respiratory depressants are avoided, and the patient is encouraged to cough and breathe deeply at frequent intervals. His position should be changed frequently, alternating the horizontal positions with low Fowler's position, which relaxes tension on the incision and favors deeper respirations; prolonged flexion is avoided.

An accurate intake-output record is essential to the detection of renal failure. Frequent urinalyses are usually ordered. Vital signs must be watched closely; marked deviations must be reported promptly, together with changes in the patient's general appearance or behavior. Leakage of bile or evidences of peritonitis must be reported immediately, since cholerrhagia if untreated will be fatal. Abdominal distention may indicate portal vein thrombosis, which is treated by the administration of anticoagulants.

In convalescence, a diet high in carbohydrate, protein, and vitamins is resumed. Activity is gradually increased as tolerated. The patient requires close medical supervision for the remainder of his life to detect recurrence of malignancy and to evaluate liver functioning.

SURGERY OF THE SPLEEN

The spleen seems to be an expendable organ in adulthood, although it functions in cellular metabolism, regulation of blood volume, and possibly antibody activity. Other functions have been assigned to the spleen but they have not been clearly or consistently proved.

Splenectomy is performed for a variety of conditions; the anatomic structure and marked vascularity of the spleen prohibit surgery within the organ. Rupture of the spleen, either spontaneous or traumatic, requires splenectomy to combat hemorrhage. Splenectomy is also performed for cysts, tumors, and some abscesses; for hypersplenism associated with

[10] *Ibid.*, p. 190.

splenomegaly, peripheral blood cytopenias, and hyperplasia of the bone marrow. Surgical procedures and/or malignant neoplastic disease of adjacent organs may necessitate splenectomy.

Preoperative and Postoperative Care

The abdominal route is most commonly used, although the spleen can be reached through a transthoracic or combined thoracoabdominal route. A variety of transverse and vertical abdominal incisions may be used, all requiring a skin preparation extending from the clavicles to and including the pubes. If a thoracic incision is to be used, the left lateral aspect of the chest, including the axilla, should also be prepared.

The patient should be in his optimal condition for elective splenectomy. Anemia is combated with transfusions of blood, a highly nutritious diet is given, and laparotomy orders are carried out in the immediate preoperative period. If the patient is undergoing emergency splenectomy, he is treated for shock and operated upon without delay.

A general inhalation anesthetic administered intratracheally allows controlled respirations should the pleural cavity be entered. Following splenectomy, transfusions of whole blood are administered until the circulation has stabilized at an adequate level. Because surgery involves the left diaphragm, there may be temporary immobility and decreased ventilation of the left lung. Therefore, oxygen may be administered early postoperatively. The activation regime is essential to the prevention of atelectasis. A transthoracic approach requires water-seal drainage and other measures described in Chapter 16. Symptoms and signs of hemorrhage and infection must be watched for.

It is of interest for the nurse to know that there are temporary though real alterations in the patient's physiology following splenectomy. These changes tend to subside in a few weeks but may persist for years; they do not seem to increase postoperative morbidity appreciably. They include an anemia, which makes the patient less resistant to hemorrhage and capable of less exertion; a leukocytosis and mild elevation of temperature without evidence of infection; lymphadenopathy; a rise in the platelet count, which may predispose to thrombosis; and an increased sedimentation rate for erythrocytes.

SURGERY FOR PORTAL HYPERTENSION

The portal vein returns blood from the spleen and other abdominal viscera to the liver. An obstructing lesion, such as hepatic cirrhosis or portal thrombosis, results in an elevation of venous pressure within the portal system. A collateral circulation is developed to relieve some of this pressure; blood is rerouted through the gastric veins to the azygos and hemiazygos veins. Gastroesophageal varicose veins develop and threaten the patient's life by rupture and exsanguination.

To prevent such a fatal episode, if liver function is compatible with the risk and a longer life, surgical attempts are made to shunt the blood directly into the systemic venous circulation. If the portal vein is thrombosed, a splenorenal shunt may be performed after splenectomy. A portacaval shunt is larger, diverts more blood, and is therefore preferable, if the portal vein is patent. (See Fig. 25.) If a shunt is not feasible, gastroesophageal resection may be performed. For poor-risk patients, transesophageal ligation, suturing, or sclerosing may be effective temporarily in controlling bleeding.

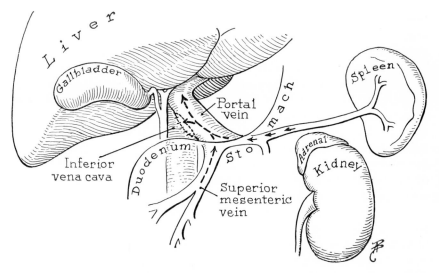

FIG. 25. Portacaval shunt. Arrows indicate the direction of blood flow. The relative locations of the left kidney and adrenal gland are illustrated.

The immediate treatment for hemorrhage is blood transfusion and traction tamponade with an esophagogastric tube containing inflatable balloons, one to exert pressure in the esophagus, the other in the stomach. A third lumen is used for hourly gastric irrigations to note the progress of bleeding; it may also be used for continuous aspiration.

The shunting procedures are performed through an incision which starts at the lateral aspect of the thorax and curves down over the anterior abdomen to the umbilicus. A portacaval shunt is performed on the right side, a splenorenal on the left. The abdomen may be drained. Water-seal drainage of the chest is instituted. It is imperative that distention be prevented to maintain the patency of the shunt; therefore, decompression therapy is used. Parenteral fluids are given. Anticoagulants and antibiotics may or may not be used. Oral intake is permitted as soon as intestinal peristalsis has resumed.

SURGERY OF THE PANCREAS

Surgical conditions of the pancreas include benign or malignant neoplastic growths, anomalies, chronic relapsing pancreatitis, calculi, cysts, abscesses, fistulas, and trauma.

Neoplasms

Pancreatic neoplasms, usually adenomatous, may involve the parenchyma or islets of Langerhans. The vast majority of patients with carcinoma of the pancreatic parenchyma have involvement of the head of the pancreas, which soon obstructs the common bile duct and/or duodenum. Because the pancreas is devoid of a true capsule and is well supplied with lymph vessels, local extension and distant metastasis occur rapidly, and the prognosis is poor. The patient experiences nagging pain, which may cause him to assume bizarre positions for relief; dorsal recumbency usually intensifies the pain. He usually reports anorexia and vomiting, weight loss, and weakness; jaundice may be present. Treatment involves *radical pancreatoduodenectomy*, in which the head of the pancreas, distal end of the common bile duct, stomach, and duodenum are removed. This involves the following procedures for reestablishment of continuity: pancreaticoenterostomy, unless the pancreatic duct is ligated; gastroenterostomy and choledochoenterostomy or cholecystoenterostomy. A defunctionalized loop of jejunum is commonly used to minimize intestinal reflux. These extensive procedures may be performed in one or two stages. The operative mortality is approximately 15 to 20 per cent, and survival after surgery ranges from a few months to a few years.

Carcinoma of the body and tail of the pancreas is treated by partial pancreatectomy and splenectomy, but the prognosis is equally poor. The symptoms are obscure and the patient is frequently inoperable when he first consults a surgeon.

Neoplasms of the islets of Langerhans usually produce hyperinsulinism, manifested by periods of apprehension, fatigue, hunger, sweating, palpitation, delirium, coma, and convulsions. The blood-sugar level is usually below 50 ml. per 100 ml. Glucose promptly relieves these symptoms; patients learn to ward off attacks by consuming large amounts of carbohydrates. Unlike the majority of patients undergoing pancreatic surgery, they may, therefore, become obese. If the tumor is found at surgery, enucleation is usually sufficient. If none is found, the tail and body are removed together with the spleen. If symptoms still persist, total pancreatectomy may be necessary.

Anomalies

The two major anomalies which commonly become surgical are *pancreatic heterotopia*, aberrant tissue growing in the gastrointestinal tract which is subject to pancreatic disease, and *annular pancreas*, an encircling of pancreatic tissue around the duodenum and common bile duct, causing obstruction. Treatment for the first is excision, for the second, a diversionary procedure, such as duodenoduodenostomy or duodenojejunostomy.

Indications for Surgery in Pancreatitis

Pancreatitis is a serious disease which progresses through three stages, namely, edema, hemorrhage, and necrosis. Acute pancreatitis may become surgical several weeks after onset for drainage of an abscess or cyst, but it is essentially a medical condition. Chronic relapsing pancreatitis is, however, usually treated surgically. The patient experiences periods of severe, upper-abdominal pain which may radiate to the back, anorexia and vomiting, weight loss, and alteration in bowel habits, with or without symptoms of paralytic ileus, obstructive jaundice, and diabetes. Pain may be so severe that drug addiction occurs. Vagotomy, sympathectomy, or splanchnicectomy, the last two procedures involving resection of sympathetic nerve fibers, is sometimes performed to relieve pain but each imposes upon the patient an additional hazard in that denervation of sensory fibers prohibits early detection of subsequent flare-ups of pancreatitis or other abdominal disease.

Surgical procedures are primarily designed to relieve intrapancreatic or extrapancreatic obstruction which may be producing pancreatitis. Abscesses and cysts are resected or drained; calculi are removed. Concurrent biliary disease is treated by cholecystectomy or choledochostomy. When the common bile and pancreatic ducts merge to enter the duodenum as a common channel, and when stricture or spasm of the sphincter of Oddi obstructs the outflow of bile and pancreatic juices, sphincterotomy may be performed. Diversionary procedures, such as pancreaticojejunostomy or choledochoenterostomy, may be necessary. Partial pancreatectomy may be performed in case of localized fibrosis or multiple calculi, or it may be necessary to establish retrograde drainage by pancreaticojejunostomy.

Pancreatic Cyst, Abscess, Fistula

A cyst is commonly manifested by pain, digestive disturbances, weight loss, and jaundice; it may be palpable. Surgical technics include excision, drainage, or *marsupialization*, i.e., evacuating the cyst and suturing the walls to the edges of the wound. External drainage necessitates the use of a catheter or T-tube attached to suction and the use of aluminum paste, or the equivalent, to protect the wound margins from excoriation. The enzymes may be replaced by oral pancreatic extract. Internal drainage, accomplished by anastomosing the cyst to the jejunum, permits both drainage and conservation of pancreatic juices, which are vital to the digestion of carbohydrates, proteins, and fats.

An abscess causes fever, leukocytosis, and a tender abdominal mass. It is treated by drainage and antibiotics.

The formation of a *fistula*, or abnormal canal, is common following external drainage procedures. Aided by continuous suction, the tract may close spontaneously over a period of time. If it persists, cauterization, excision, or anastomosis of the tract to the stomach or jejunum is warranted to reduce the danger of digestive impairment and fluid and electrolyte imbalance attendant upon prolonged loss of pancreatic juices. A cyst, abscess, or fistula may require partial pancreatectomy.

Pancreatic Trauma

Since the pancreas lies well protected in the retroperitoneal space, trauma sufficient to penetrate, rupture, or lacerate the pancreas usually is accompanied by injuries in other viscera. The pancreas is easily injured in surgical procedures performed for adjacent structures, e.g., gastric resection. As soon as shock can be treated adequately, exploratory laparotomy is usually warranted to locate and repair the injured organs. Pancreatic injuries are serious, since a tear through the ducts allows autolyzing enzymes to escape into adjacent tissues and the peritoneal cavity. Hemorrhage is another serious result of pancreatic trauma. Symptoms indicative of pancreatic trauma are those of shock, hemorrhage, and adynamic ileus accompanied by pain and rigidity of the abdominal muscles. The serum-amylase level remains high.

In repair, attempts are made to ligate and suture injured pancreatic tissue and to provide for drainage from the ducts. External drainage through a T-tube or drain with a sump pump requires continuous suction and skin protection to prevent excoriation, careful replacement with fluids, electrolytes, and pancreatic extract. Fistula formation is common after drainage and may subside spontaneously in time or may require further surgery. Internal drainage accomplished by anastomosis of the duct(s) to the stomach or intestine obviates these difficulties by allowing direct egress of pancreatic juices directly into the gastrointestinal tract. If injury is confined to the tail of the pancreas, partial pancreatectomy may be performed. Splenectomy is almost always performed in conjunction with distal pancreatectomy because these structures are in such close proximity that removal of one without trauma to the other is difficult. Hemorrhage of the pancreas may be treated by packing or by partial pancreatectomy.

Preoperative and Postoperative Care in Pancreatic Surgery

With few exceptions patients who are candidates for pancreatic surgery are poor risks either because of chronic illness associated with anorexia or vomiting, weight loss, pain, and possibly diarrhea, or because of the acute condition, such as trauma, for which they are being operated upon. In addition, the surgical procedures performed are frequently radical and prolonged. Therefore, every effort must be made preoperatively to evaluate the patient's condition and to institute necessary remedial therapy. Malnutrition and fluid-electrolyte imbalance must be corrected, diabetes controlled, hypoprothrombinemia combated, and preparations for blood transfusions made. The skin is prepared from the nipple line to and including the pubes to permit an upper abdominal transverse, paramedian, or rectus incision; occasionally a lumbar approach is used, requiring preparation of the dorsal surface instead. A general inhalation or spinal anesthetic is used.

During the first few postoperative days when gastrointestinal decompression is used, the patient is maintained on intravenous glucose in water, supplemented as necessary with vitamins B, C, and K, and sodium and potassium chloride. When peristalsis is resumed, oral intake is gradually increased to a bland, low-residue diet with a liberal amount of fluids. An enema may be given approximately 3 days postoperatively. The activation regime is initiated early.

Wound care is designed to promote adequate drainage by Penrose drains, sump pump, and/or continuous suction through a catheter. The skin must be protected from excoriation by aluminum paste, or the equivalent, and by scrupulous cleanliness. An accurate intake-output record with descriptions of the character of drainage is essential. The drains are usually removed in 3 days and sutures in 8 days. Antibiotic drugs are usually administered.

If diabetes develops following total pancreatectomy, it is usually milder than the spontaneous type; insulin is required in small doses. The patient must be taught insulin administration, urine testing, diet regulation, and skin care, as diabetes is now a permanent part of his life.

Lifelong replacement therapy with pancreatic extract, choline, and/or methionine is necessary after total pancreatectomy to prevent fatty infiltration of the liver and to combat steatorrhea and weight loss. Following partial pancreatectomy, sufficient regeneration may occur to warrant discontinuing insulin and pancreatic extract therapy.

The major immediate postoperative complications are hemorrhage, peritonitis, fistula, and obstruction of the operative stoma.

Postoperative care is incomplete without adequate teaching of the patient so that he realizes how to manage his diabetes and pancreatic insufficiency and is willing to remain under close medical supervision and follow instructions. Financial aid and occupational readjustment may be necessary to meet the expense of lifelong medication and care, and to allow the patient the satisfaction of work compatible with his strength and endurance.

SURGERY OF THE ADRENAL GLANDS

Neoplasms and hyperplasia are the major indications for surgery of the adrenal glands. Occasionally a cyst of the adrenal glands, essential hypertension, and disseminated carcinoma of the breast and prostate are treated by adrenalectomy. Trauma is uncommon because these glands lie retroperitoneally under the diaphragmatic dome where they are well protected by other viscera, fat, and the heavy dorsal musculature.

A neoplasm may arise from the adrenal cortex or medulla, may be benign or malignant, and may or may not be hormonally active. Hyperplasia may involve either the cortex or medulla.

The adrenal cortex and gonadal medulla originate from the same embryologic tissues; therefore, both adrenocortical glucosteroids and some sex hormones are produced by the adrenal cortex. Hyperadrenocorticism, whether due to hyperplasia or a tumor, is manifested by Cushing's syndrome if glucosteroids are produced in excess, and by the adrenogenital syndrome if sex hormones are excessive. Actually, these two syndromes may not be so well-defined clinically. Cushing's syndrome usually is associated with an insulin-resistant diabetes, hypertension, osteoporosis, redistribution of body fat, hirsutism, amenorrhea, impotence, and weakness. The adrenogenital syndrome is associated with masculinization or feminization, rapid growth, increased muscularity, hirsutism, and sexual precociousness. The most common cortical tumors are cortical nodule and adenoma, which are benign, and carcinoma, which has a greater tendency to cause hyperadrenocorticism.

The most common medullary tumors are neuroblastoma and pheochromocytoma. Neuroblastoma is more common in childhood but may occur in the adult. Treatment consists of excision and radiation. Pheochromocytoma produces epinephrine and norepinephrine. The patient experiences paroxysmal hypertension associated with vomiting, headache, dizziness, cold extremities, nervousness, sweating, palpitation, and precordial distress. Some patients may develop essential hypertension. Pheochromocytoma may be confused with hyperthyroidism since these patients may have an elevated basal metabolic rate. However, iodine uptake is not elevated with pheochromocytoma, a fact useful in differentiation.

Diagnostic Methods

Various diagnostic methods are used in an attempt to differentiate hyperplasia from neoplastic growth, and to identify the type of tumor; diagnosis is, however, made most accurately at surgery. Hyperplasia may respond to cortisone therapy, whereas a tumor will not. Laboratory determinations of the type of hormones being produced in excess and excreted in urine help differentiate the type of hyperadrenocorticism present. One of these tests is a 24-hour determination of the urinary output of 17-ketosteroids, which is usually increased in Cushing's syndrome because of hyperplasia or adrenocortical carcinoma. A further increase can usually be evoked by the intravenous administration of adrenocorticotropic hormone in cases of hyperplasia; there is no further response in a patient with carcinoma of the adrenal cortex. When pheochromocytoma is suspected, histamine may be administered to precipitate an attack of paroxysmal hypertension, or phentolamine (Regitine) may be used to lower the blood pressure; neither response is obtained in essential hypertension not due to tumor.

X-ray technics used to locate a tumor include the injection of oxygen into the perirenal spaces directly or through the paracoccygeal route. Occasionally lumbar aortography is performed, but this procedure involves general anesthesia and considerable risk. A tumor is usually noticed on x-ray displacing the kidney downward.

Operative Technics

The treatment for a tumor is excision, or adrenalectomy. Hyperplasia, which does not respond to hormonal therapy, is treated by total or subtotal bilateral adrenalectomy. Disseminated carcinoma of the prostate and breast may be treated empirically by adrenalectomy. Marked relief from pain is usually achieved, and there may be some regression of metastatic lesions. A general inhalation anesthetic is commonly used with endotracheal intubation to permit controlled respirations if necessary. A continuous spinal anesthetic may be used. One of several approaches to the adrenal glands may be used: transabdominal, transthoracic, posterolateral, or transcostal. The last two permit an extrapleural and subdiaphragmatic approach but require resection of the eleventh or twelfth ribs. The nurse must realize that bilateral adrenalectomy may require two extensive incisions.

Special Nursing Measures in Adrenalectomy

With adrenalectomy, a patient loses, in proportion to the amount of tissue removed, adrenocortical steroids which are essential for life. Profound physiologic changes occur in the crucial postoperative period. Fluid-electrolyte and acid-base balance may be disturbed, requiring close observation, an accurate intake-output record, and parenteral fluid and electrolyte therapy. Metabolism of carbohydrates, proteins, and fats is impaired. Capillary resistance is weakened,[11] predisposing the patient to hemorrhage. The patient is unable to excrete sodium, chlorides, and water in adequate amounts; therefore, fluid intake must be limited.[12] Hypotension demands remedial measures, such as blood transfusions and the administration of vasopressor agents. Gastrointestinal secretion is reduced; therefore minimal returns in decompression therapy should cause no alarm provided the abdomen is not distended.[13] Replacement therapy with corticosteroids is instituted preoperatively for patients with hyperadrenocorticism and postoperatively to all others undergoing adrenalectomy to combat these changes and to prevent an adrenal crisis due to acute adrenocortical insufficiency. The nurse must be vigilant in detecting symptoms of adrenocortical insufficiency manifested by headache, weakness, malaise, nausea and vomiting, hypotension, and collapse. Since corticosteroid therapy is poorly tolerated by emotionally unstable individuals with psychotic tendencies, the nurse must report any extremes in mood or unusual behavior promptly.

Early activation is instituted. Oral alimentation is resumed as soon as the patient's condition warrants intake. Other nursing measures depend upon the route used. Water-seal chest drainage and other thoracic surgery nursing measures may be indicated.

During surgery for pheochromocytoma, the patient is protected from a hypertensive crisis by an adrenolytic drug, such as phentolamine. As soon as the tumor is removed, a dilute solution of epinephrine or levarterenol is started intravenously to combat the immediate hypotension. The care for these patients is the same as that just described except that they may require a longer period of time to stabilize their blood pressures, and must, therefore, be moved with caution early in the postoperative period. Blood pressure readings must be taken every 10 to 15 minutes without fail until stabilization has occurred.

The adrenalectomized patient who has lost the majority or all of his adrenocortical tissue may experience an adrenal crisis with sudden, severe stress or with an infection. He must, therefore, have replacement therapy with corticosteroids for life and must remain under close medical supervision. He must be made aware of the symptoms of overdosage, which include edema due to sodium retention, weakness due to potassium

[11] J. D. Hardy, "Surgical Physiology of the Adrenal Cortex," Charles C Thomas, Publisher, Springfield, Ill., 1955, p. 21.

[12] *Ibid.*, pp. 18–19.

[13] *Ibid.*, p. 20.

loss, hirsutism, and hypertension. Since cortisone may mask symptoms of infection, the patient must learn to report any sign of illness to his physician promptly. He must keep his resistance high and avoid exposure to illness when possible, as he is more susceptible to infection because of his adrenalectomy. He may have insomnia for the first couple of weeks of corticosteroid therapy, but this will subside. He should be told that symptoms of hyperadrenocorticism will subside slowly to avoid undue discouragement.

SUMMARY

Surgery of the extrahepatic biliary tract is most commonly performed for cholecystitis with cholelithiasis. Other conditions requiring operative intervention include strictures of the bile ducts and neoplasms.

The preoperative preparation for cholecystectomy and choledochostomy is essentially the same as for laparotomy. Special measures usually necessary in the postoperative period include decompression and parenteral fluid therapies and care of the T-tube or Penrose drain. The activation regime is especially important because of the high abdominal incision which makes deep respirations difficult.

The liver may be repaired, incised, or partially resected in the treatment of wounds, cysts, abscesses, and neoplasms. The preoperative preparation is essentially the same as for laparotomy. The area of skin preparation depends upon whether the approach is to be transthoracic or transabdominal. Glucose may be given to fortify the liver in both the preoperative and postoperative periods. Postoperatively, decompression and parenteral fluid therapies are used. In addition, it is important to combat liver anoxia by administering oxygen and by avoiding abdominal constriction.

Splenectomy is performed in the treatment of wounds, cysts, abscesses, neoplasms, and hypersplenism. Preoperative and postoperative care is the same as that described for laparotomy. Either the transabdominal or transthoracic approach may be used.

A shunting procedure or gastroesophageal resection may be performed in the treatment of portal hypertension to prevent exsanguination due to rupture of esophageal varicose veins. A combined thoracoabdominal approach is used.

Partial or total pancreatectomy may be required in the treatment of neoplasms. A malignant neoplasm of the pancreas usually bears a poor prognosis, and surgery is more commonly palliative than curative.

Other indications for pancreatic surgery include the following: anomalies, chronic relapsing pancreatitis, cysts, abscesses, calculi, fistula, and wounds. The treatment of these conditions may entail resection of pancreatic tissue or drainage procedures. Some pancreatic wounds can be repaired.

Considerable attention must be paid in the preoperative period to improving the general condition of these patients because many are poor surgical risks. Laparotomy orders are carried out. The area of skin preparation depends upon whether an anterior or dorsal approach is to be used.

The postoperative nursing care is similar to that described for laparotomy. In addition, decompression and parenteral fluid therapies are used until intestinal peristalsis resumes. The patient who has had a total pancreatectomy will require lifelong administration of insulin and pancreatic extract. He must be taught the principles of diabetic care and must be impressed with the need to remain under medical supervision. Although a partial pancreatectomy may result in enough pancreatic insufficiency to require the administration of insulin and pancreatic extract, pancreatic regeneration frequently occurs so that in time no supplementary medications are necessary.

The postoperative period is crucial for a patient who has undergone adrenalectomy, because he has lost adrenocorticosteroids, which are essential for life. The fluid-electrolyte and acid-base balance must be closely watched and regulated by parenteral fluid therapy, which must be given with caution because the patient is unable to excrete sodium, chlorides, and water in adequate amounts. Measures to combat hypotension are necessary, especially in a patient who has had an adrenalectomy for pheochromocytoma. Gastrointestinal decompression is used until peristalsis is resumed. Replacement with corticosteroids is initiated preoperatively in patients with hyperadrenocorticism, and for all others after adrenalectomy, to combat acute adrenocortical insufficiency. This replacement therapy is necessary for the duration of the life of a patient who has undergone bilateral total adrenalectomy.

BIBLIOGRAPHY

Liver, Gallbladder, Spleen, Pancreas

ALLEN, J. G.: (1) Spleen, and (2) Mesentery, Splanchnic Circulation, Portal Hypertension, and Mesenteric Thrombosis, in "Surgery," J. G. Allen, H. N. Harkins, C. A. Moyer, and J. E. Rhoads (eds.), J. B. Lippincott Company, Philadelphia, 1957, chap. 32, pp. 741–768, and chap. 33, pp. 770–800.

BLAKEMORE, A. H.: Diseases of the Liver, in "Christopher's Textbook of Surgery," 6th ed., L. Davis (ed.), W. B. Saunders Company, Philadelphia, 1956, chap. 21, pp. 740–754.

CLIFFTON, E. E.: Diseases of the Pancreas, Clinical Symposia, Ciba Pharmaceutical Products, Inc., Summit, N.J., vol. 9, no. 2, pp. 51–78, March–April, 1957.

COLCOCK, B. P., and J. E. McMANUS: Cholecystectomy for Cholelithiasis, *S. Clin. North America*, vol. 35, no. 3, pp. 765–771, June, 1955.

COLE, W. H., and R. ELMAN: Liver, Gallbladder, Pancreas and Spleen, "Textbook of General Surgery," 6th ed., Appleton-Century-Crofts, Inc., New York, 1952, chap. 24, pp. 627–684.

COLLER, F. A., A. BLAIN, III, and G. ANDREWS: "Indications for and Results of Splenectomy," Charles C Thomas, Publisher, Springfield, Ill., 1950.

DIFFENBAUGH, W. G., and E. L. STROHL: Common Bile Duct Exploration for Stones, *S. Clin. North America*, vol. 35, no. 1, pp. 119–127, February, 1955.

DOUBILET, H.: Pancreatitis: Etiology and Management, *Spectrum Forum*, Chas. Pfizer and Company, Inc., vol. 5, no. 11, pp. 318, 321, June, 1957.

EISENBEIS, C. H., and J. W. NORCROSS: Jaundice: A Medical Review with a Surgical Viewpoint, *S. Clin. North America*, vol. 35, no. 3, pp. 747–754, June, 1955.

GANS, H.: "Introduction to Hepatic Surgery," Elsevier Publishing Company, Amsterdam and Houston, 1955.

GLENN, F.: The Liver and the Biliary System, "Christopher's Textbook of Surgery," 6th ed., L. Davis (ed.), W. B. Saunders Company, Philadelphia, 1956, chap. 21, pp. 712–754.

———: Conditions of the Biliary Tract Requiring the Consideration of Early Surgery, *S. Clin. North America*, vol. 35, no. 2, pp. 393–408, April, 1955.

McDONOUGH, F. E.: The Recognition and Medical Management of Chronic Relapsing Pancreatitis, *S. Clin. North America*, vol. 35, no. 3, pp. 775–784, June, 1955.

MacKAY, A. G., and B. E. FRECHETTE: The Surgical Treatment of Biliary Disease and Nursing Care, *Am. J. Nursing*, pp. 1062–1065, September, 1953.

PACK, G. T., and R. D. BRASFIELD: Metastatic Cancer of the Liver, *Am. J. Surg.*, vol. 90, no. 5, pp. 704–716, November, 1955.

POPPER, H.: Jaundice, *Clinical Symposia*, Ciba Pharmaceutical Products, Inc., Summit, N.J., vol. 7, no. 5, September–October, 1955.

———: Portal Hypertension, *Clinical Symposia*, Ciba Pharmaceutical Products, Inc., Summit, N.J., vol. 8, no. 6, November–December, 1956.

PUESTOW, C. B.: "Surgery of the Biliary Tract, Pancreas and Spleen," 2d ed., Year Book Publishers, Inc., Chicago, 1957.

REYNOLDS, J. T., and B. G. LARY: The Indications, Hazards and Contraindications for Division of the Sphincter of Oddi, *S. Clin. North America*, vol. 35, no. 1, pp. 129–148, February, 1955.

RHOADS, J. E.: (1) Liver, Gallbladder and Bile Passages, and (2) Pancreas, in "Surgery," J. G. Allen, H. N. Harkins, C. A. Moyer, and J. E. Rhoads (eds.), J. B. Lippincott Company, Philadelphia, 1957, chap. 30, pp. 687–713, and chap. 31, pp. 715–738.

ROUSSELOT, L. M.: Pancreatitis: Etiology and Treatment, *Spectrum Forum*, Chas. Pfizer and Company, Inc., vol. 5, no. 11, pp. 319, 321, June, 1957.

SCHWEGMAN, C. W., and W. E. DeMUTH, JR.: Acute Cholecystitis Following Operation for Unrelated Disease, *Surg., Gynec. & Obst.*, pp. 167–172, August, 1953.

SEDGWICK, C. E., and C. M. PARRISH: Portal Hypertension, *S. Clin. North America*, vol. 35, no. 3, pp. 667–677, June, 1955.

SHACKELFORD, R. T.: (1) The Pancreas, and (2) The Spleen, in "Bickham-Callander Surgery of the Alimentary Tract," vol. 2, W. B. Saunders Company, Philadelphia, 1955, chap. 5, pp. 863–966, and chap. 6, pp. 969–997.

THOMPSON, J. A., and J. R. DERRICK: The Diagnosis and Management of Acute Pancreatitis, *Am. J. Surg.*, vol. 94, no. 4, pp. 558–562, October, 1957.

WARREN, K. W.: Surgical Considerations in the Management of Chronic Relapsing Pancreatitis, *S. Clin. North America,* vol. 35, no. 3, pp. 785–798, June, 1955.

WAUGH, J. M., and G. A. HALLENBECK: The Pancreas, in "Christopher's Textbook of Surgery," 6th ed., L. Davis (ed.), W. B. Saunders Company, Philadelphia, 1956, chap. 22, pp. 756–774.

ZOLLINGER, R. M., and R. D. WILLIAMS: The Spleen, in "Christopher's Textbook of Surgery," 6th ed., L. Davis (ed.), W. B. Saunders Company, Philadelphia, 1956, chap. 24, pp. 798–808.

Adrenal Glands

"Complete Manual of Therapy with the Metisteroids," Schering Corporation, Bloomfield, N.J., 1956.

HARDY, J. D.: "Surgical Physiology of the Adrenal Cortex," Charles C Thomas, Publisher, Springfield, Ill., 1955.

HARRISON, J. H.: The Adrenal Glands, in "Christopher's Textbook of Surgery," 6th ed., L. Davis (ed.), W. B. Saunders Company, Philadelphia, 1956, chap. 23, pp. 775–795.

MARMER, M. J., B. SIMKIN, and M. H. RABWIN: The Management of Anesthesia for Adrenalectomy, *Am. J. Surg.,* vol. 94, no. 4, pp. 608–610, October, 1957.

RICHARDS, V.: Surgery of the Adrenals, *Am. J. Surg.,* vol. 89, no. 6, pp. 1212–1223, June, 1955.

SCOTT, W. W.: "Surgery of the Adrenal Glands," Charles C Thomas, Publisher, Springfield, Ill., 1954.

11

SURGERY OF THE SMALL INTESTINE AND APPENDIX

Surgery of the small intestine is performed for a variety of conditions, which may be classified as inflammatory, obstructive, neoplastic, and traumatic. These conditions may occur simultaneously and/or be interrelated. For example, inflammation accompanies neoplastic disease, and both may produce obstruction.

REGIONAL ILEITIS

The major inflammatory disease involving the small bowel is idiopathic regional ileitis. This is a chronic ulcerating disease involving the distal ileum. Extension can occur proximally along the ileum or distally into the colon. The course is marked by remissions and exacerbations. Although regional ileitis is essentially a medical condition, surgery may be performed when intractability and/or complication ensues.

Complications which bring the patient to surgery include abscess formation, strictures and intestinal obstruction, hemorrhage, and fistula. Sometimes excision of the diseased segment abates the course of the disease. Surgery, however, is seldom curative. Recurrences are common and repeated operations may be necessary. The surgeon may resect the diseased segment, including a wide margin of healthy tissue and adjacent, involved lymph nodes. He may perform instead an *ileocolostomy* by dividing the ileum at a point proximal to the diseased segment and anastomosing the ileum to the colon. This procedure diverts the fecal stream away from the diseased segment to allow healing. Preoperatively the patient's nutritional-fluid-electrolytic balance must be restored. These patients have had prolonged and repeated episodes of diarrhea, which result in severe malnutrition, weight loss, and electrolytic imbalance. They have lost much protein and blood from the exuding ulcerated ileum and will benefit from antianemic therapy, including transfusions. Immediate preparation for small-bowel surgery includes, in addition to laparotomy measures, decompression and parenteral fluid therapy. Enemas and cathartics are contraindicated for a patient with ileitis; there is hardly a need for them in view of the patient's prolonged periods of diarrhea.

Postoperatively the patient who has had a resection and end-to-end anastomosis will be cared for in the same way as the patient who has had a laparotomy. Decompression and parenteral fluid therapies are continued. The medical management is resumed early and continued for life to prevent recurrence. This includes a bland, low-residue diet; antispasmodics, sedatives, and antidiarrheal drugs; and psychotherapeutic support.

OBSTRUCTION OF THE SMALL INTESTINE

Obstruction of the small intestine is a serious surgical emergency. It is most commonly caused by one of the following: postoperative or inflammatory adhesions; carcinomatosis; incarcerated or strangulated hernia; or *intussusception,* telescoping of the intestine.

There are two major types of obstruction, namely, paralytic (or adynamic) and mechanical. Paralytic ileus, as such, is usually not treated surgically. However, it may coexist with a mechanical obstruction, which is usually treated surgically. Any condition, intraluminal or extraluminal, which destroys the patency of the intestinal canal will produce obstruction. Thus, constriction, compression, torsion, or obturation of the intestine interrupts the fecal stream and produces symptoms, the severity of which depends in large measure upon the degree of obstruction. A partial obstruction allows the escape of some stool and flatus, and therefore minimizes the danger of perforation and peritonitis. If a complete obstruction can be converted into one that is incomplete, rendering the condition less emergent, there will be more time to prepare the patient for surgery if that is necessary.

Soon after an obstruction becomes complete, distention and edema, which occur at the site, may compromise circulation. The bacterial flora increases. Unrelieved obstruction will progress to ischemia and gangrene of the bowel, toxemia, perforation, peritonitis, shock, and death. A "closed-loop" obstruction, such as is encountered in an incarcerated hernia, is particularly prone to these sequelae, there being no escape route from either end of the loop.

Symptomatology

The early symptoms of bowel obstruction are due to interruption in the passage of intestinal contents towards the anus. The character of these symptoms is determined by the site of the obstruction and the degree of completeness. Gastrointestinal contents proximal to the site of obstruction will be vomited. Therefore, the higher in the intestine that the obstruction is, the greater the degree of malnutrition, dehydration, and electrolytic imbalance. Conversely, since gas accumulates in the intestinal loops, the lower the site the greater the degree of distention. Gas and fecal material which have already passed the site of obstruction will be expelled. Therefore, the patient may have one to two stools, but thereafter he will be *obstipated*, i.e., he will pass no stool and no flatus. Peristalsis is at first increased in frequency and vigor as the body attempts to overcome the obstruction. This hyperactivity produces severe intermittent pains, usually accompanied by forceful vomiting if the obstruction is a mechanical one, or by regurgitant vomiting if the obstruction is paralytic. After a time, the bowel loses its ability to contract. Colicky pain subsides with the onset of this paralytic ileus.

Diagnostic Methods

The diagnosis of intestinal obstruction is based primarily upon the history and physical examination. Because of the nurse's intimate and repeated contacts with the patient, her observations can be of inestimable value to the surgeon in helping him to make an accurate diagnosis. The nurse must make frequent detailed reports regarding the following:

1. Vomiting: Is it forceful? regurgitant? How soon after intake does it occur? Is it preceded by nausea? by pain? What is the character of the vomitus? Does it contain digested food? undigested?

2. Distention: Is it increasing as determined by a tape measure?

3. Pain: Is it intermittent? How often does it recur? Is it subsiding? increasing?

4. Obstipation: Is the patient excreting stools? how many? what type? Is he passing flatus?

A survey x-ray film of the abdomen usually reveals a "stepladder" arrangement of the loops of small intestine and helps confirm the diagnosis.

Preoperative and/or Conservative Management

The patient may be treated conservatively or surgically. When postoperative adhesions are thought to be the cause of the obstruction, every effort is made to treat the patient without surgery, since an additional operation invites further adhesion formation. Acute mechanical obstructions, other than those due to adhesions, usually require prompt surgical intervention. The preoperative preparation is the same as the conservative management. Gastrointestinal decompression and intravenous fluids are commonly used. Analgesic drugs are used sparingly to avoid masking symptoms before the diagnosis is established.

The use of decompression in intestinal obstruction differs from that used for gastric conditions only in that a long double-lumen tube is used instead of a Levin tube. Because this tube must be allowed to pass the pyloric sphincter and travel on into the small intestine aided by peristalsis, it is not taped to the patient's face. The surgeon will insert the tube and distend the bag, usually with mercury. Maneuvering the tube past the pyloric sphincter is facilitated by positioning the patient on his right side. The surgeon may order that the nurse advance the tube a stated distance at definite intervals; this is facilitated by asking the patient to swallow as the tube is advanced. When the tube has reached the site of obstruction, as determined by fluoroscopy, it is taped to the patient's face, and the suction apparatus is connected. The surgeon may or may not order irrigations of this tube. It is the responsibility of the nurse to make an accurate report of the volume and character of the gastrointestinal returns, to ensure the functioning of the decompression system, and to promote the comfort and safety of her patient by frequent oral hygiene and position change. Complications which may ensue with an intestinal tube are those described for a Levin tube. (See pages 101 to 102.) Sometimes decompression allows the obstructed loop of bowel to disengage itself and thereby relieves the obstruction. Even without such success, decompression relieves vomiting and may relieve distention.

Parenteral fluid therapy is essential in the care of a patient with small-intestinal obstruction because his fluids and electrolytes are rapidly depleted by vomiting and decompression. Sufficient amounts of water, sodium, potassium, chlorides, and calories must be supplied to restore and maintain this patient in an adequate fluid-electrolyte and nutritional balance. He must be helped to maintain a *positive nitrogen balance,* i.e., to retain more protein than he is losing. Blood and plasma may be used, especially if the patient is in shock. To help determine whether a patient is losing more than he is gaining in this effort to combat malnutrition and dehydration, daily weights may be ordered; they may require the use of a horizontal scale. The intake-output record is another valuable guide. To ensure accuracy of the output measurements, a retention urinary catheter may be used. This also facilitates frequent urinalysis to determine electrolyte excretion and the specific gravity.

Surgical Treatment

At surgery, usually under general anesthesia, the obstruction is released, the cause corrected, and intestinal continuity is reestablished. This may entail resection of a segment of bowel if it is nonviable.

Postoperative Care

The postoperative care of this patient is identical to that described for preoperative or conservative management. Decompression and parenteral fluid therapies are continued until bowel sounds return and flatus is expelled, at which time oral intake is gradually resumed. The activation regime is instituted early. The dressing is removed by the surgeon when clips or sutures are removed. The wound may or may not require redressing. A small enema is usually ordered 3 days postoperatively and should be given without force to avoid vigorous peristalsis.

NEOPLASMS

The small intestine is not a common site for primary neoplastic growth. The majority of tumors located here are benign adenomas and polyps which are small and asymptomatic. However, they are often multiple and may bleed, producing a rather severe anemia. A polyp may initiate intussusception and cause intermittent bowel obstruction. Treatment is local resection. A frozen section may be done to rule out a malignant tumor.

Malignant tumors, though rare in the small intestine, bear a poor prognosis because of extensive lymphatic drainage. Sarcoma is the more common type. These, too, are often multiple. Treatment consists of wide resection of the involved intestine and lymphatic vessels.

These patients are prepared for surgery and given postoperative care as previously described for the patient undergoing intestinal resection and anastomosis.

WOUNDS

Wounds of the abdomen may involve the small intestine directly by compression, laceration, or penetration or indirectly by causing a paralytic ileus. The small intestine may be torn from its mesenteric attachments. Injuries to the small intestine are usually multiple and serious and commonly occur in conjunction with injury to other abdominal organs. Hemorrhage, perforation of hollow organs, peritonitis, and shock are the direct consequences of intra-abdominal trauma and demand immediate exploration and treatment.

Prior to surgery, gastrointestinal decompression is started, not only to empty the stomach but also to detect bleeding. A retention catheter is inserted into the bladder for drainage as well as to reveal bleeding into the urinary tract. Tetanus toxoid or antitoxin is administered if penetration is suspected. Antibiotics may be given. Transfusions of whole blood are started preoperatively and continued throughout surgery and the early postoperative period as necessary, for hemorrhage may be severe.

At surgery, the abdominal cavity is carefully explored, injuries are repaired if possible, or resection is carried out, bleeding points are ligated, clots are evacuated, and the peritoneal contents are aspirated. The abdomen is closed with or without drainage, as indicated. The postoperative care depends largely upon the surgery performed. Decompression and parenteral fluid therapy are usually continued until peristalsis returns.

INDICATIONS FOR ABDOMINAL ILEOSTOMY AND NURSING CARE

An abdominal ileostomy is necessary when total *colectomy* with *proctectomy*, removal of the colon and the rectum, has been performed in the treatment of ulcerative colitis, multiple polyps, and carcinoma. Occasionally multiple injuries of the colon may require a temporary ileostomy, i.e., one without a concomitant colectomy, to divert the fecal stream and allow healing.

The patient who has an ileostomy, which results in excretion of stool through an abdominal opening, requires expert nursing care and much support. Any procedure which forces the patient to alter his living habits drastically is bound to arouse both fear and anger. Diversion of the fecal stream through the anterior abdominal wall rather than through the rectum may reactivate basic personality conflicts and influence the functioning of the ileostomy. The psychologic factors underlying the adjustment of the patient with an exteriorized bowel are similar whether he has an ileostomy or a colostomy. However, the patient with an ileostomy probably has a greater problem in that his stool is excreted in the liquid state, depriving him of control over defecation. In addition, problems of nutrition, fluid-electrolyte balance, skin care, and collection of the fecal matter are all greater because the stool is liquid; however, these problems are not insurmountable.

The nursing care and teaching program for a patient with an ileostomy must center upon his major areas of need, i.e., medicophysical, socio-economic, and psychologic.[1] The paramount medicophysical needs deal with intake, output, skin care, and prevention of complications peculiar to an ileostomy. The restoration and maintenance of an adequate fluid-electrolyte and nutritional status are difficult because stool is excreted in the liquid state and transit time through the intestine may be increased. Although digestion and absorption of nutrients are accomplished primarily in the small intestine prior to the site of exteriorization, fluids and many electrolytes are absorbed in the colon. The patient, therefore, fails to benefit optimally from his intake. If the bowel is hyperactive and/or if an appreciable resection of ileum was performed, he will lose even more of his nutrients and fluid. These patients may become dehydrated and develop an electrolytic imbalance. Frequent, small feedings of a diet high in calories, protein, vitamins, and minerals help main-

[1] An excellent reference for use in patient teaching is "Manual for Ileostomy Patients," 3d ed., Q. T., Inc., Boston, 1955. (Price, $1.00.)

tain an adequate nutritional level. A liberal fluid intake should be encouraged.

For a patient who has an ileostomy, fairly frequent, liquid stools are normal. Any marked change in the frequency or consistency should be reported to the surgeon immediately. Obstipation, passage of no stool, or failure to expel flatus should arouse suspicion of obstruction. Blood, excess amounts of mucus, and pus are abnormal and must be reported promptly. An accurate record of both the intake and the output is necessary. For this procedure the patient can usually be taught to assume much of the responsibility.

At the time of skin care the stoma can be inspected for signs of bleeding, prolapse, or retraction. Evidence of such signs or reports of discomfort or pain must be brought to the surgeon's attention without delay. The surgeon may order dilatation of the stoma with a gloved finger, lubricated with a surgical jelly, to prevent stenosis. The patient can be taught to do this for himself. The nearly continuous presence of warm stool on the skin demands meticulous skin care to prevent excoriation and infection. The skin should be washed carefully and gently with a mild soap and water, rinsed thoroughly, patted dry, and protected with a moisture-repellent ointment or paste. Suction may be applied to a catheter inserted into the stoma or a temporary disposable bag may be applied to collect the stool and protect the skin. As soon as the stoma is sufficiently healed, a permanent collecting pouch is applied. There are several commercial forms of ileostomy pouches, and the patient may need to try several before he finds one that is satisfactory for him.

One type of apparatus which suits many patients is composed of a hard rubber ring which encircles the stoma and adheres to the skin; to this is attached a disposable plastic bag which can be opened at the distal end for drainage. The patient is taught how to apply the ring, change the bags, and care for the skin. The skin is carefully washed, dried, and dusted with karaya gum powder or painted with tincture of benzoin prior to the application of the ring. After convalescence, a female patient can make a bound opening in her girdle to allow the pouch to protrude and thereby avoid soilage, which would occur if the pouch were compressed.

The socioeconomic needs of this patient can hardly be separated from his psychologic needs. In fact, all needs are interrelated. For example, a patient who rejects his ileostomy will be highly resistant to a teaching program designed to help him learn how to meet his physical needs. It is imperative that the patient be helped to develop a positive approach to his problem in order to avoid an attitude and life of invalidism. He must be impressed with the fact that he is not a social outcast and can, usually, return to his previous occupation. In fact, he need be limited very little in his activities, for those who have adjusted well to this operation resume a full social life, including marriage, childbearing, working, and recreation.

APPENDICITIS

Although inflammation or perforation of any abdominal viscus can produce the symptoms of the so-called "acute abdomen," appendicitis is one of the leading causes. There has been a marked reduction in the mortality rate for appendicitis because of earlier operation and improved surgical care. The Metropolitan Life Insurance Company reported a drop in the crude death rate among its policy holders from 11.2 per 100,000 in 1937 [2] to 1.0 in 1957.[3] Much of this progress is due to the fact that the public has been educated to seek surgical treatment earlier. This testifies to the value of a vigorous program in health education, for improvements in surgical management and technics benefit most those who will accept them early.

The nurse bears much of the responsibility for health guidance as she is often the one who sees the patient first and refers him to the surgeon. It is imperative, therefore, that the nurse know and teach the following first-aid measures for undiagnosed abdominal pain: prompt referral to the physician; abstinence from oral or rectal intake, including cathartics and enemas; and rest in bed. She must know the serious complications which may ensue in persons with neglected appendicitis so that she may urge the patient to accept early surgical treatment; she must dispel the fallacious hope that "maybe this will go away" which patients tend to harbor rather than to accept the need for surgical intervention. The nurse must be able to guide the patient in health measures realistically yet optimistically so that undue fear is not generated.

Pathology and Sequelae

Appendicitis is an inflammatory process usually associated with intraluminal obstruction, although approximately 10 per cent of appendicitis cases are idiopathic. The obstruction is commonly due to a *fecalith*, hardened stool, although other foreign bodies, lymphadenopathy, or cecal carcinoma can block the appendix. Edema completes the obstruction. Mucous secretions are increased in response to irritation and accumulate in the distal portion of the appendix, causing distention and pain. Bacteria, ever-present in the appendix, multiply rapidly in the stagnant medium

[2] *Statistical Bulletin,* vol. 29, no. 1, p. 3, Metropolitan Life Insurance Company, New York, January, 1948.

[3] *Statistical Bulletin,* vol. 39, p. 4, Metropolitan Life Insurance Company, New York, January, 1958.

and suppuration occurs. Unrelieved, progressive appendicitis will eventuate in perforation, "rupture," through the ulcerated or gangrenous wall and spill bacteria-laden fecal material and pus into the peritoneal cavity.

The peritonitis which follows perforation may be localized in abscess formation, or may be generalized and fatal. Peritonitis is accompanied by hypovolemic shock, toxicity, and adynamic ileus. Septic emboli may give rise to distant abscesses. The delayed sequelae to perforation are fecal fistula and adhesion formation with subsequent bowel obstruction.

Symptomatology and Diagnosis

The patient who presents the classical symptoms of acute, nonperforative appendicitis reports an abrupt onset of generalized epigastric and periumbilical pain which later localizes in the right lower quadrant. He is more comfortable lying on his right side with his thigh flexed. Abdominal tenderness and muscle guarding can be detected by palpation. When pressure from the examining hand is suddenly released, the appendix bounces against the peritoneum, causing rebound tenderness. Pain may be referred to the left lower quadrant. Vaginal or rectal examination usually elicits pain in the right lower quadrant. Since the appendix is an extension of the cecum and is of similar anatomic construction, inflammation of the appendix often produces symptoms referrable to the gastrointestinal tract. Anorexia, nausea, and even vomiting may occur as well as constipation or, rarely, diarrhea. The patient may have a low-grade fever and a mild leukocytosis.

Diagnosis of acute appendicitis may be very difficult because the symptoms, rather than being as characteristic as described, may be extremely variable, depending upon the degree of inflammation and the stage of the pathologic process, the location of the appendix, and the age of the patient.

Any one or more of the classical symptoms may be present and with varying intensity in nonperforative appendicitis. Once perforation has occurred, symptoms of increasing toxicity develop. Although there may be a temporary respite from pain following perforation because of the appendical decompression, there soon occurs a rise in the temperature, pulse, and respiratory rates, along with an increase in the sedimentation rate and leukocyte count, especially of neutrophils. Tenderness becomes diffuse. Bowel sounds are absent. If an abscess has localized it may be palpable.

The appendix is not always stationed in the right lower quadrant. During embryonic development the abdominal organs rotate counterclockwise so that the appendix comes to rest in the right lower quadrant. Failure to complete this rotation allows the appendix to rest in an atypical location, and should the appendix subsequently become inflamed, the symptoms presented will mimic disease of the organ normally located in that area. For example, if the appendix rests in the right upper quadrant, cholecystitis will be suspected.

Even with the appendix in the right lower quadrant, symptoms vary with the position of the organ. For example, a retrocecal appendix, one lying behind the cecum, will be more tender to vaginal or rectal palpation than to abdominal palpation. The appendix may overlie a ureter and produce symptoms referable to the urinary tract. In addition, appendicitis must be differentiated from conditions affecting the ovary or fallopian tube, for example, ruptured ovarian cyst or pelvic inflammatory disease.

In the aged patient there may be few symptoms, in spite of far-advanced disease. This may be because of an increased pain threshold and/or decreased cerebral interpretation of pain. The febrile and leukocytic response may be slower. Muscle atony may obscure spasm.

Diagnosis must be made on the basis of history and physical examination. Laboratory tests serve more to rule out other diagnoses than to confirm that of appendicitis. As soon as the diagnosis is made, the patient is a candidate for operation.

Indications for Surgery

All patients with acute appendicitis require surgery. The majority will undergo an emergency appendectomy. A few will recover spontaneously but will require an elective appendectomy following convalescence to prevent recurrence. Delay in surgical intervention is hardly justifiable in view of the fact that the surgical mortality is only 0.3 per cent or less if the appendix has not perforated. The argument for early surgery is further strengthened by the high morbidity and mortality rates for perforative appendicitis.

The question of when to operate following perforation is controversial. The advent of the antibiotics has permitted early operation to drain the peritoneal cavity and/or abscesses and to remove the appendical remnant if possible. Some surgeons prefer to delay surgery until the acute phase of diffuse peritonitis is over.

Preoperative and/or Conservative Management

The preparation for emergency appendectomy involves laparotomy measures, excluding the enema and usually the bath. If the patient has eaten within the past 8 hours, gastric aspiration is necessary. The fluid-electrolyte balance is corrected, and if perforation is thought to be impending or actual, antibiotics are administered.

The conservative management is used while the patient is being observed for diagnosis or when perforation is suspected. This includes bed rest, nothing given by mouth, possibly hot or cold applications to the abdomen, and the administration of analgesics and antibiotics.

If perforation is known to have occurred, the following measures are usually ordered: elevation of the head of the bed unless the patient is in shock, decompression and intravenous fluid therapy, and the administration of antibiotics. The purpose of elevating the head of the bed is to aid the gravitation of pus to the pelvis, where drainage can be more easily performed, usually through the rectum or vagina. This position also prevents the spread of purulent material to the liver and subdiaphragmatic areas, where abscess formation is much less amenable to treatment. Surgery can be performed as soon as the patient has been prepared to withstand the procedure.

Anesthesia and Surgical Technic

The choice of anesthetic depends upon the age of the patient and his condition. Appendectomy is commonly performed under spinal anesthesia, especially for adults. A local anesthetic may be used for a patient whose condition is too poor to risk a general or a spinal anesthetic.

Through a right rectus incision or one made over McBurney's point, which lies approximately midway between the umbilicus and iliac crest, the appendix is located, ligated, and removed. The appendical stump may be crushed, buried, and/or inverted. Prophylactic appendectomy is commonly practiced in conjunction with other abdominal or pelvic surgery when the appendical area is already exposed.

Postoperative Nursing Care

The care following an uncomplicated appendectomy differs in no way from that outlined for laparotomy. Activation is initiated on the day of the operation. Full intake is resumed the following day.

If peritonitis is present, the conservative management, previously described, is resumed. Convalescence is likely to be stormy and prolonged.

SUMMARY

The major surgical conditions of the small intestine can be classified as inflammatory, obstructive, neoplastic, and traumatic.

The major inflammatory condition is regional ileitis, which is primarily a medical condition but which may require resectional or diversional surgical technics to bring the disease under control or to treat its complications.

Mechanical obstruction of the small bowel may be caused by any condition which occludes the lumen. The cardinal signs of obstruction of the small intestine include obstipation, vomiting, colicky pain, and distention. The severity of the symptoms depends upon the degree and site of obstruction. If the obstruction is complete, emergency surgery is necessary.

The majority of primary growths of the small intestine are benign and can be treated by resection. A malignant neoplasm of the small intestine may be resected but bears a poor prognosis.

Wounds of the abdomen may involve the small intestine. A patient with a penetrating wound of the abdomen requires an exploratory laparotomy, as soon as shock has been adequately treated, to control bleeding and repair or resect injured tissues.

The principles of care in the preoperative and postoperative periods are the same as for laparotomy. In addition, intestinal decompression and intravenous fluid therapies may be used.

An abdominal ileostomy is necessary when total colectomy and proctectomy have been performed and when the colon must be circumvented to allow healing. The patient with an abdominal ileostomy requires a plan for care and teaching based upon his medicophysical, socioeconomic, and psychologic needs. Such a plan requires attention to his nutritional and fluid-electrolyte needs, care of the skin and stoma, and collection of stool. The patient must be encouraged to assume responsibility for his care at a rate compatible with his physical strength and psychologic readiness.

Acute appendicitis requires an emergency appendectomy to prevent the serious consequences of perforation. The nurse shares in the responsibility to help the public understand that persistent abdominal pain must be considered due to appendicitis until some other diagnosis is made. In the presence of undiagnosed abdominal pain, the patient should be given nothing orally, should have no enema, and should rest in bed until seen by a physician.

BIBLIOGRAPHY

Small Intestine

ALLEN, J. G.: (1) Anatomy, Physiology and Treatment of Intestinal Obstruction, and (2) Traumatic, Inflammatory, and Neoplastic Diseases of the Small Bowel and the Colon, in "Surgery," J. G. Allen, H. N. Harkins, C. A. Moyer, and J. E. Rhoads (eds.), J. B. Lippincott Company, Philadelphia, 1957, chap. 36, pp. 862–898, and chap. 37, pp. 899–931.

DONATO, H., H. W. MAYO, and L. H. BARR: Peroral Barium in Partial Intestinal Obstruction, *Surgery*, vol. 35, no. 5, pp. 719–723, May, 1954.

EADE, G. G., D. METHENY, and V. O. LUNDMARK: An Evaluation of the Practice of Routine Postoperative Nasogastric Suction, *Surg., Gynec. & Obst.*, vol. 101, no. 3, pp. 275–279, September, 1955.

JAFFE, L.: The Patient and His Ileostomy, *Am. J. Nursing*, p. 68, January, 1954.

KIEFER, E. D.: Recurrent Regional Ileitis, S. *Clin. North America,* vol. 35, no. 3, pp. 801–807, June, 1955.

PRIESTLY, J. T., and E. S. JUDD: The Alimentary Canal—The Duodenum, Jejunum, Ileum and Appendix, in "Christopher's Textbook of Surgery," 6th ed., L. Davis (ed.), W. B. Saunders Company, Philadelphia, 1956, chap. 20, pp. 632–653.

WAGNER, D. H.: Intestinal Intubation Techniques, Safeguards, Complications, S. *Clin. North America,* vol. 35, no. 1, pp. 151–157, February, 1955.

Appendix

ALLEN, J. G.: (1) Appendicitis and the Acute Abdomen, and (2) Peritoneum, Peritonitis, and Intra-abdominal Abscesses, in "Surgery," J. G. Allen, H. N. Harkins, C. A. Moyer, and J. E. Rhoads (eds.), J. B. Lippincott Company, Philadelphia, 1957, chap. 34, pp. 802–839, and chap. 35, pp. 841–861.

BANCROFT, F. W.: Forty Years' Experience in Acute Appendicitis, S. *Clin. North America,* vol. 35, no. 2, pp. 411–426, April, 1955.

COLLINS, D. C.: A Study of 50,000 Specimens of the Human Vermiform Appendix, *Surg., Gynec. & Obst.,* vol. 101, no. 4, pp. 437–445, October, 1955.

12

HERNIA

The lay person may consider a hernia, or "rupture," as merely an inconvenience. The physician realizes that a hernia is a surgical condition which if complicated bears a high rate of mortality. The annual sale of *trusses*, or "supports," which exceeds 1,000,000 in the United States, indicates the number of people with hernias that have not been operated upon. A hernia is potentially very serious, and the public must be educated to seek surgical repair early.

PATHOGENESIS

A *hernia* can be defined as a bulging or protrusion of an organ or a part through the wall which normally contains it. There must be a pre-existing defect in the containing wall to allow herniation. This defect may be a *congenital* weakness, or it may be *acquired*, as by trauma or surgery. Initially, the majority of hernias are potential, i.e., the defect is present but strain or stress is required to force the contents of the underlying cavity to protrude. As the organ leaves its normal confines, it usually pushes the serous membrane lining the cavity ahead of it, forming the *hernial sac*. At first, the contents of the hernial sac can usually be returned to the cavity normally containing it by gentle manipulation, or *taxis*. Such a hernia is termed *reducible*. Following repeated episodes of herniation, inflammatory adhesions may form between the organ and the sac, preventing the reduction of the hernia. The hernia has then become *irreducible*, or *incarcerated*, i.e., imprisoned. After incarceration, edema at the neck of the sac may compress the hernial contents and occlude the blood supply, resulting in necrosis of the contained organs. Such a hernia is termed *strangulated*. Both the incarcerated and strangulated hernias are accompanied by intestinal obstruction when loops of intestine are caught in the hernial sac. An irreducible hernia, therefore, is a condition urgently requiring surgical intervention. (See Fig. 26.)

148

COMMON TYPES OF HERNIAS

A hernia can occur from any of the major cavities of the body but is much more common in the abdomen. This is probably because of the accessibility of the abdomen to surgery and trauma, to the relative mo-

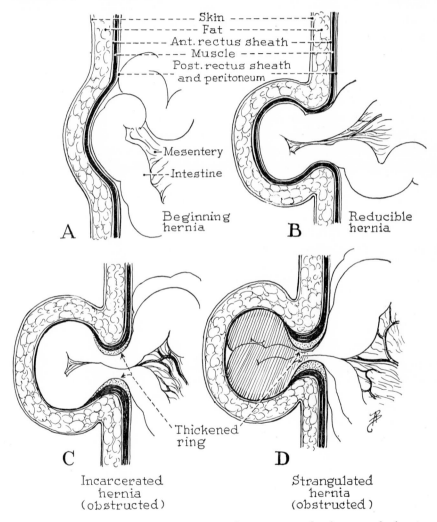

Fig. 26. Herniation. This diagram illustrates the progressive development of a hernia. (A), (B) Reducible; (C) incarcerated. Note the distention of the proximal loop of intestine and uncompromised blood supply. (D) Strangulated. Note the greater degree of distention and the compromised blood supply to the shaded portion of intestine contained within the sac.

bility of the intestines, and to the construction of the abdominal wall, which contains several anatomically weak areas, e.g., the inguinal canal, femoral opening, and the umbilicus.

Inguinal Hernia

The inguinal hernia is the most common of all hernias in both sexes and all ages. It is nine times more common in the male than in the female, probably because the testes descend *in utero* from the abdominal cavity into the scrotum, passing through the inguinal canal. Normally the peritoneal sac, or processus vaginalis, which is pushed ahead of the testes, enveloping that organ in its descent, is obliterated behind the testes at birth. If the sac fails to close, a patent canal is left, through which intestinal loops can be forced by a crucial strain. In the female the broad ligament that helps support the uterus passes through the inguinal canal to the labium majus. In the male, an inguinal hernia may be related to *cryptorchidism*, failure of the testes to descend, in which case there is a patent canal but no obliteration of the undeveloped sac.

TABLE 5   INCIDENCE OF HERNIA *

Type	Percentage
Indirect inguinal	56
Direct inguinal	22
Femoral	6
Ventral and incisional	10
Umbilical	3
Esophageal hiatus	1
Others	2
Total	100

* Reprinted with permission from H. N. Harkins, Hernia, in "Surgery," J. G. Allen, H. N. Harkins, C. A. Moyer, J. E. Rhoads (eds.), J. B. Lippincott Company, Philadelphia, 1957, chap. 39, p. 982. The percentage of incidence is based upon the author's personal observations and readings relative to hernioplasties performed.

The vast majority of inguinal hernias are classified as *indirect* and occur at birth or in early adulthood. The hernia passes through the abdominal inguinal ring, traverses the inguinal canal beside the spermatic cord or broad ligament, and emerges at the subcutaneous inguinal ring. The hernia may lodge within the inguinal canal as an *incomplete* hernia, or may descend into the scrotum or labium majus as a *complete* hernia.[1]

[1] The student is encouraged to review the anatomy of the inguinofemoral region at this point in order to understand the text more fully. An excellent reference is "Blakiston's New Gould Medical Dictionary," 2d ed., McGraw-Hill Book Company, Inc., Blakiston Division, New York, 1956, plates 4, 7, 9, and 39.

A *direct* inguinal hernia protrudes through Hesselbach's triangle, the area bounded by the inferior epigastric artery, the rectus abdominis, and the inguinal ligament. This hernia extends out through the subcutaneous inguinal, or external abdominal, ring. The bladder is commonly contained within the hernial sac. The incidence of direct hernia increases with age, probably because of relaxation of overlying muscles. This hernia is rare in females. The recurrence rate, even with careful surgery, is higher than with indirect hernia.

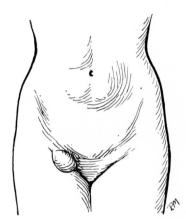

Fig. 27. Drawing showing the appearance of a femoral hernia.

Femoral Hernia

The femoral hernia (Fig. 27) accounts for only 6 per cent of hernias in the groin but is more apt to become strangulated. This hernia is more common in females, probably because of the difference in inclination of the pelvis and because of pregnancies. The weakness is more commonly congenital than acquired, but the hernia usually does not develop until middle age. The hernia travels through the femoral ring into the femoral canal, which is the passageway for the femoral vein, artery, and nerve. It lodges in the subcutaneous tissues of the *fossa ovalis*, an opening in the deep fascia of the thigh which allows the passage of the saphenous vein. Although this hernia is usually small and painless, its tendency to become strangulated makes early repair imperative.

Ventral, or Incisional, Hernia

A ventral, or incisional, hernia is acquired when the deep musculo-aponeurotic and fascial layers fail to remain in apposition owing to faulty healing, interference with the nerve supply, inadequate closure, infection, and/or prolonged drainage. It is differentiated from dehiscence and subsequent evisceration by the fact that the superficial tissues remain intact in an incisional hernia. These same factors, however, contribute to all three conditions: malnutrition, especially with inadequate protein and vitamin C levels; obesity; abdominal distention; and severe coughing.

The incidence is relatively high, ranging from 0.5 to 8 per cent. Incisional hernia seems to occur more often when vertical rather than transverse incisions are used. However the use of the transverse incision is relatively new, and since the majority of surgeons seem to favor the vertical incision, the rate of incisional hernia would be correspondingly greater. Those who favor the transverse incision feel that it facilitates closure and healing because there is less interference with the nerve supply to the abdominal wall, because it does not cut across the aponeurotic and fascial fibers which run in a transverse direction, and because it better withstands intra-abdominal pressures.[2] Surgeons who prefer the vertical incision seem to feel that greater operative exposure is possible.

An incisional hernia is usually incarcerated and may become strangulated. Repair, which is difficult, consists of obliterating the hernial sac and reinforcing the area. A drain may or may not be used.

Umbilical Hernia

The umbilical hernia occurs primarily in infants but may also occur in adults who are obese or pregnant. Because of its tendency to become strangulated, an umbilical hernia in an adult requires immediate repair.

Rarer Hernias

A few hernias which occur less frequently will be defined, as the nurse will have occasional experience with them. A combination of both a direct and an indirect inguinal hernia on the same side is termed a *pantaloon,* or *saddle-bag, hernia* because it straddles the deep epigastric vessels.

A *sliding hernia* is one in which a viscus, such as cecum or bladder, becomes adherent to the herniating organs, forming part of the wall of the sac but not actually entering the sac. In repairing such a hernia, the surgeon must recognize that a sliding hernia is present and must avoid injury to the adherent organ.

Richter's, or *Littre's, hernia* is one in which only part of the circumference of the bowel is caught in the constricting ring. This type is prone to early gangrene and peritonitis.

The *hiatus hernia* involves stomach herniating into the thoracic cavity and will be described in the next section dealing with thoracic surgery.

SYMPTOMATOLOGY

Except for the protrusion, which can be seen and palpated, a reducible hernia usually produces few symptoms. Many hernias are discovered in

[2] B. A. Nelson, Laparotomy Incisions, *J. Kansas M. Soc.,* vol. 55, p. 9, January, 1955.

routine physical examinations. The patient with an inguinal hernia may complain of a heavy or dragging sensation in the groin. The physician can elicit an *impulse,* i.e., a sensation communicated to the examining finger when the patient coughs. After reduction of the hernia, the aperture can usually be felt.

If the hernia has become incarcerated and strangulated, there will be extreme tenderness over the tense, inflamed hernia. The overlying skin may be discolored. No impulse can be elicited by the examiner. Symptoms of intestinal obstruction, increasing toxicity, and perhaps peritonitis will be manifested.

PREOPERATIVE MANAGEMENT AND CARE

The basic principles of preoperative medical management and nursing care are similar regardless of the type of abdominal hernia. Because the patient with a hernia already has a defect in his abdominal wall, it is important to raise his reparative processes to an optimal level before surgical repair to help ensure healing without dehiscence, incisional hernia, or recurrence. The patient undergoing elective herniorrhaphy (*herni + orrhaphy,* repair of) has time for adequate preparation, which favors uncomplicated healing. This is one of the major reasons for encouraging the repair of a hernia when it is first detected, since the patient undergoing emergency surgery for an incarcerated or strangulated hernia must forego the benefits of optimal preparation. All the factors important in the healing process must be considered (see Chapter 3). The patient's nutrition must be optimal, especially his protein and vitamin C levels. The obese patient must reduce. All concurrent conditions which increase the intra-abdominal pressure must be treated prior to herniorrhaphy. Such conditions are constipation; benign prostatic hypertrophy, which causes straining on urination; respiratory diseases, which cause coughing; and intra-abdominal tumor.

The immediate preparation for elective herniorrhaphy is similar to that for laparotomy. It is especially important to empty the intestine and bladder because the proximity of these organs to the field of surgery renders them, if distended, accessible to trauma and obscures the operative field. The stomach must be empty, not only to prevent regurgitation and aspiration but also to reduce the possibility of postoperative vomiting with its attendant increase in intra-abdominal pressure.

The skin preparation for inguinal herniorrhaphy includes the area from the costal margins to and including the perineum and anterior thigh on the affected side. Ventral herniorrhaphy requires the same skin preparation as for laparotomy.

The patient undergoing elective herniorrhaphy requires considerable reassurance and support in his decision to undergo surgery. The care of the patient with a herniorrhaphy has been altered considerably in the past few years because of improved methods of preoperative preparation and surgical repair. Strict bed rest in Fowler's position, tight binders, nothing taken by mouth, and minimal exertion by the patient have given way to early activation and intake, with no binders unless especially indicated. Patients who have had experience, directly or indirectly, with the former regime will require an explanation of the newer concepts of care to allay their fears and gain their much-needed cooperation.

ANESTHESIA AND REPAIR

Either general or local anesthesia can be used for hernia repair, which is called *herniorrhaphy, herniotomy,* or *hernioplasty.* Local anesthesia, either regional or spinal, has the advantage of producing no excitement stage or vomiting in the recovery period.

There are several classical procedures for hernia repair. The choice of the procedure depends upon the type and location of the hernia, the size of the defect, and the condition of the patient. Common to all repairs is the reduction of the hernia, providing the contents are known to be viable, high ligation with or without excision of the sac, and repair of the defect. If there are bilateral hernias, repair is made first on the larger one; the second hernia is operated on at a later day.

Large, recurring hernias present difficulties in repair and usually require the use of a reinforcing material such as tantalum or nylon mesh, or fascia lata to close the defect. The recurrence rate after herniorrhaphy is high, approximating 7 to 30 per cent, probably in part because of the patient's delay in seeking surgical treatment.

In some long-standing hernias the intestines have been carried in the hernial sac for such a long period of time that the abdominal cavity can not contain them when reduction is attempted. In such a case it is said that the intestines have lost their "right of domain." Special procedures must be employed to facilitate reduction. Pneumoperitoneum, which enlarges the abdominal cavity and relaxes the hernial ring, or phrenic nerve crush, which enlarges the abdominal cavity by allowing the diaphragm to rise, or even intestinal resection may be necessary.

When incarceration or strangulation complicates a hernia, emergency surgery is necessary and usually for a very ill patient. Complete intestinal obstruction almost always occurs. Gangrene of the intestinal wall with perforation and peritonitis, which occurs with unrelieved strangulation, contribute to the patient's toxic and moribund condition. The fluid and electrolyte balance is rapidly corrected, along with the use of intestinal decompression, and surgery is performed as soon as the patient's condition allows.

At surgery, the hernia sac is usually opened, and the contents are carefully inspected for viability. If viable, the contents of the hernial sac are reduced, and the defect in the abdominal wall is repaired. If necrosis is present, the involved segment will require resection, followed by an end-to-end anastomosis and repair of the defect. In known cases of strangulated femoral hernias, some surgeons carefully resect the hernial sac with its contents en masse without opening the sac, to prevent contamination of the abdominal cavity.

POSTOPERATIVE NURSING CARE

The two major concerns postoperatively are the prevention of wound infection and increased intra-abdominal pressure, both of which threaten the stability of the wound closure, inviting disruption or herniation. It is usually sufficient to leave the original dressing in place until sutures are removed on the seventh day, providing the dressing is kept clean and dry. To prevent increased intra-abdominal pressure, attention is directed toward the relief of urinary retention and abdominal distention. Urinary retention is common following herniorrhaphy because of the necessary exposure, and sometimes manipulation, of the bladder. Encouraging fluid intake and activation aids the patient to void. Catheterization may have to be resorted to temporarily. As soon as peristalsis returns, a full diet is encouraged. The early resumption of an adequate oral intake seems to stimulate peristalsis and prevent distention. A mild cathartic or low enema is usually ordered on the third postoperative day to relieve distention and prevent constipation. The activation regime is initiated on the day of surgery or the following day to encourage elimination and to prevent respiratory and vascular complications.

If the hernia was incarcerated or strangulated, nursing care will be as outlined in Chapter 11 dealing with intestinal obstruction and surgery.

Sometimes scrotal hematoma, epididymitis, or orchitis follows a herniorrhaphy. These conditions may occur with hemorrhage into the scrotum or with a tight closure of the subcutaneous ring constricting the spermatic cord. The patient will have swelling and tenderness of the scrotum. A scrotal support usually alleviates symptoms, and the patient should be instructed in its use. Warm, moist dressings, antibiotics, and incision and drainage may be necessary.

The patient always shares in his recovery and, therefore, must be instructed in what is expected of him. He must understand why it is so important for him to turn and breathe deeply. He must realize that moderate activity is desirable but that he must not strain at elimination nor attempt to lift or push heavy objects.

DISCHARGE INSTRUCTIONS

The surgeon will instruct the patient regarding his care following discharge from the hospital. The nurse must know what those instructions are in order to answer the patient's questions, clarify points of doubt, and ascertain that the patient really understands the instructions.

Usually the only restriction imposed on the patient by a herniorrhaphy is the avoidance of straining, lifting, or pushing for at least 6 weeks. The surgeon probably will inform the patient that recurrence is not uncommon and that regular medical supervision is, therefore, necessary. The patient should be taught the factors that contribute to herniation in order to avoid another hernia if possible. The surgeon may prescribe exercises to strengthen the abdominal wall and instruct the patient when to start them. Correct posture with the abdominal wall held in is important. Obesity should be avoided, the infiltrating fat weakens tissues. Lifting, when necessary, should not be done with the abdominal wall relaxed. A patient who has had a hernia should never do heavy lifting and may, therefore, have to change his occupation. Constipation and other chronic conditions which increase the intra-abdominal pressure must be treated.

NONOPERATIVE TREATMENT OF HERNIA

Two nonoperative measures should be reserved for the use of the patient who is too poor a risk to justify surgery. One of these treatments is the wearing of a truss, a heavy support designed to keep a hernia reduced. This should be applied next to the skin with the patient in the dorsal recumbent position and with the hernia reduced. It must be worn all the time that the patient is out of bed. The skin underlying the truss may become excoriated. The truss may slip, allowing the hernia to become incarcerated. A truss is an awkward, fairly expensive apparatus which is a poor substitute for surgical repair but which may be necessary for some patients. The public should be taught that a truss never cures a hernia, that it is at best only a support, and that early surgery is the only way to cure a hernia.

If a truss is necessary, it must be fitted to the patient and he must know how to apply it and how to protect the underlying skin. He must realize that the truss must never be applied to an irreducible hernia. Close medical supervision is necessary. The patient should be told that if his hernia becomes irreducible he should notify his physician, go to bed, and lie in dorsal recumbency with knees flexed. An ice bag may be applied, with the physician's permission, to minimize edema.

The other method of treatment consists of injecting the neck of the sac with a sclerosing solution after the hernia has been reduced. The aim of the treatment is to produce an inflammatory reaction and subsequent fibrosis which closes the neck of the sac. However, this treatment is losing favor with surgeons because it is hazardous and often ineffective. Blind injection of the hernial sac may injure adjacent structures, such as the intestine, and deaths due to peritonitis have been reported. Complete obliteration of the sac is often difficult to accomplish and may be only temporary. Recurrence after 6 to 12 months is not uncommon. When the injection method is used, the wearing of a truss is mandatory until the sac is obliterated.

SUMMARY

Hernias occur most commonly from the abdominal cavity in the inguinofemoral area through congenital or acquired defects in the abdominal wall.

Early surgical repair is necessary to prevent the serious complications of intestinal obstruction, incarceration, and/or strangulation.

The primary aims of preoperative and postoperative medical and nursing care are to raise the patient's reparative powers to an optimal level and to prevent increased intra-abdominal pressure.

Recurrence is not uncommon. The patient should be thoroughly instructed, before discharge from the hospital, regarding factors which predispose to herniation and how to avoid them.

BIBLIOGRAPHY

ENQUIST, I. F., and C. DENNIS: The Management of Strangulating External Hernias, S. Clin. North America, vol. 35, no. 2, pp. 429–438, April, 1955.

GALLAGHER, W. B., and R. H. SEGNITZ: Intestinal Obstruction Due to Incarcerated External Hernia, Am. J. Surg., vol. 93, no. 5, pp. 771–776, May, 1957.

GUY, C. C., C. Y. WERELIUS, and L. B. BELL, JR.: Five Years' Experience with Tantalum Mesh in Hernia Repair, S. Clin. North America, vol. 35, no. 1, pp. 175–188, February, 1955.

HARKINS, H. N.: Hernia, in "Surgery," J. G. Allen, H. N. Harkins, C. A. Moyer, and J. E. Rhoads (eds.), J. B. Lippincott Company, Philadelphia, 1957, chap. 39, pp. 980–1025.

LEMMER, K. E., and S. R. WATSON: Inguinal Hernia, Am. J. Nursing, pp. 1471–1475, December, 1953.

McNEALY, R. W., and J. A. GLASSMAN: Experience with Vitallium Plates in the Repair of Hernias, Surgery, vol. 27, no. 5, pp. 752–761, May, 1950.

McVAY, C. B.: Hernia, in "Christopher's Textbook of Surgery," 6th ed., L. Davis (ed.), W. B. Saunders Company, Philadelphia, 1956, chap. 19, pp. 502–554.

RYAN, E. A.: An Analysis of 313 Consecutive Cases of Indirect Sliding Inguinal Hernias, Surg., Gynec. & Obst., vol. 102, no. 1, pp. 45–58, January, 1956.

THOREK, P.: Some Surgical Aspects of Inguinal Hernia, What's New (Abbott Lab.), no. 187, pp. 14–17, 1955.

WATSON, L. F.: "Hernia," 3d ed., The C. V. Mosby Company, St. Louis, 1948.

13

SURGERY OF THE COLON AND RECTUM

Surgery of the colon is performed primarily in the treatment of carcinoma, precarcinomatous lesions, and complications of chronic inflammatory processes. Rectal surgery is indicated for neoplastic disease as well as for conditions peculiar to that area and described subsequently.

COLORECTAL CARCINOMA

No other site in the body bears so high a mortality rate for carcinoma in men and women combined than does the colorectal area, and yet two-thirds of these tumors, usually adenocarcinomas, are within reach of the examining finger or proctosigmoidoscope and offer a good prognosis for cure if excised early. Early detection depends upon regular, complete physical examinations, since carcinoma characteristically has an insidious onset and may present vague symptoms or no symptoms until growth is extensive.

Symptomatology

Carcinoma of the descending and sigmoid colon tends to cause intestinal obstruction early because the lumen of the colon is smaller in these areas and the stool is formed. Rectal carcinoma, however, rarely causes obstruction. The most common signs and symptoms of colorectal carcinoma are changes in bowel habit; bleeding with subsequent anemia, weight loss, and weakness; pain; tenesmus if the carcinoma is rectal; and, sometimes, a palpable mass. Changes in bowel habit, the most common symptom, include constipation and/or diarrhea. The diarrhea may be the result of mucous erosion of the tumor, lying usually within the sigmoid or rectum, which permits passage of a liquid, mucoid stool. The stools may become ribbonlike in passing through a partially obstructed lumen. Bleeding is more likely to be occult in right-sided carcinoma and, therefore, to escape detection until a severe anemia is manifested together with weakness and weight loss. Left-sided carcinoma is commonly evidenced first by bright red blood in or on the stool. This may be attributed to bleeding *hemorrhoids,* sacculation of engorged veins. Indeed, hemorrhoids may themselves signal carcinoma inasmuch as they are the result of venous stasis, one of the causes of which is neoplastic growth.

Diagnostic Methods

The presumptive diagnosis, made on the basis of history and physical findings, is confirmed by biopsy. If the lesion is in the sigmoid colon or rectum, the biopsy specimen is obtained through a *sigmoidoscope.* This is an illuminated, rigid, hollow instrument which allows direct visualization of the distal intestinal tract and is, therefore, invaluable in the detection of carcinoma and precarcinomatous lesions, such as polyps. Sigmoidoscopic examination should be performed at regular intervals for all persons forty years of age or older.

A sigmoidoscopic examination can be extremely trying for the patient, especially if he has rectal and/or colonic spasm, which is aggravated by the instrumentation and apprehension. Much of the success of this examination depends upon the nurse, whose responsibility it is to prepare the patient, the equipment, and the environment. The preparation of the patient begins with the physician's explanation of the examination and why it is necessary. Enemas are usually ordered to be given until returns are clear. The nurse must see that these enemas are given without excess heat or soap, if soapsuds are ordered, since both irritate the mucous membranes and produce an inflammatory reaction. Time must be allowed for thorough evacuation to ensure clear visualization. When the sigmoidoscopic procedure is performed primarily for the purpose of obtaining specimens for culture, the enemas may be omitted. Some restriction of oral intake may be ordered to avoid vomiting due to apprehension and to ensure a clear lower intestinal tract.

The nurse is responsible for checking the equipment to be sure that all needed supplies are assembled and that the instrument's light and battery are in working order. She should not have to leave the patient to gather supplies once the procedure has been started. The room should be darkened to facilitate visualization through the sigmoidoscope.

Immediately prior to the examination the patient should empty his bladder to avoid injury to that organ or incontinence. The physician will position the patient on his side, on his knees and left shoulder, or on a table especially designed for this examination. The nurse must see that the patient is made to feel as secure and comfortable as possible in whatever position is used, that he is draped properly, and that his privacy is assured. She will attend the patient closely throughout the examination, observing his condition, encouraging relaxation, and diverting his attention as much as possible. After the procedure, the patient should be allowed to rest prone for a few minutes before attempting to walk. After a brief rest, however, walking should be encouraged to help him expel the air which enters the intestinal tract by way of the sigmoidoscope. If a biopsy has been performed, the patient may be kept in bed for a few hours and observed for symptoms of hemorrhage, which infrequently occurs. Although the terms *sigmoidoscopy* and *proctoscopy* are used interchangeably, the latter requires the use of an instrument which is shorter, designed to reach no higher than the rectosigmoidal junction. The care of the patient is the same with both procedures.

A barium enema may be used to delineate the tumor and establish the site. However, when obstruction is suspected, rectal barium is used with caution, and oral administration is prohibited, because of the danger of converting a partial obstruction into a complete one.

Treatment

The treatment for colorectal carcinoma is wide excision, under general anesthesia, of the involved tissues, the extent of surgery depending upon the site and amount of involvement. Cancer of the cecum and the ascending colon requires a *hemicolectomy*, excision of half the colon, intestinal continuity being reestablished by anastomosis of the ileum to the transverse colon. If the neoplasm is in the transverse colon, wide resection of that segment with an end-to-end anastomosis or a combined abdominoperineal resection may be necessary. In this latter procedure, through an abdominal incision, the descending segment is loosened from its attachments, or mobilized, and excised from the transverse colon, which is exteriorized, creating a permanent colostomy. Lymph node dissection is completed, and the abdomen is closed. Next the posterior perineum is widely excised, and the freed intestinal segment is removed through the perineal wound. Usually, the perineal area is packed and allowed to heal by secondary intention. Sometimes it is possible to perform a *Bacon's procedure* for carcinoma low in the sigmoid colon or in the upper rectum. This entails resection of the distal intestinal segment with a "pull-through" of the proximal intestine, which is secured at the level of the preserved anal sphincters. A colostomy is thereby obviated.

Sometimes a temporary colostomy is performed to allow for elimination when an inoperable neoplasm is obstructing the descending and sigmoid colon, to decompress the patient who is completely obstructed prior to excision of a low colorectal tumor, or to bypass the lower intestinal tract to allow healing following trauma. Through a small incision a loop of colon, usually transverse, is lifted from the abdominal cavity and held in place by a glass rod inserted under the loop. (See Fig. 28.) The loop of intestine may be opened at the close of the operation or after a day or more. A temporary colostomy has two loops, the *proximal*, leading to the stomach, and the *distal*, leading to the rectum, whereas a permanent colostomy has only the proximal loop, the distal segment having been removed. A temporary colostomy may be closed surgically after its purpose has been fulfilled.

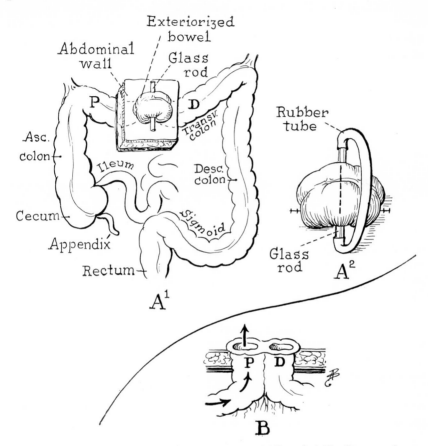

Fig. 28. Temporary transverse colostomy. Inserts (A^1) and (A^2) illustrate the retaining rod in place. Insert (B) illustrates the proximal and distal loops designated in (A^1) and (B) by P and D, respectively.

Preoperative Care and Teaching

Because these patients tend to be within the older age groups, it is important to keep them active preoperatively and to ensure their proper nutritional and fluid intake. If time permits, a high-caloric, low-residue diet may be ordered. In addition, antibiotics and/or sulfonamides are commonly ordered to reduce the bacterial flora of the intestinal tract.

Prior to surgery, the patient is instructed by the surgeon so that he knows what type of anesthesia and operation to expect. He is then prepared as for a laparotomy, with the additional measures necessary for colonic surgery. The immediate preparation for colorectal surgery aims to reduce peristalsis to a minimum and to have the tract as empty and clean as possible. Therefore, the patient is given nothing orally, being sustained instead by parenteral fluids; decompression therapy may be substituted, using a long intestinal tube. An enema is usually given, which may or may not be ordered to be repeated until the returns are clear.

The skin preparation for right hemicolectomy, or resection of the transverse colon, includes the abdomen from the nipple line to and in-

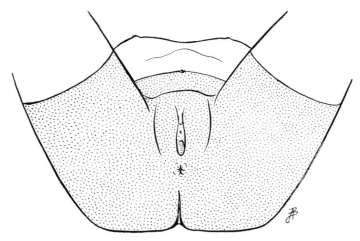

FIG. 29. Area of skin preparation for perineal surgery. Note that the skin is prepared from the umbilicus to and including the pubic and perineal areas and buttocks and the superior half of each thigh.

cluding the pubes. (See Fig. 29.) For a carcinoma in the left colon, skin preparation is made of both the abdomen and the perineum, including a margin of at least 6 in. around the anal opening, in the event that a combined anterior-posterior resection may be necessary.

Care Following Hemicolectomy, or Segmental Resection

Following a hemicolectomy, or segmental resection with anastomosis, the intestinal tract is kept at rest by decompression therapy and the prohibition of oral intake, while parenteral fluids are used to maintain the nutritional, fluid, and electrolyte balance. An accurate intake and output record is necessary. Urinary retention must be relieved. When bowel sounds return, decompression therapy is discontinued, and a small, low enema may be given. Alimentation is resumed gradually after the integrity of the anastomosis has been assured. The activation regime is especially important, since the majority of these patients are in the older age groups. Early complications which may ensue include dehiscence, peritonitis, stenosis at the site of the anastomosis, as well as hermorrhage, shock, atelectasis, and thrombosis. Later, fistulas and/or adhesions may form. A patient who has been operated upon for carcinoma requires close medical supervision for the remainder of his life to detect possible recurrence early.

Care of the Patient Undergoing an Abdominoperineal Resection

A right hemicolectomy, or resection with anastomosis, in itself imposes no restrictions upon a patient's way of living, once he has recovered. This is not the case when an abdominoperineal resection is necessary, as will be illustrated by this discussion of Mr. Fred Witt. This 78-year-old patient has been brought to the hospital by his son directly from his physician's office, where the provisional diagnosis, "partial bowel obstruction due to carcinoma of the sigmoid," was made. He has passed no stool and only occasional flatus in 4 days.

The nurse notices in assisting this quiet, white-haired patient to bed that he is small, underdeveloped, and poorly nourished. His abdomen is moderately distended. His thin, dry skin feels warm. He seems weak and in a moderate amount of distress. His temperature, pulse, and respirations are 100°F.–120–28; blood pressure is 150/80 mm. mercury.

The son tells the nurse that this patient is a widower and a retired businessman. Although Mr. Witt receives a monthly pension which augments his social security, the major burden of the expense of hospitalization must be borne by this married son, with whom he lives. This fact has imposed upon the patient a further sense of indebtedness. Mr. Witt embraces no formal religious doctrine. He cannot see how he can ever accept the operation proposed by his physician.

The diagnosis is confirmed in the hospital by the surgeon, who further notes a palpable rectal mass, blood on the examining finger, and absent bowel sounds. Biopsy reveals carcinoma. The patient is scheduled for operation on the day following admission, which leaves the nurse only 24 hours to help this patient accept the idea that this operation is both necessary and hopeful. She realizes that Mr. Witt probably has fears about the anesthesia, pain, and death, but that he is even more concerned about living with the colostomy after recovery. She realizes, too, that in this case it is better to delay detailed teaching until after surgery when more time can be allowed for the patient to grasp the instruction. His paramount need now is to be given hope for a satisfying life after recovery. To this end she encourages Mr. Witt to tell her about his grandchildren, to whom he is devoted; she refers to his activities with them after convalescence. This discussion provides Mr. Witt with an outlet and he begins to refer with hesitancy to his immediate concerns. The nurse senses that Mr. Witt would like the services of a clergyman, although he professes no formal religion, and asks the hospital chaplain to see the patient. The chaplain, too, makes reference to visits after surgery, reinforcing the feeling that Mr. Witt will survive and will be cared for. There is a well-rehabilitated patient on the clinical division who is almost ready for discharge. With the permission of the surgeon, this patient is allowed to visit Mr. Witt and talk with him. Admittedly this is an ideal situation, which might or might not be duplicated in a hospital situation. The nurse's ingenuity will be taxed when such help is not available or when the patient can not be led so quickly to accept reassurance. However, community clergymen are always available when there is no hospital chaplain; the nurse, too, should be prepared to lend spiritual strength to her patients.[1] Notice that the nurse did not say, "There now, don't you worry; you'll be all right." Instead she opened channels of communication and provided the patient with positive, reassuring experiences, all the while administering physical care to promote comfort and security—which is her unique contribution.

Postoperatively, Mr. Witt's care must be designed to hasten his recovery from anesthesia and surgery, prevent complications, and help him become as fully rehabilitated as possible. The nurse, along with the other members of the health team, will continue to be supportive and reassuring, gradually relinquishing to Mr. Witt the responsibility for his total care as he shows evidence of capability. His desire to live a normal, independent life is to be stimulated fully. His program of rehabilitation follows.

The Rehabilitation of the Patient Who Has a Colostomy

One of the most challenging and rewarding experiences of surgical nursing is the rehabilitation of the patient who has a permanent colostomy. The problems of such a patient are not unlike those of the patient who has an ileostomy. However, the patient with a colostomy does not have to contend with the problem of lifelong semiliquid stools and consequent deprivation of control over his defecation. This very fact imposes upon both patient and nurse a greater responsibility for a hygienic program designed to effect a normal way of living.[2]

Initially, the nurse must consider the patient's motivation and readiness to learn. She must consider his situation in life and the roles he plays. For example, a young person who is the father of four children and who feels that he is loved and needed will probably accept the procedure and participate actively in his rehabilitation. It is quite different for an older

[1] G. Westberg, "Nurse, Pastor and Patient," Augustana Press, Rock Island, Ill., 1955.

[2] An excellent reference for use in patient teaching is "Care of Your Colostomy," published by the American Cancer Society, Inc., New York, 1956.

patient who may be alone and dependent upon society for maintenance. A person who could not really accept himself before surgery will hardly be able to accept a colostomy satisfactorily. First then, the patient must be able to accept himself, his diagnosis, and his colostomy. The nurse can be substantially aided in bringing the patient to a point of readiness to learn by enlisting the aid of a person who has already adjusted well to a colostomy. Such a person can discuss with the patient the problems of colostomy care in a most realistic manner. More important, this person can serve as one with whom the patient can identify. In some cities there are colostomy clubs composed of people who have had this procedure.[3] These people gather to discuss their common problems, to socialize, and to render the type of service just described. They help the new patient to realize that his situation is neither unique nor hopeless.

The major areas of need in a program of rehabilitation are similar to those described for the patient with an ileostomy, i.e., psychologic, medicophysical, and socioeconomic. Psychologic needs have been given priority in this discussion of the rehabilitation of a patient with a colostomy since so much of the responsibility for an adequate adjustment rests with the patient. In other words, a colostomy can be well-regulated, whereas an ileostomy can not. The degree of success achieved in regulation is usually directly proportional to the patient's desire to control his defecation and to resume an independent status.

The surgeon prepares the patient for a colostomy by explaining what it is, how it functions, and why it must be performed. In spite of this instruction, however, the patient may be unable to comprehend just what is to happen, or he may be unable to accept the fact that a colostomy is necessary. Such a patient may, therefore, assert postoperatively that no one told him what the operation would be and refuse to participate in rehabilitation. To prevent this negative reaction it is important that clear channels of communication be established preoperatively and that the patient be encouraged to talk about the feelings he has regarding the impending surgery. This provides the health team with many opportunities to clarify and reinforce the original teaching. Occasionally, the

---

[3] It has been the author's privilege to observe the highly successful progress of The Colostomy and Ileostomy Rehabilitation Guild, Inc., of Saint Paul, Minn. This group was organized under the direction of Miss Dorothy Schneider, a young nurse who recognized the need for bringing these patients together for the purpose of sharing and solving thir mutual problems. The following excerpt from a letter written by a member indicates the degree of encouragement patients derive from such a group: "To me the meeting of the C and I Club is the most important day of the month. To one who has recently returned from the darkness, it's an inspiration and certainly a promise toward a brighter future. Each individual appears to be enjoying life perhaps better than before surgery."

Similar groups have been organized in New York, Boston, Philadelphia, Los Angeles, and Minneapolis.

surgeon may deem such preoperative instruction a greater risk than none and will instruct the relatives accordingly, delaying detailed explanation to the patient until after the operation. The nurse must realize that the surgeon is the one who bears the responsibility for deciding how much explanation the patient needs and can accept. Therefore, the teaching program must be planned in conference with the surgeon. Sometimes the emergency nature of the condition requiring a colostomy limits the amount of explanation that can be given preoperatively. Usually, the more the patient knows about a colostomy preoperatively, the more easily he will be able to make the necessary adjustments in his living. Teaching must be done within a framework of realistic optimism. Of course the patient's life will be handicapped somewhat, but he must be impressed with his ability to control defecation and to have a full and useful life.

One of the ways by which defecation can be controlled is by adherence to a slightly constipating but highly nutritious diet. The patient must avoid foods to which he formerly was sensitive and those which produce a loose stool, gas, or odors. In an effort to overcome the liquid stools which are characteristic of a new, unregulated colostomy, the patient may develop the habit of insufficient food and fluid intake. He must be assured that his stools will become more solid in time. He must be impressed with the need for maintaining a liberal fluid intake and an optimal nutritional level.

Adherence to the prescribed diet and the avoidance of excessive physical and emotional stress are necessary in helping the patient to achieve regularity based on his preoperative pattern of defecation, e.g., one stool daily without intermittent drainage. To help him establish this pattern, colostomy irrigations may be ordered. They are given as an enema each day at the same time. Since rehabilitation is designed to return the individual to the community able to function at his optimal level, all the colostomy teaching must be done with the patient's usual living habits in mind. This applies especially to the colostomy irrigations. The nurse must consider at what time of day the patient has been in the habit of defecating in order to reestablish this pattern with irrigations. She must in addition consider the patient's schedule. (See page 12.) For example, a patient who does not have the time or opportunity to irrigate his colostomy in the morning might well tend to this matter in the evening. Regularity is the keynote, regardless of the time of day. The patient will learn how much time he must allow for adequate drainage after a colostomy irrigation and will plan his activities accordingly. For example, a man might irrigate his colostomy, attach a bag to collect the returns, and shave while the colostomy is draining.

The procedure for colostomy irrigation need not be given in detail, but a few essential principles will be pointed out:

1. The new colostomy requires only 350 to 500 ml. warm water or normal saline solution for the irrigation, which is administered without force through a small catheter (No. 16 Fr. or 18 Fr.). Gradually the

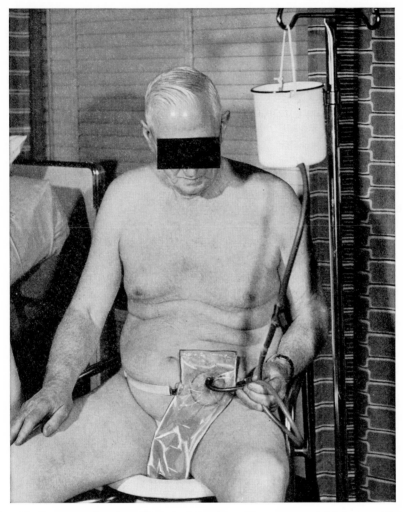

FIG. 30. Patient performing colostomy irrigation with a commercial irrigator. (*Courtesy of Colostomy Appliance Laboratory, Chicago.*)

amount of solution can be increased to 500 or 1,000 ml.; it is then administered through a larger tube (No. 20 or 22 Fr.).

2. The surgeon will indicate whether the proximal or distal segments, or both, should be irrigated. If there is any doubt regarding the identity of the segments, the surgeon should be consulted.

3. Force must never be exerted in the introduction of the catheter. This procedure can be facilitated by lubricating the catheter tip well and by allowing some solution to flow as the tube is being inserted.

4. The reservoir of solution must hang no higher than 1 to 1½ ft. above the stoma.

5. If the irrigation is not returned after 20 or 30 minutes, gently massage the abdomen, have the patient change his position, or encourage him to laugh or cough. If these measures fail, give a second, smaller irrigation. If the irrigation still does not return, the solution must be siphoned back and the surgeon notified.

6. The stoma may need dilatation, as in an ileostomy. The surgeon usually teaches the patient how to do this, or he may ask the nurse to demonstrate the procedure.

7. The distal loop may be irrigated with solutions of antibiotics or sulfonamides, or with plain water, to prevent stasis and consequent infection, or to prepare the loop for reestablishment of intestinal continuity. The patient will then require a bedpan as well as an irrigation receptacle.

8. The use of a commercial colostomy irrigator is to be encouraged (Fig. 30). This appliance consists of a plastic cup which fits over the colostomy stoma and is held in place by a belt. A disposable sheath is attached to the cup and hangs between the patient's thighs into the toilet. The catheter is introduced into the colostomy through an opening in the irrigator cup. After the solution has flowed in, the catheter is removed, and the opening in the cup is closed. The irrigation returns flow down through the sheath and into the toilet, thus obviating the psychic trauma associated with soiling during the irrigation.

9. Some surgeons may prefer not to use irrigations, relying instead upon a colostomy pouch. (See Fig. 31.) Some patients may regulate themselves without the aid of irrigations. For these reasons, an irrigation may not always be ordered. In some patients the use of a pouch encourages dependence on the apparatus and laxity in adhering to the colostomy diet. Pouches are usually disposable. If they are not, it is imperative that they be kept clean and aired frequently; the patient should have at least two. A permanent pouch should not be washed with disinfectant solutions, as they may cause severe burns of the stoma. It is imperative that suction not be created by the pouch as herniation may result.

The integrity of the skin surrounding the stoma is maintained with greater ease as the stools become more solid. The patient should be made to understand that his stools will be liquid at first, that this is expected, and that he will be kept clean. He will learn to wash the area carefully after each elimination, dry well, and powder. A moisture-repellent ointment or aluminum powder may be necessary early and at any time that the area becomes excoriated, but the constant use of an ointment for a prolonged period of time may cause maceration and is to be avoided.

Dressings must be changed frequently for a patient with a new, unregulated colostomy; for this measure there is no substitute. Dressings need not be voluminous and should not merely be reinforced. They must be completely removed, skin care given, and reapplication made by "nesting" the stoma in fluffed gauze over which an absorbent pad is placed. After the colostomy has been regulated by diet and irrigations, it is sufficient for the patient to wear a soft tissue held in place by a colostomy belt or modified elasticized support.

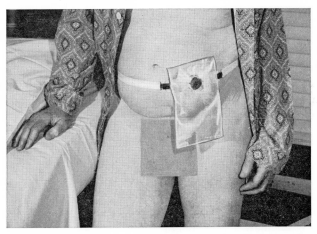

FIG. 31. Patient wearing one type of colostomy pouch which may be used early postoperatively or in times of stress. A modification of this type of pouch may be worn by the patient with an ileostomy. (*Courtesy of Colostomy Appliance Laboratory, Chicago.*)

At first the nurse will assume complete care of the colostomy, which includes observation of the stoma and surrounding skin to detect excoriation, prolapse, retraction, stenosis, and unusual drainage; irrigations; dressing changes; and skin care. She will teach the patient the principles underlying this care and help him gradually to assume complete responsibility for his colostomy. Many pamphlets are available that can be used in teaching the patient who has a colostomy. Some hospitals have their own lists of printed instructions.

Perineal Wound Care

The goal in the management of the perineal wound is promotion of healing from within outward by granulation tissue. Premature closure of the superficial tissues is prevented by packing, which is inserted at surgery and either withdrawn gradually or replaced with smaller amounts daily. Irrigations of the wound are commonly ordered to keep the area clean and odor-free. An oxidizing solution is usually used. Gradually, as granulation occurs, the amount of solution is decreased, as is the size of the irrigating catheter. Sitz baths are usually ordered to be taken several times a day—as a method of applying heat, as well as for their cleansing effect. The patient must understand how to take sitz baths safely and effectively at home if these treatments are to be continued after discharge.

ACUTE COLONIC OBSTRUCTION

Colorectal carcinoma may escape detection until the occurrence of complete intestinal obstruction, which is manifested by colicky pains, obstipation, and distention. Vomiting is rare if the ileocecal valve is competent. Impaction of stool can also obstruct the colon, a fact that the nurse must remember in meeting the needs of the bedfast patient. A third condition, which, although rare, does cause obstruction, is *volvulus*, a twisting of the colon, usually of the sigmoid portion.

Diagnostic Methods

Diagnosis of colonic obstruction is made by x-ray, which usually reveals a markedly distended bowel framing the abdomen. X-ray may reveal the site and cause of the obstruction. Primarily to determine whether the obstruction is complete or incomplete, oil may be administered orally, followed by enemas. The principle underlying this procedure is that a substance which can be administered orally, remain unchanged by the intestinal tract, and be recognizable when passed rectally can demonstrate that the obstruction is partially open. Mineral oil is such a substance. The patient is given an ounce or more of oil (the dose may later be repeated) orally or through the decompression tube, which is clamped for ½ hour. The oil also acts to soften feces, which may then pass the obstruction. Warm saline or tap-water enemas are given at regular intervals to encourage elimination of the oil. The enema can also be used to help determine the site and degree of obstruction if the amount of solution taken and the amount returned are noted accurately. To illustrate, if only 200 ml. can be taken, the obstruction is probably low in the sigmoid colon; if more is taken, the site is higher. If 500 ml. can be taken, but only 300 ml. returns, then the other 200 ml. has probably passed through a partially open obstruction. The enema sometimes serves a therapeutic purpose, too, by reducing the inflammation present, thereby converting a complete obstruction into an incomplete one.

It is absolutely essential that the nurse who carries out this procedure understand its purpose thoroughly. It can be seen, for example, that to administer the oil rectally, rather than orally, would completely defeat the purpose of the procedure. It is equally important that the enemas be administered by a nurse who can give them skillfully, enabling the patient to take as much of the solution as possible in order to gain a true index of the site of the obstruction. A 2-qt. enema is given, as this is the approximate capacity of the normal adult colon. Since soap would emulsify oily returns, warm normal saline solution or tap water is used. The use of an oily lubricant on the rectal tube is avoided; water is often sufficient lubricant if the tube is inserted with care. Since the nurse must measure and observe the returns accurately, a bedpan should be provided rather than allowing the patient the use of the toilet.

The following facts must be recorded:

1. Administration of mineral oil: time, amount, route
2. Administration of the enema
a. The exact amount taken
b. The exact amount returned
c. Presence of oil on the surface of the returns
d. Passage of flatus
e. Passage of stool
f. Abnormal constituents, such as blood, pus, or parasites

The passage of oil, flatus, or stool demonstrates that the obstruction is partial rather than complete, indicating that there is time to prepare the patient more adequately for surgery, should that be necessary.

Preoperative Care and Nursing Responsibilities

Medical measures instituted during the period of diagnostic evaluation serve to prepare the patient for surgery, which must be performed immediately if the obstruction is complete or may be delayed to allow for more adequate preoperative preparation if the obstruction is incomplete. These measures include prohibition of oral intake and administration of parenteral fluids. Enemas and antibiotic drugs may be ordered. Analgesia, if used at all, is mild, to prevent masking symptoms during this period of evaluation.

The nurse's observations are very important in helping the surgeon to evaluate the patient's condition and to determine the time for surgical intervention. Frequent determinations of the degree of abdominal distention must be made, using a tape measure for accuracy. Pain must be noted and described fully. The occurrence of vomiting or the passage of stool or flatus must be reported promptly. A fall in blood pressure or rise in temperature, pulse, and respirations portends strangulation and/or perforation and requires the surgeon's immediate attention.

Treatment

A complete obstruction of the colon is a surgical emergency requiring immediate decompression by cecostomy or colostomy to prevent perforation and fatal peritonitis. Definitive surgery is usually delayed until the patient can be more adequately prepared, except in the case of obstruction due to volvulus, which urgently requires surgical correction to prevent strangulation of the intestine.

If the patient has an incomplete obstruction, definitive surgery is carried out as soon as he has been adequately prepared.

CHRONIC INFLAMMATORY CONDITIONS

In general, chronic inflammatory diseases of the colon, such as diverticulitis and ulcerative colitis, are treated medically by diet, drugs, and rest. Both diseases are marked by remissions and exacerbations occurring over a period of years. When complications ensue, surgical intervention becomes necessary. These complications, the direct result of inflammation and ulceration, include hemorrhage; obstruction; perforation; abscess, sinus, fistula, and stricture formation; and intractability.

Diverticulitis

Diverticulitis is superimposed upon *diverticulosis,* a condition marked by multiple permanent outpouchings of the intestinal mucous membrane through a fragmented muscular wall of the colon. These pouches are shaped like a tear drop and may, therefore, collect particles of stool, which by causing irritation give rise to ulceration, bleeding, and perforation. Diverticulosis is far more common than *diverticulitis,* inflamed diverticula, and is usually asymptomatic. Diverticulitis, on the other hand, gives rise to many variable symptoms. Usually some abdominal discomfort is present. The patient may pass frequent, loose stools of decreased caliber, or he may have frank diarrhea; he may even be constipated. He may report a sensation of rectal urgency. Rectal bleeding may be the only sign. He may or may not have chills, fever, vomiting, and/or a palpable abdominal mass.

Although the entire colon may be affected, the sigmoid is the most common site. Resection and anastomosis can be curative if the process is not in the acute stage and is localized. Because of the chronicity of diverticulitis and the invalidism it imposes, some surgeons advocate resection prior to the occurrence of any complications. Once complications ensue, definitive surgery must await measures to combat the complications. For example, if the colon is obstructed, the patient must first have a colostomy to divert the fecal stream and to decompress the colon. A subsequent resection of the sigmoid colon is then carried out. Abscesses must be drained prior to resection. However, in good-risk patients the surgery may be performed all at once rather than in stages. Carcinoma must be ruled out in patients who have diverticulitis, because both entities favor the sigmoid colon and can manifest the same symptoms.

The nursing care for a patient undergoing segmental resection and anastomosis for diverticulitis is designed to meet the needs of a patient who usually is in the older age group and who may have been chronically ill for many years. Malnutrition may be marked, increasing the surgical risk and likelihood of postoperative shock, dehiscence, and delayed healing. Intravenous administration of blood and protein may be necessary before and after surgery. Tissue turgor is likely to be poor, requiring excellent skin care and frequent turning to prevent decubiti. The activation regime is especially important in these patients to prevent pulmonary and vascular stasis. Continued medical supervision will be necessary, as remaining diverticula may also become inflamed.

Ulcerative Colitis

The patient who comes to surgery for treatment of ulcerative colitis usually has been chronically ill for many years. However, he tends to be considerably younger and more acutely ill. The definitive treatment for ulcerative colitis is radical extirpation of the purulent, ulcerated, and necrotic colon. A permanent ileostomy may be established a month or two prior to the total colectomy and proctectomy. However, the ileostomy and total colectomy can be carried out safely in one stage in many patients. Surgery can effect a cure in a high percentage of patients, and the operative mortality is relatively low.

The nursing care must be geared to meet the needs of a patient who is usually emaciated and anemic, who may have skin and arthritic involvement, and who probably is an extremely dependent personality who reacts excessively to all stimuli. He will tax the patience of the nurse, but her accepting, optimistic attitude alone will have definite psychotherapeutic value. Life is not, nor has it been, very satisfying to such a patient. He will need considerable encouragement to accept the ileostomy and colectomy. He, too, must remain under close medical surveillance, probably for the remainder of his life.

POLYPOSIS

The majority of colorectal polyps are either potentially or actually malignant adenomas. These tumors, which may be pedunculated and/or sessile, are most commonly located in the anorectum, although they may be found throughout the colon. They vary in size and are usually multiple. Although the majority are asymptomatic, they may produce bleeding, mucous discharge, change in bowel habit, and/or abdominal discomfort. Diagnosis is made by sigmoidoscopy and roentgen-ray studies using barium and air-contrast media.

Treatment depends primarily upon the location and degree of malignancy, potential or actual. Polyps located within reach of the sigmoidoscope may be *fulgurated,* i.e., destroyed by electrical current, or excised through this instrument. If histologic studies reveal adenocarcinoma, an abdominoperineal resection with proctosigmoidectomy is carried out. Polyps located within the colon are reached by colectomy and sterile coloscopy. If the polyp is definitely benign, polypectomy may be adequate treatment, but the patient must undergo repeated observation by sigmoidoscopy for the remainder of his life. However, the malignancy potential for polyps of the colon is high, and treatment is usually more extensive, ranging from segmental resection to total colectomy with an ileostomy.

COLORECTAL INJURIES

The management of wounds of the colon and rectum is essentially the same as that described for abdominal injuries in the preceding chapter. An additional consideration is the possibility of a colostomy to divert the fecal stream from the injured segment of large intestine. While this would probably be an emergency procedure with limited time for emotional preparation, it is also usually a temporary measure, which makes the adjustment far easier. As with trauma anywhere in the body, the treatment of shock and hemorrhage takes priority over definitive measures to repair the structures involved.

HEMORRHOIDS

Hemorrhoids, or "piles," one of the most common afflictions of mankind, have been defined variously as vascular tumors, vascular enlargements, and anorectal varicose veins. Anal infection extending into the hemorrhoidal plexuses and relaxation of the overlying mucous membranes or skin are thought to be contributory factors. For practical purposes, hemorrhoids may be thought of as masses of inflamed venous plexuses bulging through the rectal mucosa or anal skin. They are probably aggravated by such factors as prolonged straining, portal obstruction, and pregnancy. (See Fig. 32.)

Symptomatology

Hemorrhoidal disease may be asymptomatic, but acute, disabling episodes may also occur. Symptoms depend primarily upon the location of the hemorrhoid(s). Internal hemorrhoids originate above the pectinate line and are covered with rectal mucous membrane which is insensitive, being supplied only with visceral innervation. These hemorrhoids bleed and may produce a hypochromic anemia. They protrude into the anal canal, sometimes presenting through the anal opening, initially with defecation and later with any strain. At first reducible, they later remain

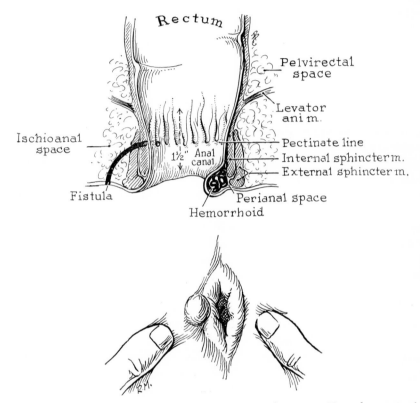

Fig. 32. (Above) Section of the anorectum, coronal section. Note the anatomic relationships, the fistula, and the external hemorrhoid. (Below) Drawing to show the appearance of an external hemorrhoid.

prolapsed and soil the patient's clothing with a bloody, mucous discharge. External hemorrhoids originate below the pectinate line and are covered with anal skin which is supplied with somatic innervation and is, therefore, very sensitive. External hemorrhoids more frequently become thrombosed, causing exquisite pain.

The major complications of hemorrhoidal disease are the formation of multiple, infected thrombi; ulceration; strangulation and gangrene, occurring when the sphincters contract on the prolapsed tissues. Hemorrhoidal disease may signal carcinoma higher in the intestinal tract and, therefore, requires a thorough investigation to rule out this more serious lesion.

Indications for Surgery

Surgical intervention is indicated for hemorrhoids which recur, cause severe anemia, or prolapse. Since any untreated rectal condition associated with mucous drainage may cause *pruritus*, itching, with all its attendant physical and emotional complications, surgery may be the treatment of choice for all hemorrhoids in good-risk patients. The injection method of treatment, using a sclerosing solution, is usually reserved for poor-risk patients.

Preoperative Care

Hemorrhoidectomy can be accomplished with less risk and greater satisfaction if delayed until after the acute stage has subsided. Edema and inflammation are reduced by the following measures: the application of heat in the form of warm, moist compresses or sitz baths; bedrest; and the production of a soft stool by liberal fluid intake, a soft, low-residue diet, and mineral oil. An external thrombosed hemorrhoid may be treated briefly with bedrest, ice packs, and anodynes prior to spontaneous or surgical evacuation of the clot. This procedure is inadequate as definitive therapy, as another thrombus may form. A skin tag may remain after inflammation has subsided, causing annoyance and pruritus, and, therefore, may require excision.

The immediate preparation for hemorrhoidectomy depends upon the type of hemorrhoid and choice of anesthetic. Little preparation is necessary for removal of external hemorrhoids under local anesthesia other than an enema the night before, restriction of oral intake for a few hours preoperatively, cleansing and shaving the perianal region, and administering a sedative. Prior to the removal of internal hemorrhoids, enemas are usually ordered to be given until clear the night before surgery to allow for thorough evacuation, with or without catharsis; oral intake is restricted for several hours; and an antisecretant drug is ordered if general anesthesia is anticipated. For the preparation of both types of patient, a tub bath is advisable to ensure thorough cleansing of the operative site. The perineum and a margin of at least 6 in. around the anus are shaved. The bladder must be emptied prior to surgery because of the proximity of this organ to the field of operation. All nursing procedures involving the anal region must be performed skillfully, gently, and with finesse. The rectal tube must be inserted very carefully to avoid injury, even perforation, of the edematous anal canal. The nurse must realize that the patient is under duress because of the nature of his ailment.

Anesthesia and Surgical Technic

Both internal and external hemorrhoids are treated most satisfactorily by removal, prior to the development of complications if possible. The lithotomy position may be used, or the patient may be placed in a prone position, flexed at the hips with buttocks elevated. General, low-spinal, caudal, or local-infiltration anesthesia may be used. The surgeon may use ligature excision with a scalpel or with an electrosurgical cutting unit which employs a high-frequency current to incise the tissues and effect hemostasis simultaneously. The use of this electrosurgical cutting unit is freely employed in many types of surgery, and the nurse should understand the underlying principles.[4] Electrical currents conducted between two electrodes meet with resistance when in contact with certain metals, air, or tissues, all of which conduct poorly; heat is generated in the resistance, and this heat is employed to destroy tissues. The term *electrocauterization* refers to destruction of tissues by applying the heated tip of the electrode directly to the tissues; in such a manner a colostomy is opened or an ulcer of the anal wall cauterized. *Fulguration* means destruction of tissues by a shower of sparks transmitted to the tissues through air; this is the method of removing some rectal polyps and benign tumors. *Electrocoagulation* is achieved by placing one electrode in the tissues while maintaining the other at a short distance to transmit deep heat and control bleeding. A *thermal cutting unit,* which is an electrically heated knife, may also be used.[5]

Postoperative Care and Teaching

The major aims of postoperative care are the prevention of complications and the promotion of healing. In order to postpone defecation until healing has been initiated, the patient is instructed not to attempt defecation for 2 days. The formation of a soft stool which can be easily passed on the third postoperative day is encouraged by a soft, low-residue diet, liberal fluid intake, oral doses of mineral oil once or twice daily, all started on the day of operation. A low oil enema may be given through a small catheter and with extreme gentleness on the third postoperative day. A low enema is given by holding the reservoir only high enough to permit the solution to flow and by administering less than 200 ml. solution. Narcotics may be necessary early postoperatively, supplanted later by milder analgesics, unless a long-lasting, oil-soluble anesthetic has been injected into the operative site.

The most common early complications are hemorrhage and infection.

[4] Adapted with permission from A. Cantor, "Ambulatory Proctology," 2d ed., Paul B. Hoeber, Inc., New York, 1952, pp. 77–78.

[5] *Ibid.,* p. 82.

Dressings must be observed for evidence of excessive or bright-red drainage. The compression dressing and packing, if used, are removed in 24 hours, after which the dressings must be changed frequently to keep them clean and dry. Infection is further prevented or minimized by the administration of antibiotics and by keeping the area scrupulously clean and dry. Irrigations or sitz baths, therefore, are given several times daily, especially following defecation.

Urinary retention is very common following surgery of this area because the lower urinary system and anorectum share the pudendal nerve supply and basic external musculature. Therefore, spasm of the anal sphincter is associated with urethral spasm, and retention results. Early ambulation, a liberal fluid intake, and measures to relieve anal sphincter spasm help to relieve retention. Sometimes the spasm is relieved by sitz baths and the patient can be encouraged to void in the tub. Bladder catheterization should be resorted to only if all other measures fail.

Stricture or stenosis are late complications more easily prevented than treated. The buttocks are separated by gauze which is removed by irrigation in 24 hours. Manual dilatation of the area may be performed regularly by the surgeon after the fifth postoperative day.

Inasmuch as prolonged straining and constipation are thought to play a role in the formation of hemorrhoids, the patient should be taught the value of prompt attention to the stimulus for defecating, regularity in establishing the habit, activity, a liberal fluid intake, and a well-balanced diet which contains fresh fruits and vegetables in generous amounts. He must learn not to be overly concerned about his elimination and to avoid dependence upon cathartics and enemas. Of course it is understood that this "bowel training" must await healing of the site of operation. Benign prostatic hypertrophy which necessitates straining to void should be corrected surgically.

Throughout the postoperative period the nurse must realize that this patient probably suffers more than one with visceral surgery because of the extremely sensitive area of operation, which must be dilated by stools and examination, both of which the patient fears. The anal area is very important in psychologic development, and conflicts in this area, having escaped resolution in normal development, may produce intense guilt feelings. The patient requires open channels of communication, empathy, and gentle care. Compounding his problems emotionally, while relieving them physically, is the practice of injecting a long-lasting local anesthetic to relax the sphincters and relieve pain. This treatment, combined with the administration of mineral oil to produce a soft, lubricated stool, may make defecation involuntary. The nurse and others who give personal care must realize that the patient can not help but soil his bed and must not add to his problems by assuming a judgmental attitude. The patient is discharged with instructions to continue sitz baths, mineral oil, and a low-residue diet. He may return to light work in approximately 10 days to 2 weeks if the hemorrhoids were internal, sooner if they were external. Prolonged standing is to be avoided. Close medical supervision is necessary, since late complications may occur.

ANAL FISSURE

Anal fissure (Fig. 33) is another condition which may require surgical intervention. This is actually a longitudinal ulcer through the anal wall due to infection and trauma, such as tears from childbirth, and the passage of hard stool and the residue of rough foods.

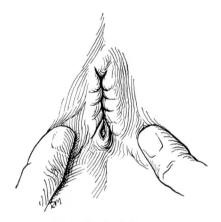

FIG. 33. Anal fissure.

The symptoms are cyclic episodes of exquisite pain and muscle spasm, initiated by defecation and lasting for an hour or more in some patients. There may be slight bleeding with defecation. Pruritus may develop. The patient becomes increasingly more constipated because of his fear of pain associated with defecation.

Palliative therapy is similar to that already described for the patient with acutely inflamed hemorrhoids: moist heat is applied, measures to produce a soft, lubricated stool are used, and the area is kept scrupulously clean. The use of toilet tissue is avoided; irrigations or baths and thorough, gentle drying with surgical wipes are used instead. If healing does not occur, the ulcer is widely excised together with its associated anal crypts and anal papillae. At the same time the external sphincter is relaxed by dilatation to promote healing. Postoperative care is as outlined following hemorrhoidectomy.

ANORECTAL ABSCESS AND FISTULA

Anorectal abscess and fistula formation can be considered as a continuation of the same process, originating, usually, in an infected anal crypt, or pocket, located in the pectinate line. (See Fig. 32.) In seeking egress, the pus burrows through the tissues, forming a fistulous tract which may open into the perianal, ischiorectal, or pelvirectal spaces to set up secondary abscesses. The fistula may communicate with the external environment through the rectal mucosa or through the anal, perianal, or perineal skin.

The patient who has an anorectal abscess usually experiences severe, throbbing pain, aggravated by sitting or walking, although pain may be minimal if the abscess is located in the tissues adjacent to the rectum. Chills, fever, malaise, and prostration are usually marked. There may be a palpable mass.

Whether the abscess ruptures spontaneously or is incised for drainage, the formation of a fistula is almost inevitable. A fistula is marked by periodic, spontaneous emissions of purulent exudate accompanied by an abrupt cessation of pain.

Incision and drainage is usually an emergency procedure allowing minimal preparation. The area is cleansed and shaved. Antibiotic therapy may be initiated. An enema may or may not be ordered. The choice of anesthesia determines the need for additional measures. Low-spinal, caudal, or general anesthesia may be used. Following incision and drainage, the abscess cavity is packed with iodoform gauze which is changed daily. Warm, moist dressings and/or sitz baths are used several times daily until the fistulotomy is performed in approximately 1 week. In *fistulotomy*, the tract is probed, unroofed, and cureted; adjacent anal glands and the external opening are excised. It may be necessary to incise the external sphincter to reach the fistula. Incision of the sphincter in one place will not produce incontinence. The packing inserted between the cut ends of the sphincter for hemostasis must be removed in 24 hours. Postfistulotomy nursing care is similar to that outlined for both hemorrhoidectomy and fissurectomy. Sometimes a chronic, fibrotic, fistulous tract requires fistulectomy.

RECTAL PROLAPSE AND PROCIDENTIA

Rectal prolapse can occur with varying degrees of severity. The mucosa may prolapse with chronic strain and atony; this is repaired by excision and anastomosis. A more severe type of prolapse, which is actually an intussusception of all layers of the rectal wall, is called a *procidentia*.

Repair is made through the abdominal and/or perineal routes by resection of the involved segment and anastomosis, followed by repair of the pelvic floor.

PILONIDAL CYST

A *pilonidal cyst* is a fluid-filled sac, found in the sacrococcygeal region of young adults. This cyst is thought to be an embryonic rest in development because ectodermal structures, such as hair and skin, are found therein. *Pilonidal* means "nest of hair," being derived from the Latin

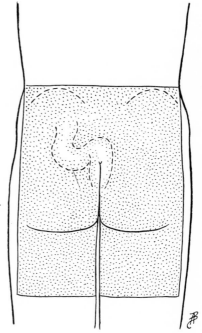

FIG. 34. Area of skin preparation for excision of a pilonidal cyst.

pilus, hair + *nidus*, nest. Communicating with the skin through one or more openings, the cyst readily becomes infected, especially if subjected to trauma, and pain and swelling develop. If the cyst ruptures spontaneously, or is incised for evacuation, a chronic draining sinus results. Therefore, the preferred treatment is complete excision or *saucerization*, i.e., partial excision, to prevent a recurrence of the acute stage or the development of a sinus. Preoperative preparation includes an enema, abstinence from oral intake, sedation, voiding, and shaving of the area from the midlumbar area to the midthighs. (See Fig. 34.)

Surgery is performed with the patient in the prone or partially inverted position and under spinal or local anesthesia. One of three procedures may be used: (1) saucerization, (2) excision with primary closure of the overlying skin, or (3) excision without closure, allowing the wound to heal by secondary intention. Although the use of antibiotics may permit surgery for an infected cyst, in which case an open procedure is used, many surgeons prefer to treat the patient first with warm, moist compresses, sitz baths, liberal fluid intake, bed rest, and antibiotics.

The postoperative care for the patient who has had an excision and closure is relatively simple. The youthful patient is soon ambulatory, and diet is not restricted. The pressure dressing is left undisturbed until retention sutures are removed in approximately 3 days. The dressings must be kept clean and dry and the patient observed for signs of wound infection or bleeding. The patient should be instructed not to lie on the site that has been operated on. A mild cathartic may be ordered the first day postoperatively to prevent straining at defecation; a low enema is usually ordered to be given on the third postoperative day. If the cyst has been saucerized or excised without closure, a petroleum-jelly pack will be left in place for 3 days, when warm saline irrigations, warm, moist compresses, and/or sitz baths are initiated. The pressure dressing is re-applied after each irrigation or bath and is soaked off with each treatment to avoid disturbing the granulating area. Analgesia is necessary for a few days postoperatively. Urinary retention is common after spinal anesthesia; therefore, bathroom privileges are allowed as soon as the patient has recovered from the anesthetic, and a liberal fluid intake is encouraged. The patient is discharged from 5 to 10 days postoperatively and allowed to return to light work in a couple of weeks. Healing may not be complete for another month; therefore, he must remain under close medical supervision and must protect the operated site.

SUMMARY

Conditions which may require resection of the colon, in part or in whole, include carcinoma, diverticulitis and ulcerative colitis, polyposis, and injuries.

The preoperative care of a patient undergoing colonic surgery includes special measures to empty the intestinal tract and to reduce the bacterial flora. Such measures include prohibition of oral intake with maintenance of fluid-electrolyte-caloric balance by intravenous therapy, institution of decompression therapy, administration of enemas, and the use of chemotherapy. These same measures are continued in the early postoperative period.

A permanent colostomy, necessitated most commonly by carcinoma of the descending colon and rectum, requires a plan of rehabilitation based upon the psychologic, medicophysical, and socioeconomic needs of the patient. Once the patient has accepted the idea of having a colostomy, he can be taught self-care, which includes attention to diet, skin care, elimination, and the prevention of complications.

Anorectal surgery is performed in the treatment of hemorrhoids, anal fissure, anorectal abscess and fistula, and rectal prolapse. Pilonidal cyst, located in close proximity to the anorectum, requires nursing measures similar to those described for the care of the patient undergoing anorectal surgery.

Preparation for anorectal surgery consists of measures to allay apprehension, reduce inflammation, and promote cleanliness of the area. Because of the area involved, the patient is likely to have considerable physical and psychologic distress. The nurse must be especially careful to be tactful and gentle in meeting the needs of this patient.

Postoperative care is designed to promote healing, minimize pain, and prevent infection. Sitz baths are commonly used to meet these three objectives. Measures are used to assist the patient to pass soft, well-lubricated stools after the third postoperative day.

Many opportunities for health teaching will be presented in the care of patients with anorectal disease. Constipation contributes to the development of many of these conditions which require surgical intervention, and may, if unrelieved, cause a recurrence. Therefore, the patient must be taught hygienic measures to promote normal defecation.

BIBLIOGRAPHY

Colon

ALLEN, J. G.: Anatomy, Physiology, and Treatment of Intestinal Obstruction; Traumatic, Inflammatory, and Neoplastic Diseases of the Small Bowel and the Colon; and Tumors of the Colon and the Rectum, in "Surgery," J. G. Allen, H. N. Harkins, C. A. Moyer, and J. E. Rhoads (eds.), J. B. Lippincott Company, Philadelphia, 1957, chap. 36, pp. 862–898, and chap. 37, pp. 899–931 and 933–955.

BACHRACH, W. H.: Medical Treatment of Ulcerative Colitis, Clinical Symposia, Ciba Pharmaceutical Products, Inc., Summit, N.J., vol. 7, no. 4, pp. 103–118, July–August, 1955.

BACON, H. E.: Cancer of the Colon, Rectum and Anal Canal, Am. J. Surg., vol. 94, no. 4, pp. 567–572, October, 1957.

CATTELL, R. B., and B. P. COLCOCK: Ulcerative Colitis: Selection of Cases for Surgical Treatment, S. Clin. North America, vol. 35, no. 3, pp. 817–822, June, 1955.

————, D. H. MACKENZIE, and B. P. COLCOCK, Cancer of the Colon and Rectum, S. Clin. North America, vol. 35, no. 3, pp. 823–831, June, 1955.

COLLER, F. A.: "Cancer of the Colon and Rectum," American Cancer Society, Inc., New York, 1956.

GASTON, B. H., and J. H. MULHOLLAND: Treatment of Penetrating Abdominal Wounds, S. Clin. North America, vol. 35, no. 2, pp. 463–469, April, 1955.

GREEN, W. W.: Diverticulitis of the Colon, Am. J. Surg., vol. 94, no. 2, pp. 282–289, August, 1957.

KIEFER, E. D.: The Management of Chronic Ulcerative Colitis, S. *Clin. North America*, vol. 35, no. 3, pp. 809–816, June, 1955.

McMILLAN, F. L.: Trends in the Surgical Treatment of Diverticulitis of the Colon, S. *Clin. North America*, vol. 35, no. 1, pp. 159–173, February, 1955.

MOBLEY, J. E., M. B. DOCKERTY, and J. M. WAUGH: Bleeding in Colonic Diverticulitis, *Am. J. Surg.*, vol. 94, no. 1, pp. 44–51, July, 1957.

PATTERSON, H. A.: The Management of the Complications of Diverticulitis of the Colon, S. *Clin. North America*, vol. 35, no. 2, pp. 451–462, April, 1955.

Psychological Effects of Colostomy, *The Psychiatric Bulletin,* Smith, Kline, and French Laboratories, vol. 7, no. 2, pp. 23–24, Spring, 1957.

RANKIN, F. W.: Surgical Treatment of Chronic Ulcerative Colitis, *Clinical Symposia,* Ciba Pharmaceutical Products, Inc., Summit, N.J., vol. 7, no. 4, pp. 121–130, July–August, 1955.

SECOR, S. M.: New Hope for Colostomy Patients, *Nursing Outlook,* vol. 2, pp. 642–643, December, 1954.

STRENGER, G.: Elective Resection for Sigmoidal Diverticulitis, *Am. J. Surg.*, vol. 94, no. 4, pp. 577–583, October, 1957.

WELCH, C. E.: The Alimentary Canal—The Colon, in "Christopher's Textbook of Surgery," 6th ed., L. Davis (ed.), W. B. Saunders Company, Philadelphia, 1956, chap. 20, pp. 654–668.

Anorectum

CANTOR, A. J.: "Ambulatory Proctology," 2d ed., Paul B. Hoeber, Inc., New York, 1952.

FEIGENBAUM, H. A.: Excision of Acute Pilonidal Cyst Abscess, *Am. J. Surg.*, vol. 94, no. 4, pp. 636–637, October, 1957.

NESSELROD, J. P.: The Alimentary Canal—The Anal Canal and Rectum, in "Christopher's Textbook of Surgery," 6th ed., L. Davis (ed.), W. B. Saunders Company, Philadelphia, 1956, chap. 20, pp. 669–684.

PORTES, C.: Surgery for Anorectal Disease, in "The Recovery Room," M. S. Sadove and J. H. Cross (eds.), W. B. Saunders Company, Philadelphia, 1956, chap. 10, pp. 295–302.

SALVATI, E. P., and M. S. KLECKNER: Urinary Retention in Anorectal and Colonic Surgery, *Am. J. Surg.*, vol. 94, no. 1, pp. 114–117, July, 1957.

SWINTON, N. W.: Sigmoidoscopic Examination, S. *Clin. North America*, vol. 35, no. 3, pp. 833–845, June, 1955.

——— and W. L. MATHIESEN: The Treatment of Rectal Prolapse and Procidentia, S. *Clin. North America*, vol. 35, no. 3, pp. 847–852, June, 1955.

STUDY GUIDE FOR PART TWO

1. Assume that you are a public health nurse visiting Mrs. White following the birth of her son. You learn that she is concerned about her husband, who has a duodenal peptic ulcer but makes no consistent effort to follow his physician's orders. Mr. White tells you, "I cannot see any reason for following these orders all of the time since the pain comes and goes anyway." What are the reasons which would prompt you to urge Mr. White to consult with his physician for clarification of the need for medical treatment?

2. A patient undergoing gastric resection for carcinoma would probably have what orders regarding intake in the preoperative period? in the postoperative period?

3. What nursing measures are necessitated by the use of gastrointestinal decompression therapy?

4. What factors are important for the nurse to consider in planning for the postoperative care of a geriatric patient?

5. *a.* Outline the preoperative nursing care for a patient undergoing cholecystectomy.

   b. What are the most important postoperative nursing measures for this patient who returns to the clinical division with a T-tube in place?

6. What are the most important nursing measures for a patient who has had a partial hepatectomy?

7. List the major indications for splenectomy.

8. What is the relationship between portal hypertension and gastro-esophageal varicose veins? What is the purpose of performing a portacaval shunt?

9. *a.* List the major indications for surgery of the pancreas.

   b. Outline a plan of rehabilitation for a patient undergoing total pancreatectomy.

10. What instructions must be given to a patient who is being discharged following subtotal adrenalectomy?

11. You have been notified that a patient is being admitted to your clinical division with the diagnosis, "acute intestinal obstruction."

    a. What are some of the conditions which may obstruct the small intestine? the colon?

    b. How do the symptoms of a complete obstruction of the ileum differ from those presented by a complete obstruction of the descending colon?

    c. How does the physician determine whether an obstruction is partial or complete?

    d. What therapeutic measures are instituted immediately for a patient with an acute obstruction of the small intestine?

12. Outline a teaching program for a patient with an abdominoperineal resection. Identify the major areas of need from the day the patient is told that he must undergo this surgery through to the day of his discharge. Indicate how this patient can be helped to become well rehabilitated.

13. What are some of the factors which contribute to herniation? To what extent can a hernia be prevented?

14. A neighbor consults you regarding the advisability of buying a new truss for her eleven-year-old son who has an inguinal hernia. Identify

the teaching needs in this situation and consider how you might answer her.

15. What are the first-aid measures for undiagnosed abdominal pain?

16. Why is the practice of "watchful waiting" dangerous in acute appendicitis?

17. *a.* What are the most common indications for surgery of the anorectum?

　　b. What nursing measures are especially important in the preparation of a patient for anorectal surgery?

　　c. Outline the nursing care and teaching necessary in the postoperative period.

Part Three

CARE OF THE PATIENT UNDERGOING
SURGERY OF THE NECK AND THORAX

14

SURGERY OF THE THYROID GLAND, TRACHEA, AND NECK

Neoplasia and hyperplasia constitute the most common indications for surgery of the thyroid gland. Radical neck dissection is performed in the treatment of metastatic carcinoma. A tracheostomy may be necessitated by complications of thyroidectomy or by radical neck dissection.

NONTOXIC SURGICAL CONDITIONS OF THE THYROID GLAND

Because the thyroid gland overlies the trachea, an enlargement, whether due to neoplasm or goiter, may cause compression symptoms and even asphyxia. The enlargement is usually visible and/or palpable, but if the growth extends downward behind the sternum, it may escape detection and treatment entirely and asphyxiate the patient.

A neoplasm is excised not only to prevent or relieve compression but also to differentiate the benign neoplasm from one that is malignant. The benign tumor can usually be removed easily and completely, leaving the unaffected portions of the gland intact. Incomplete removal of the tumor will result in recurrence. A tumor is usually detected by palpation. The patient may report a sensation of "a lump in the throat," and symptoms of compression may be present. The most common of the benign tumors affecting the thyroid gland is the adenoma.

A malignant neoplasm may produce these symptoms, but, more commonly, only a solitary nodule is palpable within or near the gland. Diagnosis is confirmed by a frozen section. Treatment is wide excision of the thyroid gland and adjacent tissues, including the lymph nodes but preserving the recurrent laryngeal nerves and parathyroid glands. The most common of the malignant neoplasms involving the thyroid gland as the primary site are papillary and nonpapillary carcinomas and sarcoma.[1]

---

[1] G. Crile, Jr., and R. W. Schneider, The Thyroid and Parathyroid Glands, in

189

Papillary carcinoma is a slow-growing tumor which occurs primarily in young adult women. The nonpapillary neoplasms, usually affecting persons over forty years of age, include the angioinvasive type, which, by name, involves the blood vessels; and medullary carcinoma and adenocarcinoma, which tend to metastasize early by way of the bloodstream. All nonpapillary carcinomas bear a poor prognosis. The most malignant neoplasms are sarcoma and undifferentiated carcinoma, which grow rapidly, causing pressure, pain, and hoarseness. Metastasis occurs early; the prognosis is very poor.

Diagnostic Methods

A patient undergoing surgery for the removal of a space-occupying lesion is evaluated preoperatively by certain measures designed to determine the type and extent of the lesion and to rule out toxicity. A chest x-ray is helpful in determining the presence of a substernal thyroid gland, metastatic carcinoma, or thyroid cysts, as well as in evaluating the condition of the heart and lungs.

Often the radioactive iodine uptake is determined preoperatively. Radioactive iodine, given to the patient in the form of a colorless, tasteless drink, is concentrated by thyroid tissue. A Geiger counter can then be used to determine locations of greatest concentration. This helps to outline the size of the thyroid gland and to detect aberrant thyroid tissue. The patient is prepared for this procedure by an explanation of what will be done and the assurance that the procedure is painless. This determination is usually carried out in the laboratory with the patient in a fasting condition. No aftercare is necessary; the patient is not rendered radioactive, and no precautions need be observed. The radioactive iodine uptake is determined by measuring the difference between the dose given and that excreted in the urine.

Since a patient who is markedly toxic due to an excessive secretion of thyroxin can not be operated on without great risk, it is important that the physician detect hidden or overt toxicity before surgery. To this end a determination of the basal metabolic rate (B.M.R.), or more than one determination, is made. This measure of the number of calories burned for energy while the patient is fasting and at rest gives a rough index of the thyroid gland's activity. The normal range lies within plus or minus 10 to 15. Toxicity is evidenced by a marked elevation in the B.M.R., decrease in blood-cholesterol level, electrocardiographic changes, and symptoms such as tachycardia, tremor, sweating, weakness, and weight loss. A toxic patient must be brought to a normal state of thyroid activity, *euthyroidism,* by medical measures before surgery can be performed.

"Christopher's Textbook of Surgery," 6th ed., L. Davis (ed.), W. B. Saunders Company, Philadelphia, 1956, chap. 13, p. 343.

In addition to these procedures, a laryngoscopy may be performed preoperatively to evaluate the condition of the vocal cords. One very real danger in a thyroidectomy is damage to one or both of the recurrent laryngeal nerves, which course behind the thyroid gland to innervate the vocal cords; therefore the surgeon may wish to establish the preoperative conditon of the larynx. This procedure is performed with a laryngeal mirror usually under a local anesthetic. It is painless, with no preparation required other than restriction of oral intake before and for 2 hours after the examination, and possibly the use of a sedative and antisecretory drug. Restricting intake after this examination prevents aspiration while the throat is anesthetized.

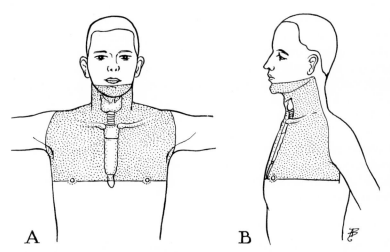

Fig. 35. Area of skin preparation for surgery of the neck.

Preoperative Preparation for Thyroidectomy

The immediate preoperative preparation for the patient who is to have a thyroidectomy for neoplasm or goiter is the same as that for laparotomy. Oral intake is withheld for several hours preoperatively, an enema is given if a general anesthetic is anticipated, ambulation is encouraged until the preoperative medication is given, and the cardinal signs are recorded and observations made of the patient's condition. The skin preparation includes the mandible from ear to ear, the anterior and lateral surfaces of the neck, the anterior chest to the nipple line, and both axillae. (See Fig. 35.) Such an extensive area is prepared in case a wide resection of tissues should be necessary.

When the diagnosis is uncertain, as with a neoplasm, and the patient realizes that the differentiation between benign and malignant tumor will be made at surgery, she is likely to be extremely apprehensive. The cooperative efforts of the entire health team will be required to allay anxiety. Such a patient needs to be reminded that she has a capable surgeon and that early adequate treatment has effected countless numbers of cures. The patient may fear disfigurement, since surgery is to be on an exposed surface of the body; she should be told that scarring will be minimal with the newer technics of operating and suturing.

Surgical Technics

Surgery may be performed under general or local anesthesia. A local anesthetic has the advantage that the patient remains conscious and can speak as directed during surgery to help the surgeon identify and preserve the recurrent laryngeal nerves. On the other hand, it is a trying procedure for the patient, especially if a total thyroidectomy is being performed or if she must wait through a frozen section worrying about the diagnosis; for these patients a general anesthetic is usually given. As previously stated, the entire thyroid gland together with expendable adjacent structures will be removed if a malignant neoplasm is encountered; if the neoplasm is benign, a total lobectomy will be done. If a goiter is compressing the trachea or esophagus, that portion necessary to relieve compression will be removed. A drain will be left in the site of operation. A compression dressing will be applied to obliterate *dead space*, the area left after excision of a structure, and to prevent an accumulation of serous fluid in the wound.

Postoperative Care and Observations

The postoperative care of the patient who has had a thyroidectomy centers upon the recognition of complications which immediately threaten the patient's life. The nurse must know the symptoms and the emergency treatment for asphyxia due to hemorrhage or injury to the recurrent laryngeal nerves. A small amount of blood can compress the trachea; therefore, any sign of hemorrhage demands immediate investigation and treatment. If the patient complains of an increasing sensation of fullness in the neck, has a rapid pulse, is restless, or seems dyspneic or cyanotic, the surgeon must be notified and the wound examined immediately. If there is bulging of the neck, the sutures must be released and the clot evacuated. Hemorrhage may be due to faulty hemostasis during surgery or to the slipping of a ligature when the patient begins to drink and talk, for swallowing moves the structures that have been operated on.

Injury to both recurrent laryngeal nerves causes the vocal cords to meet in the midline, obstructing the airway. Asphyxia ensues unless an emergency *tracheostomy* is performed. This operation entails a vertical incision into the trachea below the cricothyroid cartilage and the insertion of an artificial airway into the trachea below the larynx. (See Fig. 36.) If one nerve has been traumatized, hoarseness and dyspnea will result. Fortunately trauma to the recurrent laryngeal nerves is a rare complication and is usually temporary unless the nerve has been severed. A *hematoma*, blood clot, compressing the nerve will be absorbed. If the nerve has been ligated, the surgeon can release the ligature. If the nerve has been severed, an end-to-end anastomosis may be done, but it is rarely followed by recovery of function. These procedures require the strain of an additional operation for the patient.

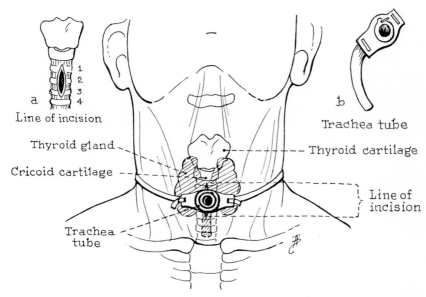

Fig. 36. Tracheostomy. This diagram illustrates the tracheostomy tube in place. Note the inserts, which show the site of incision and the tracheostomy tube in detail.

It can readily be seen then why the nurse must be vigilant for signs of respiratory distress or voice changes, observe cardinal signs at frequent intervals, and have suture-removal and tracheostomy sets available postoperatively.

A third complication peculiar to a patient who has had a thyroidectomy is *parathyroid tetany*, due to the inadvertent removal or disruption of blood supply and function of the three or four parathyroid glands which underlie the thyroid. Their function is the regulation of the amount of ionized calcium used in circulation. Since calcium controls muscle irritability, a deficit causes a characteristic *carpopedal spasm*, or tetany. The first symptoms are numbness and tingling in the extremities, followed by intermittent, painful, tonic spasms of the muscles of the fingers and toes. Intravenous calcium gluconate is used to relieve carpopedal spasm when parathyroid dysfunction is temporary. When the parathyroid glands have been permanently destroyed or completely removed, it is necessary to administer A.T.10 (dihydrotachysterol, vitamin D, and calcium) for the remainder of the patient's life.

In addition to observing the patient's condition for detection of these complications, the nurse can take certain measures that promote comfort and recovery. Motion of the head and neck must be minimized for the first few postoperative hours, and the patient must be in a position which favors neck relaxation and respirations. Therefore, the head is stabilized between sandbags or pillows, with the patient in dorsal recumbent semi-sitting position. When the patient is turned from side to side for care and activation, the head must be firmly supported.

The activation regime, modified as described above, is necessary to prevent pulmonary and circulatory stasis. Coughing and deep breathing will be painful for these patients; the nurse must be very persuasive to overcome the patient's fear and reluctance to cooperate in activation. Excessive coughing, of course, is to be discouraged. Ambulation the day of surgery is usually ordered. The patient will need to be encouraged to walk erect to overcome the tendency to protect the area by holding the neck in a flexed position.

Because swallowing is painful early postoperatively, the patient is usually given a liquid diet after nausea has subsided. She must be encouraged to maintain an adequate oral fluid intake to maintain kidney function and obviate the need for continued intravenous hydration and nutrition.

Usually no medications are required other than analgesics for nontoxic patients. If a total thyroidectomy was performed, lifelong medication with thyroid extract will be necessary to prevent the symptoms of *myxedema*, hypothyroidism. Analgesic drugs should be given rather freely early postoperatively to relieve pain and apprehension. A sense of compression in the neck is a frightening experience; until edema subsides and a lighter dressing is applied, these patients usually appear extremely apprehensive and uncomfortable. They can be made more comfortable with frequent oral hygiene, attention to position change and skin care, and a reassuring attitude on the part of the health team.

The compression dressing will be replaced by a lighter covering a few hours postoperatively if bloody drainage is present. The drain is usually removed in 24 hours. Sutures or clips will be removed in 3 to 4 days, after which no dressing may be needed. The patient must be reassured that the swelling will subside and that the scar will fade and contract until it is nearly invisible.

Discharge instructions are minimal; the patient is reminded to return to her surgeon for follow-up observations. Full activity is usually resumed as the patient's strength returns.

TOXIC GOITER

Another indication for thyroidectomy is *toxic goiter,* or *hyperthyroidism,* a condition in which an excess amount of thyroxin is being produced and is overstimulating metabolism. An adenomatous goiter may also become toxic. If this hyperfunctioning of the thyroid gland is not relieved, the strain on the heart and liver may prove fatal.

The symptoms of toxic hyperthyroidism are those of a very rapid metabolism. Temperature, pulse, and respirations are increased. In spite of an enormous appetite, weight loss is rapid because all food consumed is burned for energy. The blood-cholesterol level is decreased. Muscular weakness is marked; a fine tremor of the extended hands is evident. Emotional instability may be pronounced. The patient soon exhibits an *exophthalmos,* bulging eyeballs, caused by retention of water in the orbital fat pad and an increased amount of fat, which, unfortunately, seems not to be relieved by surgery. Exophthalmos is seen in diffuse hyperplastic goiter, too, but is absent with toxic nodular goiter.

Preoperative Management

A prolonged period of medical management must precede the thyroidectomy because these patients tolerate surgery, or any strain, poorly—a fact to remember when a patient with toxic hyperthyroidism must undergo any emergency operation. Therefore, the aim of medical management in preparation for surgery is to reduce the functioning of the thyroid gland to normal. A graph of daily weight, temperature, pulse, and respirations, together with repeated determinations of the basal metabolic rate, and evaluations of muscular strength and emotional stability all guide the physician in his therapy. Antithyroxin drugs, such as propylthiouracil, will be administered. Propylthiouracil interferes with the synthesis of thyroxin and is effective in reducing the B.M.R. However, it is a toxic drug which causes increased friability and vascularity of the thyroid gland. Therefore, it must be stopped 1 week preoperatively or administered with iodine, which counteracts this effect. Propylthiouracil can cause agranulocytosis; secondary infections can, therefore, occur readily. An iodine preparation, such as Lugol's solution, is effective in reducing the size and activity of the thyroid gland, because iodine is necessary for the production of thyroxin; a deficiency in available iodine causes the thyroid gland to undergo compensatory hyperplasia.

A diet high in carbohydrates, protein, minerals, and vitamins is necessary to build up depleted reserves. A liberal fluid intake must be encouraged. Physical and mental rest is achieved both at home and in the hospital with the help of sedatives and an environment which encourages calmness and emotional stability. The immediate preparation for surgery is the same as that outlined for the patient about to undergo thyroidectomy for a neoplasm.

Postoperative Care

The postoperative care is similar to that outlined for the patient who has had a thyroidectomy for neoplasm. A blood transfusion may be necessary, depending upon the amount of blood lost in surgery. Oxygen will probably be used the first few hours because of previous heart strain. An additional complication occasionally met early after any type of surgery in a patient who has had toxic hyperthyroidism is *thyroid crisis*. This condition is rarely encountered in a patient who has had time to be well prepared preoperatively, but it is often fatal in spite of the heroic measures used to combat the symptoms. The patient evidences a physiologic storm with all cardinal signs markedly increased, pronounced agitation and delirium, and diarrhea and vomiting. Treatment consists of oxygen by tent for its cooling effect, intravenous fluids with iodides, sedatives, and alcohol sponges.

After thyroidectomy the patient is discharged with instructions to remain under medical surveillance, because of the tendency for toxic hyperthyroidism to recur. Full activity is resumed as the patient gains strength, usually in a few days. If a total thyroidectomy was performed, the patient must be placed on thyroid medication to prevent the symptoms of myxedema. If a subtotal thyroidectomy was performed, iodine medication is given to prevent recurrence.

TRACHEOSTOMY CARE

The care of the patient with a tracheostomy is encountered not only with post-thyroidectomy complications which threaten asphyxia but also preparatory to or following extensive resection of oral-pharyngeal and neck tissues. The major indication for a tracheostomy is obstruction of the upper airway, evidenced by crowing respirations with suprasternal and substernal chest retractions, cyanosis, and rapid pulse. The tracheostomy may be permanent, as when a laryngectomy is necessary, or temporary until the edema of resection has subsided. Frequently the artificial airway is created prior to surgery to allow the patient to adjust to breathing through a tracheostomy tube. The operation is performed under a local anesthetic, or in an extreme emergency with none. A double set of curved silver, silver-plated, or plastic tubes is inserted into the trachea through the neck incision. To prevent dislodgement, the outer cannula is securely fastened in place with tape which encircles the neck and is tied in square knots on each side of the tube; the inner cannula is locked into place.

The inner cannula is removed at frequent intervals for cleaning with a detergent to prevent an accumulation of mucus from reducing the size of the lumen. Soda bicarbonate solution may be used to dissolve the mucus. Frequent suctioning of the tracheostomy tube, usually through the outer cannula, is required to keep the airway patent. Suctioning is done for an adult patient with a No. 16 to 18 French-size, whistle-tip catheter inserted 3 in., the approximate length of the cannula; the suction machine is then turned on, and the catheter is rotated gently. The surgeon may order the insertion of the catheter beyond the cannula to stimulate coughing, which further aids in the expulsion of mucus. Steam inhalations or aerosol Alevaire early postoperatively may be necessary to moisten the inspired air and loosen mucus. A thin layer of moistened gauze is sometimes placed over the opening to filter, warm, and moisten the inspired air. The patient's life depends upon the patency of the airway. Nothing must obstruct the lumen within or without. Suctioning, though done at frequent intervals, is restricted to 5 to 10 seconds at a time. Compression dressings are watched lest they slip and occlude the opening; bedding must not cover the neck. The skin around the tracheostomy must be kept scrupulously clean and dry to prevent irritation and infection. It is necessary to have a sterile duplicate tracheostomy tube and forceps without teeth readily available in case the first set is coughed out. The airway can be held open with forceps until the surgeon inserts the new tracheostomy set.

The tracheostomized patient is rendered aphonic, so the thoughtful nurse provides a pad and pencil for communication, ensures the functioning of the signal system, and reassures the patient through this trying time by frequent visits to his bedside. If the larynx is intact, and the surgeon permits it, the patient can speak by holding his finger over the opening. If the larynx has been removed, esophageal speech can be learned.

The patient with a temporary tracheostomy will be *decannulized*, have the tube removed, at once or after a trial period of corking the tube to determine the adequacy of the airway. The opening closes without sutures in a short time.

The rehabilitation of the patient with a permanent tracheostomy requires that he be taught in detail how to remove and clean the inner cannula, how to suction if necessary, and how to change the neck tape and care for his skin. All these procedures should be taught early in front of a mirror, with the patient being encouraged to assume increasing responsibility for his care. He should have a second tracheostomy set always available in case the first set is dislodged. However, in time a fistula is created, so that there is less danger of asphyxiation.

The patient must be helped to plan ahead. He will have to adjust his clothing so that the tracheostomy tube is not occluded but is protected. He must exercise care in bathing or showering; swimming is prohibited. His diet must avoid dry, crumbly food which might be aspirated through the tube. Speech therapy may be advisable. The new tracheostomy patient is a candidate for teaching by a successfully rehabilitated tracheostomized person. Such a person can best help the patient overcome feelings of depression and hopelessness, encourage him to assume self-care, and counteract a tendency to withdraw because of the appearance of the tracheostomy and loss of voice. Some cities have rehabilitation groups organized for these patients.

RADICAL NECK DISSECTION

Radical neck dissection is performed in the treatment of metastatic carcinoma which is primary in the head and neck area. The cancer may originate in the thyroid, salivary glands, or in the larynx. It may have spread from oral or pharyngeal growths, but metastasis must be confined above the level of the clavicles in an accessible area for this surgery to be effective.

The patient with intraoral cancer first presents himself for examination when he discovers a "lump" in the neck. Since early cancer is asymptomatic, pain is usually absent. Cancer of the intrinsic larynx will produce hoarseness early in the disease. The diagnosis is made on the basis of the history; careful examination of the head and neck area including the use of a mirror to visualize the larynx, hypopharynx, and nasopharynx; and digital palpation of the entire oral cavity, base of the tongue, and the tonsillar areas. Aspiration biopsy of lymph nodes suspected to be involved with metastatic cancer confirms the diagnosis in more than three-fourths of the cases of metastatic squamous cell carcinoma.

The treatment of metastatic cancer with the primary growth in the head and neck area depends upon the successful control of the primary site as well as of the metastasis. Both the primary and metastatic growths may be dealt with surgically, preferably at the same time. If the primary growth has previously been controlled by surgery or irradiation, the metastatic disease to the neck requires a radical neck dissection on the side in which there is histologic proof that metastatic cancer is present.

Indications for such extensive resection of tissues are as follows: there must be definite clinical evidence of metastasis in the cervical lymphatic vessels, with a reasonable chance for complete extirpation of all involvement; there must be no evidence of distant metastasis below the clavicles; either the primary lesion must have been controlled or its excision must have been contemplated with the neck dissection; surgery must offer a better chance of cure than irradiation therapy.[2]

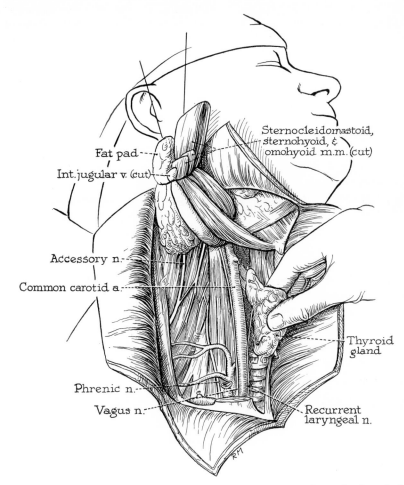

Fat pad

Int. jugular v. (cut)

Sternocleidomastoid, sternohyoid, & omohyoid m.m. (cut)

Accessory n.

Common carotid a.

Thyroid gland

Phrenic n.

Vagus n.

Recurrent laryngeal n.

FIG. 37. Appearance of the surgical site toward completion of a radical neck dissection. The thyroid gland is about to be removed.

Preoperative Preparation

The candidate for radical neck surgery requires a great deal of emotional support, for apprehension freely accompanies the diagnosis of cancer and the extensive procedures necessary to effect a cure. Spiritual

[2] Hayes Martin et al., Neck Dissection, *Cancer,* vol. 4, no. 3, p. 446, May, 1951.

guidance helps the patient immeasurably in accepting therapy and in maintaining a hopeful attitude. In addition, diversional activities, such as reading, are important in helping the patient to focus attention outside himself.

Because a cancer involving the hypopharynx may be associated with dysphagia, malnutrition may be present. Every effort is made preoperatively to improve the patient's nutritional status and to restore and maintain his fluid-electrolyte balance. A high-caloric diet is served in frequent small amounts; vitamins are supplemented. Soft-to-liquid foods are handled more easily than solid ones. Tube feedings may be necessary. Mouth care after feedings helps to reduce the associated infection and to counteract pain and anorexia. Malnutrition and dehydration will cause a decrease in total blood volume and hemoglobin. Preoperative transfusions of whole blood to correct the red cell mass deficit will reduce operative shock. Blood replacement during the procedure will reduce postoperative shock and improve wound healing.

If infection is present, as with oral-pharyngeal tumors, the use of antibiotics in conjunction with mouth care is necessary preoperatively. Rest is important, but the hazards of bed rest, namely, pulmonary and circulatory stasis, weakness, constipation, decubiti, and emotional depression, must be prevented by the activation regime. Since the majority of these patients are in the fifth, sixth, and seventh decades of life,[3] activity is even more essential.

The immediate preparation for surgery is similar to that outlined for the patient undergoing thyroidectomy for neoplasm. The skin preparation is extended, however, to include 2 in. around the ear on the affected side.

Surgical Technic

Under nasotracheal anesthesia, and/or intravenous sodium pentothal, a double Y incision is made lateral to the midline extending from the mandible to the clavicle. The skin flaps are reflected, and through this incision the contents of the anterior and lateral triangles of the neck are resected. The primary neoplasm is resected in continuity with the neck dissection; associated lymph nodes, lymph-bearing fascia, adipose and areolar tissue, sternomastoid and omohyoid muscles, submaxillary salivary gland, internal jugular vein, and the spinal accessory nerve are removed. This en bloc dissection spares the common and internal carotid arteries, and the phrenic, vagus, and hypoglossal nerves.[4] (See Fig. 37.) During surgery, an airway is kept open through a nasotracheal tube, with

[3] *Ibid.*, p. 443.
[4] *Ibid.*

a pharyngeal pack in the hypopharynx for intraoral surgery, or a trache-ostomy. Long cigarette drains are placed beneath the closed skin flaps to prevent an accumulation of serum in the operative site. A head and neck compression dressing is applied to ensure apposition of the skin flaps, to obliterate the dead space, and to reduce serum seepage. The endotracheal tube is left in place until the patient has reacted from anesthesia.

Postoperative Care and Teaching

The plan for postoperative care and teaching is directed toward maintaining an adequate airway, meeting needs for nutrition and hydra-tion, preventing complications, and rehabilitating the patient. Frequent suctioning of the nasal and oral-pharyngeal passages, and/or trache-ostomy, is necessary to clear the airway and prevent aspiration of secre-tions. During recovery from anesthesia, the patient is placed in semi-Fowler's position to aid respirations and decrease the danger of aspira-tion. Coughing is encouraged to prevent atelectasis. The free use of narcotics is contraindicated because they depress the cough reflex. Mild analgesics are adequate for the relief of headache and discomfort; indeed, there is very little pain in the operative area because all the associated sensory fibers have been cut at the time of surgery.

Needs for fluids and electrolytes are met by intravenous fluids during surgery and immediately postoperatively if necessary. Tube feedings are required when there is an intraoral suture line or when edema and pain prevent swallowing. Tube feedings are started on the first postopera-tive day; 300 to 400 ml. formula is given every 2 to 4 hours, alternating with 100 ml. water. The patient is instructed on the first postoperative day in tube feeding himself; if tube feedings will be necessary after healing of the intraoral suture line, the patient must be instructed in the removal, cleansing, and insertion of the feeding tube. Without an intra-oral suture line the majority of patients can start oral intake the day after surgery. The food must be highly nutritious, liquid-to-soft in consistency, and attractively served in frequent small amounts.

Postoperative Complications. One major complication to be prevented is infection, especially with a combined dissection, because of the rich oral bacterial flora. Oral irrigations and sprays with a salt and soda solution, at room temperature, or with equal parts of hydrogen peroxide and saline solution, followed by a saline mouth spray, are given at least three times a day after feedings. Simultaneous suctioning at the time of pressure spraying of the solutions prevents aspiration of the fluid. A pack of zinc peroxide paste may be applied to the oral suture line, after mouth care, to provide the prolonged release of nascent oxygen, which reduces the number of anaerobes in the mouth. Antibiotic drugs administered parenterally may be necessary postoperatively. In the absence of infection or fistula formation, the pressure dressing is changed every other day, starting on the second postoperative day. At the same time the drains will be shortened; they will probably be removed by the fourth to sixth postoperative day, when a lighter dressing will suffice.

Other complications which may be encountered after radical neck dissection include salivary fistula, chylous fistula, chylothorax, pneumothorax, carotid "blowout," and transient facial edema especially with a bilateral radical neck dissection. If a salivary fistula occurs, the tract must be kept clean of saliva and food particles; the patient is given tube feedings exclusively. Meticulous mouth care is practiced until the fistula closes. At the time of mouth care the patient may be given sips of water which return through the fistula and serve as an irrigation. Pressure dressings to a small fistulous area aid closure of the tract; large fistulous tracts are benefited little by pressure dressings. The tract usually closes spontaneously in 7 to 10 days with the treatment outlined. Usually the later the fistula occurs after surgery the smaller it is and the more rapid the closure.

A chylous fistula is recognized by milky drainage. It occurs in left-side dissections because of inadvertent opening of the thoracic duct. If noticed at surgery, the duct is immediately ligated with a nonabsorbable suture. If the fistula is noted postoperatively, pressure dressings and tamponading with Gelfoam will lead to spontaneous repair in a few days. A low-fat diet is given during this period.

Pneumothorax, an infrequent but serious complication, occurs most commonly with median dissections, which include thyroidectomy or the removal of bulky metastasis behind the clavicle. This may lead to the more serious mediastinal emphysema and tension pneumothorax. Surgical repair and decompression of the collapsed lung by closed drainage of the pleural space are necessary and should be carried out as soon as the condition is recognized. (See Chapter 17.)

A carotid blowout is the most serious complication of a radical neck dissection. The artery may have been weakened by surgery, previous x-ray therapy, or infection, or it may have been eroded by tumor. Death is almost certain, but fist pressure to the site of bleeding, blood replacement, and then ligation of the common carotid are often lifesaving. The external carotid artery can be sacrificed if necessary without complication. The common and internal carotid arteries, on the other hand, are vital. Prophylactic ligation to prevent spontaneous blowout is associated with a 10 to 20 per cent mortality rate owing to cerebral anoxia; approximately 30 per cent of these ligations are followed by hemiparesis, since the common and internal carotids are the major arteries supplying the brain.[5]

Facial edema occurs with simultaneous bilateral radical neck dissection. This is first noticed at the end of surgery, reaches its peak in 4 to 6 days, and subsides in 2 weeks. Faulty hemostasis of the superior internal jugular stump can be treated with pressure and tamponading for 3 to 4 days, but bleeding from the distal stump near the subclavian vein requires immediate religation of the stump.

Horner's syndrome occurs rather infrequently and is due to injury to the cervical sympathetic trunk posterolateral to the carotid sheath. This syndrome, which may be temporary but is usually permanent, is characterized by ptosis of the eyelid, constriction of the pupil, and absence of perspiration. Another annoying but not disabling complication is a shoulder droop due to sectioning of the spinal accessory nerve at the time of radical neck dissection.

Shock or chronic respiratory disease may indicate the need for oxygen immediately postoperatively. The majority of these patients are elderly, and concomitant heart disease and emphysema are, therefore, fairly common. The activation regime is especially important to prevent complications in the elderly patient. Ambulation for all patients begins the first postoperative day. Diversional therapy is especially important for patients following radical neck dissection to help them through the early postoperative period, when they are likely to be apprehensive and uncomfortable.

Rehabilitation. The program of rehabilitation is intensive. Because there is so much for the patient to accept and learn, teaching must begin early to allow time for all facets of care to be thoroughly understood. Instruction in tube feeding, mouth care, and tracheostomy care is begun early, and the patient is encouraged to assume full responsibility for these procedures before discharge from the hospital. A prosthesis may be needed, such as a rubber obturator or upper denture plate, to cover defects in the palate and thereby aid speaking and eating. These are used as soon as healing permits while the patient is still hospitalized. He must learn how to remove, clean, and reapply the prosthesis. It must be removed for oral irrigations, which may continue at home. Thorough but gentle toothbrushing and mouthwashes or gargles may take the place of irrigations. Heating devices and hot beverages must be avoided, because pain and thermal sensations may be lost on the side that has been operated on. The patient needs to be impressed with the need for close medical supervision after discharge to ensure maintenance of his optimal condition and

[5] C. Moore, Pre- and Postoperative Care in Major Mouth and Neck Surgery, *Am. J. Surg.*, vol. 90, no. 6, p. 918, December, 1955.

for the early detection of recurrent disease. If a total laryngectomy was necessary, the patient will need to receive speech therapy to learn to substitute the esophagus for his vocal cords. With esophageal speech the patient swallows air and forms the words as he belches. He may prefer to use a reed larynx or an electrolarynx. While his voice will not sound normal, his speech will be intelligible and allow communication, which markedly aids in making a satisfactory adjustment.

SUMMARY

Surgery of the thyroid gland is most commonly performed in the treatment of neoplasia and hyperplasia, toxic or nontoxic. The location of the thyroid gland overlying the trachea makes removal of a space-occupying lesion mandatory.

The patient usually undergoes an extensive preoperative evaluation to determine the extent and type of lesion and the presence of toxic hyperthyroidism. A toxic patient must be brought to a state of euthyroidism preoperatively; this may require a prolonged period of medical management.

The thyroid gland may be removed in part or in whole, depending upon the lesion. If a total thyroidectomy must be performed, lifelong medication with thyroid extract is necessary.

The major postoperative complications include hemorrhage, injury to the recurrent laryngeal nerve(s), and parathyroid tetany. Thyroid crisis is a fourth complication which may occur with toxic hyperthyroidism.

A tracheostomy may be necessitated by complications of thyroidectomy which threaten asphyxia, or by radical neck dissection. The plan for nursing care and teaching centers upon maintaining a patent airway, keeping the tube clean, preventing infection, and providing for nonverbal communication.

Radical neck dissection is performed in the treatment of metastatic carcinoma. Preoperative measures to improve the patient's nutritional status and reduce intraoral infection are very important.

Postoperative care is designed to maintain a patent airway, meet needs for nutrition and hydration, prevent and treat complications, and assist the patient in his rehabilitation. The patient may need instruction in tube feeding, mouth care, tracheostomy care, and use of a prosthetic device, especially if surgery was extensive enough to require this care following discharge from the hospital. Speech rehabilitation will be necessary if a laryngectomy was performed.

BIBLIOGRAPHY

BARTELS, E. C.: Medical Management of Hyperthyroidism, *Seminar,* Sharp and Dohme, Division of Merck and Company, Inc., Philadelphia, vol. 18, no. 1, pp. 2–7, 27–28, Spring, 1956.

BEAHRS, O. H., J. D. GOSSEL, W. H. HOLLINSHEAD: Technic and Surgical Anatomy of Radical Neck Dissection, *Am. J. Surg.,* vol. 90, no. 3, pp. 490–516, September, 1955.

COHEN, M., and G. E. MOORE: Malignant Lesions of the Thyroid, *Surgery,* vol. 35, no. 1, pp. 62–76, January, 1954.

CONLEY, J. J.: Tracheotomy, *Am. J. Nursing,* pp. 1078–1081, September, 1952.

COPE, O.: Thyroid, Thymus, and Parathyroids, in "Surgery," J. G. Allen, H. N. Harkins, C. A. Moyer, and J. E. Rhoads (eds.), J. B. Lippincott Company, Philadelphia, 1957, chap. 26, pp. 536–568.

CRILE, JR., G.: Radioactive Iodine in Treating Thyroid Disease, *Am. J. Nursing,* p. 825, July, 1954.

———— and R. W. SCHNEIDER: The Thyroid and Parathyroids, in "Christopher's Textbook of Surgery," 6th ed., L. Davis (ed.), W. B. Saunders Company, Philadelphia, 1956, chap. 13, pp. 339–345.

GREENE, J. S.: Speech Rehabilitation Following Laryngectomy, *Am. J. Nursing,* pp. 153–154, March, 1949.

HISLOP, R.: Nursing Care of Patients with Mouth or Throat Cancer, *Am. J. Nursing,* pp. 1317–1319, October, 1957.

HUBAY, C. A., and R. D. EVANS: Hyperthyroidism, *Am. J. Nursing,* pp. 1206–1210, October, 1955.

JAMES, A. G.: The Diagnosis of Cancer of the Head and Neck, *Postgrad. Med.,* vol. 17, no. 6, pp. 449–452, June, 1955.

———— and B. J. PIATT: Radical Neck Surgery, *Am. J. Nursing,* pp. 930–934, August, 1953.

MARTIN, H. E., B. DELVALLE, H. EHRLICH, and W. G. CAHAN: Neck Dissection, *Cancer,* vol. 4, no. 3, pp. 441–499, May, 1951.

———— and H. EHRLICH: Nursing Care Following Laryngectomy, *Am. J. Nursing,* pp. 149–152, March, 1949.

MOORE, C.: Pre- and Postoperative Care in Major Mouth and Neck Surgery, *Am. J. Surg.,* vol. 90, no. 6, pp. 911–918, December, 1955.

MORFIT, H. M.: Surgical Treatment of Cancer of the Extrinsic Larynx and Hypopharyngeal Walls, *Surgery,* vol. 37, no. 2, pp. 229–241, February, 1955.

SALTZSTEIN, H. C.: Diagnosis of Tumors of the Neck, *Am. J. Surg.,* vol. 89, no. 5, pp. 937–954, May, 1955.

UTENDORFER, R. W.: Total Parotidectomy for Mixed Tumor, *Am. J. Surg.,* vol. 91, no. 2, pp. 159–163, February, 1956.

15

THE SURGICAL TREATMENT OF CARCINOMA OF THE BREAST

The breast is the most common site for carcinoma among women, with a yearly mortality exceeding 20,000 in the United States alone. Since the breast is readily accessible for examination, and since early detection plus adequate treatment can effect a cure, it is essential that women be trained in methods of self-examination and that they develop a healthy attitude toward this practice. Undue concern with too-frequent examination can be crippling emotionally; wise observation of breast-tissue changes with prompt reporting of alterations to the physician can be lifesaving.

SELF-EXAMINATION OF THE BREAST

Once a month, immediately following the menstrual period, every woman should examine her breasts by observation and palpation. She will thereby learn to recognize the normal appearance and feeling of her breasts, so that changes will be more readily detected. A painless lump, or palpable mass, is the most common early symptom of breast carcinoma and is often discovered accidentally. The examination is performed after the menstrual period because many breasts become engorged, tender, and lumpy prior to menstruation. Cystic disease of the breasts is common among women and is accentuated prior to menstruation, owing to hormonal influences. Chronic cystic mastitis is often bilateral and diffuse, whereas a tumor is solitary.

The examination [1] begins with the woman seated before a mirror. (See Fig. 38.) With arms relaxed at the sides, she should study the contour of the breasts to determine any change since the last examination. Next,

---

[1] This method of self-examination has been adapted from publications of the American Cancer Society, Inc., New York.

with arms raised above the head, she should determine whether the
breasts are symmetrical, whether the nipple line is even, and whether
there is puckering or dimpling of the skin. She should then examine the
nipples, noting discharge, retraction, or scaliness of the areola. Following this observation, she should lie flat on her back with a small pad
under the chest on the side to be examined first, with the arm raised

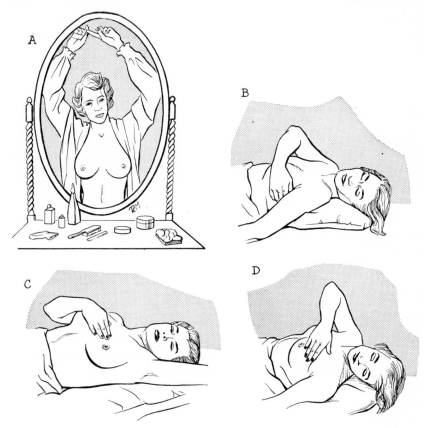

FIG. 38. Self-examination of the breast. (A) Inspection before a mirror. (B) Palpation of the axilla. (C), (D) Palpation of all quadrants of the breast.

above her head. In this position the breast tissue is thinned and flattened
against the chest wall so that a lump or thickening can be more easily
detected. With the flat of her fingers she should gently palpate the breasts
and sides in a systematic pattern to ensure complete coverage of all
breast tissue. The inner half of the breast is palpated while the arm is
raised; the outer half with the arm down at the side. The axilla should be
palpated with the arm extended above the head, and again down at the

side, because metastasis to the axilla, the most common site, would be revealed by a mass in that area. It is important that the woman be gentle and avoid using her fingertips, as she could conceivably press the sub-cutaneous tissue into a mass simulating a lump, or might spread carcinoma if it is present. Should a lump or any other abnormality be detected she should report immediately to her physician for evaluation and treatment. If her findings are negative she should accept this reassurance and abstain from self-examination until the following month. All women over thirty-five years of age should be examined by their physicians once or twice yearly in addition to monthly self-examination because the in-cidence of breast cancer increases with age, even beyond the menopause.

INCIDENCE

Carcinoma of the breast occurs most commonly in middle-aged women, although men occasionally are also affected. The incidence is greater in women who have had prolonged irritation or infection of the breasts, and in those who have never performed the function of lactation. Cancer of the breast occurs with greatest incidence in the upper outer quadrant of the breast. The upper inner quadrant, nipple area, lower outer quadrant, and lower inner quadrant are affected with decreasing incidence in that order.

PATHOLOGY

To understand the pathology involved in breast cancer it must be recalled that the mammary gland overlying the pectoralis major and minor muscles is composed of fat and loose areolar tissue interspersed with acini and ducts, which converge at the nipple. This gland is richly supplied with lymphatic vessels, which facilitate metastasis. (See Fig. 39.) As the cancer grows, invasion of the skin with fibrosis causes the skin to pucker, resembling an orange peel. If this process involves the nipple, it will be drawn inward, or retracted; it may cause the nipple to point toward the site of the cancer. Intraductal carcinoma may cause a discharge from the nipple.

Metastasis occurs through the lymphatic and hematogenous routes. The axillary lymph nodes on the affected side are first involved. The lungs and pleura, liver, bone, opposite breast, adrenal glands, brain, and ovaries are the most common additional sites for metastatic involvement. Once distant metastasis has occurred, the prognosis for life is poor. Pallia-tive irradiation therapy is then instituted.

CONFIRMATION OF DIAGNOSIS

It is imperative that a palpable mass in the breast be subjected to immediate surgical biopsy for histologic diagnosis. This procedure should be performed under general anesthesia with the patient prepared for a radical mastectomy in the event that the report from the frozen section reveals a malignant neoplasm. Aspiration biopsy is unwarranted when

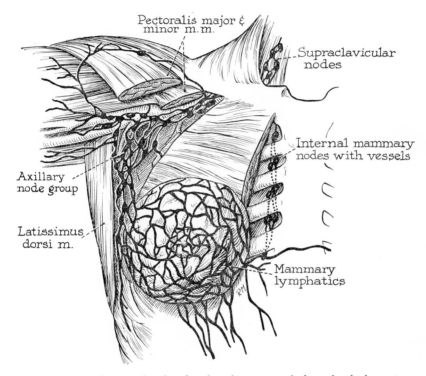

Fᴵɢ. 39. Drawing showing the abundant lymphatic network through which carcinoma of the breast can metastasize.

breast cancer is suspected because the local anesthetic may distort the specimen or allow it to be missed altogether; valuable time may be lost in preparing a patient for a radical mastectomy following a biopsy performed as a minor procedure.

PREOPERATIVE PREPARATION

In order to reduce emotional trauma postoperatively, the patient should be made aware before surgery of the fact that it may be necessary to remove her breast. The usual measures prior to a general anesthetic are carried out; namely, administering sedation and an antisecretory drug and emptying the gastrointestinal tract and bladder. The surgical skin preparation includes the area from and including the neck to the anterior superior iliac crest, on the affected side, extending 3 in. beyond the midline anteriorly and posteriorly, the axilla, and upper arm. (See Fig. 40.)

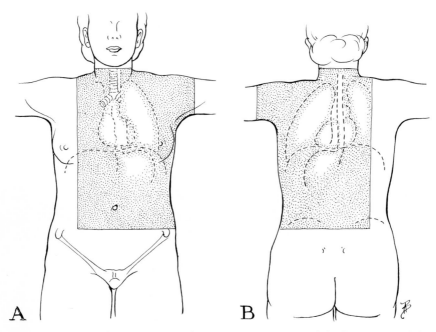

Fig. 40. Area of skin preparation for mastectomy (A) or left thoracotomy (B). Note the relative relationships of the left lung, heart, esophagus, and diaphragm.

SURGICAL TECHNIC

If the diagnosis of carcinoma is confirmed by frozen section, an *extensive*, or *radical*, *mastectomy* is performed. This procedure involves removal of the affected breast, pectoralis major and minor muscles, lymphatic vessels, and axillary lymph nodes. Such extensive surgery occasionally necessitates skin grafting to close the surgical defect. If the report is negative, the benign neoplasm or cyst is removed.

Occasionally a *simple mastectomy*, excision of only the affected breast tissue, is performed to remove a far-advanced ulcerating neoplastic involvement, thereby making the patient more comfortable.

POSTOPERATIVE CARE AND TEACHING

The early postoperative care is similar to that described for laparotomy. Shock and hemorrhage may occur and require blood transfusions. Analgesics are usually necessary early because of the extensive incision. A full diet is resumed as soon as tolerated.

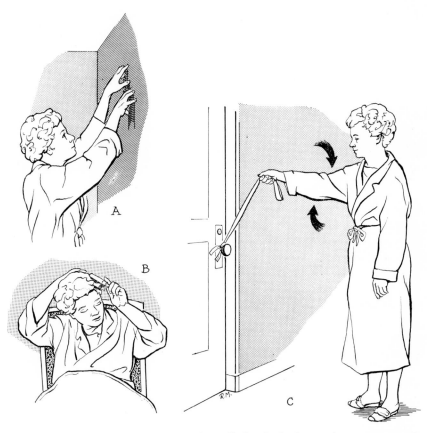

FIG. 41. Postmastectomy exercises. (A) Wall hand climbing: the patient stands facing the wall, with toes as close to the wall as possible and feet apart; she then places the palms on the wall at shoulder level; by flexing the fingers, she advances hands up the wall until arms are full extended and then works hands down to the starting point. Each time this exercise is repeated, the patient is encouraged to climb a little higher until full extension is accomplished. (B) Hairbrushing encourages flexion and elevation of the affected arm as well as abduction of the shoulder joint. (C) Rope twirling provides for rotation of the affected shoulder joint. All these exercises are started early postoperatively and are repeated several times daily as ordered.

The two major postoperative concerns are the prevention of wound infection and the promotion of function of the arm on the affected side.

Wound Care

The care of the wound will depend somewhat on the type of dressing applied and the type of drainage instituted. Some surgeons insert drains into the affected area and apply a compression dressing to control the accumulation of serum, obliterate the dead space, and hasten adherence of the skin flaps. Others insert a catheter to which suction is applied for the first few postoperative days. A light dressing or none may be used when catheter drainage is instituted. (A separate small incision is often preferred for the insertion of drains and catheters because such a wound closes spontaneously following removal of the drain and does not interfere with the healing of the major incision.) When suction is not used, drainage will be copious early postoperatively, and the nurse will need to reinforce saturated dressings to prevent infection. Saturation will occur in the axilla and posteriorly where drainage gravitates.

Activity

Early postoperatively the patient is placed in dorsal recumbency with the affected arm abducted at the shoulder joint, internally rotated, and flexed at the elbow; the forearm is elevated. Early passive motion of the arm, supplanted as soon as possible by active motion, is instituted to prevent the disabling complications of lymphedema and ankylosis. Lymphedema, more easily prevented than treated, occurs because removal of the axillary lymph nodes interferes with drainage of lymph from the arm. Exercising the arm improves circulation and aids the veins in assuming the function of draining lymph from the forearm. (See Fig. 41.) When activity is not encouraged, the arm may become markedly edematous; amputations have sometimes been required because of the weight of such an extremity. Exercise also strengthens the deltoid muscle and prevents ankylosis of the shoulder joint. These patients require much encouragement to exercise; they naturally tend to immobilize the arm to prevent pain. The patient must be encouraged to raise her arm and to put her shoulder joint through its full range of motion several times daily. Such laborious exercises are performed more willingly when a purpose is evident, e.g., brushing hair and cleaning teeth using the affected arm. After discharge from the hospital, the performance of routine household duties exercises the arm effectively, but heavy lifting and pushing are, of course, contraindicated.[2] (See Fig. 42.)

[2] Several excellent pamphlets are available for use of patients in rehabilitation following mastectomy. Written in lay terminology, they answer many questions which patients may be reluctant to ask the nurse or surgeon. One of the most helpful of

The patient who has had a radical mastectomy is an excellent candidate for reassurance by a well-rehabilitated breast amputee. The breast is intimately feminine, and women who must have a mastectomy not uncommonly become profoundly depressed. This mood usually lifts as healing ensues and the patient realizes that she is not really handicapped, that a well-fitting prosthesis will restore her contour, and that surgery has probably eradicated the neoplasm, or has at least lengthened her

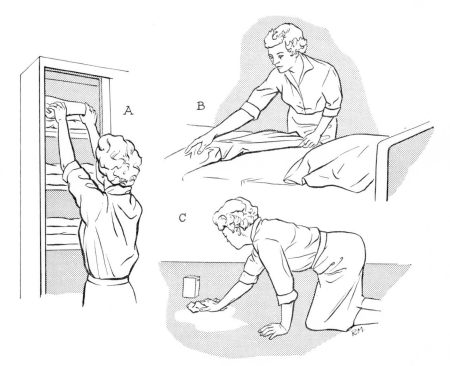

FIG. 42. In the home the affected arm can be put through the full range of motion in the course of routine daily tasks. The exercises learned in the hospital will be continued more readily if they are associated with the performance of daily living activities.

life and made it more comfortable. The prosthesis can be fashioned from soft padding or foam rubber inserted into the brassiere. A commercial product is available, made of plastic and filled with fluid to conform more nearly to normal breast alterations in contour with positional changes. This prosthesis approximates the normal weight of a breast and helps to prevent the tendency for the patient to hold her shoulder higher on the affected side. The prosthesis should be kept clean. The

these is "Help Yourself to Recovery," published by the American Cancer Society, Inc., New York, 1957.

plastic, fluid-containing form must be protected from extremes in temperature. The patient can be fitted for a prosthesis in a surgical supply house or in a large department store.

She must realize that she must remain under medical supervision for life to detect recurrence or metastasis. The remaining breast must be examined monthly by the patient as before. However, it is especially important for this patient to be helped to develop an objective attitude toward self-examination since she is more apt to become overly concerned. Here again a well-adjusted person who has learned to face the problem of mastectomy can help the patient immeasurably. Spiritual support also is very important for patients who have had mutilating yet life-saving surgical procedures.

SUMMARY

The breast is the most common site for carcinoma among women. The only hope for cure lies in early detection and extensive resection.

Early detection is possible when women learn to examine their breasts once monthly, and when all those over thirty-five years of age are examined by their physicians once or twice a year.

Some of the more common signs of breast carcinoma are a lump in the breast or axilla, a change in the contour or size of a breast, puckering of the skin, and nipple changes such as retraction, discharge, or rash.

Confirmation of the diagnosis is made by frozen section under general anesthesia with the patient prepared for an extensive mastectomy should a report of carcinoma be returned.

The postoperative care is similar to that described for a laparotomy, with emphasis upon the detection of hemorrhage and prevention of infection in the extensive wound. Rehabilitation is achieved by helping the patient to accept the surgical result, by teaching exercises designed to prevent complications and to promote function of the affected arm, and by fitting a prosthetic device which restores the normal breast contour. The patient must remain under medical surveillance for life.

BIBLIOGRAPHY

ALEXANDER, S. E.: Nursing Care of a Patient after Breast Surgery, *Am. J. Nursing,* pp. 1571–1572, December, 1957.
"Cancer Nursing," A joint project of the National Cancer Institute, U.S. Public Health Service, Federal Security Agency, and the New York State Department of Health, New York State Department of Health, Albany, 1950, pp. 48–51.
HAAGENSEN, C. D.: "Carcinoma of the Breast," American Cancer Society, Inc., New York, 1950.
———: "Diseases of the Breast," W. B. Saunders Company, Philadelphia, 1956.

HIGGINBOTHAM, S.: Arm Exercises after Mastectomy, *Am. J. Nursing*, pp. 1573–1574, December, 1957.

LEWISON, E. F.: "Breast Cancer," The Williams & Wilkins Company, Baltimore, 1955.

MACDONALD, I.: The Breasts, in "Christopher's Textbook of Surgery," 6th ed., L. Davis (ed.), W. B. Saunders Company, Philadelphia, 1956, chap. 14, pp. 348–388.

POPMA, A. M.: Cancer of the Breast, *Am. J. Nursing*, pp. 1570–1571, December, 1957.

SMITH, G. W.: When a Breast Must Be Removed, *Am. J. Nursing*, pp. 335–339, June, 1950.

SUGARBAKER, E. D., and L. Wilfrey: Cancer of the Breast, *Am. J. Nursing*, pp. 332–335, June, 1950.

16

SURGERY OF THE LUNGS AND MEDIASTINUM, I

Thoracic surgery has been made feasible by several developments in medicine and allied fields. Anatomy and physiology are better understood. Improved methods of diagnosis by roentgenography and by tests of heart and lung function permit earlier detection and treatment of surgical conditions of the chest. Improvements in methods of anesthesia, refinements in surgical technics, and the advent of potent pharmaceutic adjuncts combine to reduce morbidity and mortality rates to reasonable levels. Current research will enlarge the scope of thoracic surgery and extend its benefits to an increasing number of persons.

Surgery of the thoracic cavity is most commonly performed for conditions affecting the lungs and mediastinal structures, including the heart, great vessels, and esophagus.

Conditions which may require pulmonary surgery are numerous and varied but can be classified broadly as neoplasms; infections, including bronchiectasis, tuberculosis, empyema, and abscesses; and wounds of the chest wall and/or lung producing pneumothorax or hemothorax.

PREOPERATIVE EVALUATION

The lungs are vital organs. Consequently, a careful preoperative evaluation is necessary prior to the performance of any procedure which affects the combined power of the lungs to function. On the basis of this evaluation, which includes cardiorenal-respiratory functioning, the surgeon determines the procedure of choice for the specific type, location, and extent of disease. He must evaluate not only the surgical risk but also the respiratory risk, i.e., if the patient can survive the operative procedure, which may include collapse or removal of a lung in part or in whole, will a sufficient amount of functioning lung tissue be left to maintain him without the development of severe dyspnea?

Diagnostic procedures which may be performed prior to elective pulmonary surgery include x-ray studies, sputum examinations, pulmonary function tests, and bronchoscopy. Special roentgenographic methods permit the lung to be viewed through various planes and from several angles, thereby aiding the physician to locate the lesion and evaluate the extent of disease.

Sputum Examination

Sputum is examined for bacteria, fungi, and tumor cells. The specimen is best collected early in the morning before oral intake. The patient must be instructed to raise sputum by deep coughing rather than merely to expectorate saliva. A single specimen, three consecutive specimens, or a 24-hour collection may be ordered. The total volume or weight of sputum may be ordered. Since sputum may contain viable organisms, the nurse must use appropriate measures of medical asepsis in collecting these specimens to protect herself and laboratory personnel.

Pulmonary Function Tests

There are numerous tests of pulmonary function. *Spirometry* utilizes an instrument into which the patient breathes to obtain a measurement of the volume of air inhaled and exhaled. Commonly this method is used to measure *vital capacity,* the volume of air that can be expired after a maximum inspiration. Normally the vital capacity of an adult ranges between 3 to 4½ liters per minute. The *maximum breathing capacity,* a measure of the maximum volume of air that can be brought to the alveoli and removed in 1 minute, is approximately 100 to 150 liters. Figures substantially below these normal values suggest inoperability. These tests as described measure the combined pulmonary function. Endobronchial catheterization permits the measurement of pulmonary function for each lung separately.

Bronchoscopy

The insertion of a bronchoscope through the oral pharynx and trachea into a bronchus permits several diagnostic procedures. The bronchi can be inspected. Secretions can be aspirated or bronchial washings performed for bacteriologic and cytologic examination. If a neoplasm is within reach of the bronchoscope, a biopsy can be made. In addition, a *bronchogram* can be made by instilling a water-soluble or oil-soluble contrast medium into a bronchus to outline the distal tract for roentgenographic study. Bronchoscopy is performed for therapeutic purposes also, such as removal of a foreign body, dilatation of a stricture, or aspiration of secretions. Bronchoscopy is a trying procedure for the patient. Since a local anesthetic is used and the patient's cooperation is essential for the safe and effective use of the bronchoscope, adequate explanation must be given so that he understands what is to be done and what is expected of him preoperatively and postoperatively. Although actual surgery may not be performed, the term "preoperative" is used, and the procedure is commonly performed in the operating room. The patient often fears that

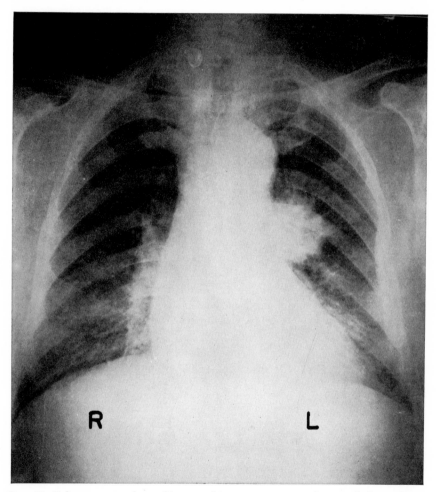

Fig. 43. Pulmonary neoplasm. Note in this roentgenogram the rounded neoplastic mass in the left lung field.

an operation will be performed; if this is not the intention, he must be reassured that only an examination will be carried out. Preoperative medication usually includes a sedative, a narcotic, and an antisecretant. Cocaine, or a derivative, is the anesthetic usually used for bronchoscopy. The nurse must realize that this drug may cause fatal overstimulation of the central nervous system when used in large amounts or in sensitive individuals. The preoperative barbiturate helps prevent such a reaction. Postoperatively, the nurse must watch for the following symptoms, which indicate a cocaine reaction: a rapid, weak pulse which later becomes slow and weak; breathing that at first is rapid, becoming slow and shallow and eventuating in Cheyne-Stokes respirations; overactivity and convulsions; talkativeness, confusion, and delirium; pale, moist skin; dilated pupils; and occasionally vomiting and/or diarrhea. The parenteral administration of a barbiturate when the patient first evidences excitement or a fast pulse usually helps prevent the reaction from being fatal. The surgeon must be notified immediately if any of these symptoms develops. Because the local anesthetic abolishes the cough reflex, oral intake is restricted for several hours before and after the procedure. Nothing should be given to eat or drink postoperatively for approximately 2 hours, until the nurse is assured that the patient can swallow and cough. If a bronchogram was performed, the contrast medium must be removed from the bronchial tree by postural drainage.

Postural Drainage. This procedure utilizes various positions to facilitate drainage of the bronchial tree by gravity. The effective use of postural drainage to remove the contrast medium and secretions requires a knowledge of the bronchial anatomy and an understanding regarding which segments of the bronchial tree are to be drained. Therefore, the physician must direct the nurse regarding the positions to be used. A high-sitting or erect position drains the superior lobe of each lung; a left side–lying, moderate Trendelenburg position facilitates drainage from the middle lobe of the right lung; the lower lobe of each lung is drained by inverting the patient over the edge of the bed with his hands supported on a low footstool or chair, or by placing him in shock position. These positions are maintained for 5 to 15 minutes several times daily as tolerated, and the patient is encouraged to cough into a receptacle.

SURGERY FOR PULMONARY NEOPLASM (Fig. 43)

Bronchogenic Carcinoma

Neoplastic disease of the lung is more commonly malignant than benign. Bronchogenic carcinoma is the most common of the malignant neoplasms and is steadily increasing in incidence. In 1954 this disease ranked as the most common cause of death due to cancer, claiming 22,000 lives. The vast majority of patients are men between the ages of forty and seventy. Although the exact cause of pulmonary carcinoma has not been determined, the following factors are thought to be contributory: prolonged, excessive cigarette smoking; the inhalation of certain fumes and dusts;

and radiation. The classification of primary malignant neoplasms of the lung based upon the predominant cell type is as follows: 50 per cent or more are epidermoid or squamous cell tumors and offer the best prognosis with early, adequate treatment; approximately 30 per cent are anaplastic or undifferentiated and bear the poorest prognosis; approximately 20 per cent are adenocarcinomas, which account for one-third to one-half of the lung cancers in women. All may metastasize early through the lymph and blood streams and not uncommonly result in cerebral metastases. They may invade the mediastinal structures and chest wall. Metastasis from other organs to the lungs is relatively common and usually inoperable.

Symptomatology. There are no early symptoms of bronchogenic carcinoma. One of the first symptoms to be manifested is a dry, hacking cough which later becomes productive but remains disproportionately severe in relation to the amount of sputum. This cough is usually associated with hemoptysis, anorexia, and weight loss. Recurring episodes of pneumonitis with fever are common. Dyspnea and chest discomfort usually occur late.

Diagnostic Methods. Carcinoma can be diagnosed more readily in the lung than in any other internal organ since x-ray almost always reveals the neoplasm even before symptoms occur. Nevertheless, in some series over one-half the lesions are inoperable by the time the patient consults a surgeon. The necessity for x-rays of the chest at regular intervals is obvious, and the nurse should encourage this practice in herself and others. Cancer cells may be found in sputum and/or bronchial washings. Biopsy obtained through a bronchoscope, or occasionally by thoracotomy, is the most accurate method of diagnosis.

Treatment. The treatment of choice for a primary malignant neoplasm of the lung is *pneumonectomy*, removal of a lung and visceral pleura, with wide excision of regional lymph nodes, although *lobectomy*, removal of a lobe, may be sufficient. Radiotherapy may be used for palliation.

Bronchial Adenoma

This is the most common of the relatively rare benign tumors affecting the lung. Bronchial adenoma is a slow-growing neoplasm which, although initially benign, has malignant potential and may metastasize after many years. Patients are usually between twenty and forty years of age. The most common symptoms are those of bronchial obstruction and ulceration, i.e., cough, hemoptysis, and dyspnea. Lobectomy is usually adequate, but pneumonectomy may be necessary.

All tumors of the bronchi and lungs should be removed, even if known to be benign, because they interfere with pulmonary function. Simple enucleation, segmental resection, lobectomy, or pneumonectomy may be the procedure of choice.

SURGERY FOR PULMONARY INFECTIONS

Bronchiectasis (Fig. 44)

In this disease of unknown etiology, irreversible dilatation and sacculation of the bronchial tree occur. Collections of sputum pool in these

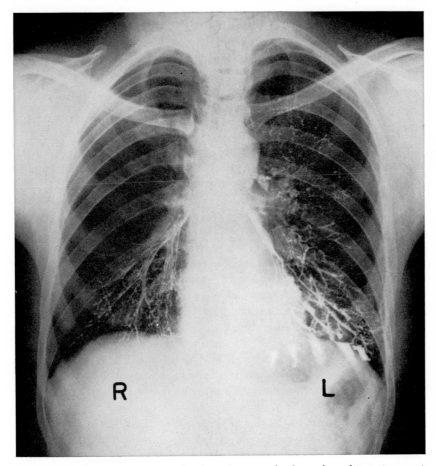

FIG. 44. Bronchiectasis. Note in this bronchogram the large bronchiectatic sacs in the left lower lobe; the right lung field appears to be normal.

dilated bronchial segments, which become infected, and reduce the efficiency of the lungs by mechanically blocking the exchange of respiratory gases. Contributing even more directly toward reducing the efficiency of pulmonary function are the recurrent episodes of interstitial pneumonia, which accompany bronchiectasis and result in fibrotic destruction of the parenchyma. The patient develops a chronic paroxysmal cough, which in time becomes productive of copious amounts of foul, purulent sputum. This cough is frequently accompanied by hemoptysis, which may amount to blood-streaked sputum of hemorrhagic proportions. Weight loss, exertional dyspnea, and chest pain are common in advanced stages.

Bronchiectasis is a disease of youths, who seldom survive beyond the third or fourth decade without adequate medical and surgical therapy. This disease imposes upon its victims a serious socioeconomic and emotional strain because the nature of the symptoms invites social ostracism and depression. Gainful employment may not be possible, yet the expenses incurred in a chronic illness such as this are high.

The diagnosis is confirmed by bronchography. The treatment of choice is segmental resection or, if necessary, lobectomy. If all the diseased lobes or segments can be removed, bronchiectasis is curable.

Pulmonary Tuberculosis

The patient with pulmonary tuberculosis may require surgical intervention as a part of his total therapeutic program. Although not curative in itself, surgery does help to arrest the disease, i.e., to render the lesion inactive and noninfectious in a large percentage of carefully selected, well-prepared patients.

Pathology and Symptomatology. Tuberculosis is a long-term, usually debilitating, systemic disease which commonly has pulmonary manifestations and is communicable. Tubercle bacilli usually reach the lung by inhalation, but the organisms can be swallowed and then be carried to the lung or to other parts of the body by the blood or lymph streams. Following inoculation of the lung parenchyma, an exudative lesion develops, associated with hilar lymphadenitis. This area of pneumonia is then infiltrated and walled off by phagocytic leukocytes allowing liquefaction, absorption, fibrosis, and calcification of the lesion. This primary lesion, or Ghon tubercle, usually remains quiescent and noninfectious. In some persons, especially those with low resistance, a secondary infection later develops. Whether this is because of breakdown of the primary lesion or reinfection is a matter of controversy. The center of the lesion undergoes liquefaction, caseation, and cavity formation. The open cavity remains a source of virulent tubercle bacilli, causing repeated reinfection.

The onset of pulmonary tuberculosis is usually insidious, with increasing fatigability, weight loss, and evening elevation of temperature, but in some patients there are no symptoms. In some young adults the only indication of pulmonary tuberculosis is pleural effusion. Hemoptysis, mild or severe, may be the first sign. In some patients the onset is acute, marked by cough and fever. As the disease progresses, increasing amounts of sputum are produced, resulting in anorexia and protein loss; emaciation ensues. Night sweats occur in all stages of tuberculosis.

Diagnostic Methods. The presumptive diagnosis is made by x-ray studies and confirmed by culturing the acid-fast tubercle bacilli from sputum and/or bronchial or gastric washings. Histopathologic studies of the lesion may be necessary. Since these bacilli elaborate an endotoxin to which the body becomes sensitive, a tuberculin skin test can be performed. This test is limited in value as a diagnostic tool, however, because it reveals only that the person has a primary lesion; it gives no indication of the activity of the disease, a positive tuberculin test resulting whether the lesion is quiescent or active. Hematologic studies are indicative only of a systemic infection: the leukocyte count and sedimentation rate of erythrocytes usually rise; a hypochromic anemia may develop.

Indications for Surgical Intervention. Surgery is indicated when medical management alone is not able to free the patient from systemic symptoms, make the sputum negative, resolve lesions, and close cavities.

Surgical treatment requires that the disease first be controlled by the administration of antituberculosis drugs and that the lung which is *contralateral*, i.e., on the opposite side, be either free from disease or responding to treatment.

Preoperative Management and Nursing Care. A period of 2 to 6 months of medical management is necessary to prepare the patient for surgery. Surgery is accomplished with greater safety when the patient is free from systemic symptoms and when the sputum has been converted to negative and reduced in volume to a minimum preoperatively. This state is achieved for the majority of patients by the use of antituberculosis drugs, such as streptomycin, para-aminosalicylic acid, and isoniazid. The patient should be encouraged to expectorate secretions; postural drainage may be instituted.

Bed rest, a nutritious diet, and a liberal fluid intake are essential. The hazards of bed rest and inactivity must be combated with excellent skin care, frequent turning, coughing and deep-breathing exercises, and active motion of the extremities. Attention must also be directed toward meeting the patient's needs for spiritual reinforcement; diversional, occupational, and physical therapies; vocational rehabilitation; and education in matters pertaining to self-care and the protection of society. The combined efforts of all members of the health team are necessary to support a patient effectively through this long-term illness. Inasmuch as no surgical procedure can eradicate every trace of this disease, this program outlined for the preoperative period must also be followed for several months postoperatively. Isolation precautions should be observed until the patient is no longer infectious.

Surgical Technics. The over-all aims of surgery in the treatment of pulmonary tuberculosis are to achieve a permanent arrest of the disease, to prevent complications and the spread of tuberculosis, to preserve the function of the uninvolved lung tissue, and to hasten the patient's return to useful activity.

To achieve these ends the diseased tissue may be resected or collapsed. Pulmonary tuberculosis frequently affects both lungs, with scattered lesions undergoing varying degrees of activity. Therefore, surgical treatment is directed toward the eradication of the most active lesions, which are serving as foci of reinfection.

Resection. Considerable lung tissue can be resected without producing pulmonary insufficiency provided the remaining tissue is healthy and capable of expanding to fill the pleural cavity. Several types of resection are used, depending upon the extent of the lesion. A small area can be excised in a *wedge resection.* A segment, which is the portion of lung tissue supplied by a bronchiole, can be removed in *segmentectomy.* Lobectomy or even pneumonectomy may be necessary. Contrary to the practice of extensive resections for carcinoma, in pulmonary tuberculosis no tissue is removed in excess of that necessary to achieve an arrest of the disease.

Pulmonary resection is a major procedure, and certain criteria must be met before this method of treatment is chosen. The patient must be able to withstand major thoracic surgery. The disease process must be localized, and all reversible lesions must have undergone resolution. The remaining lung tissue must be capable of reexpansion and adequate functioning. The patient must be free from systemic symptoms and active endobronchial disease.

The types of patient for whom resection is especially advocated are young persons, who have a longer anticipated period in which to experience a recurrence; women of childbearing age whose disease is likely to become reactivated during pregnancy; those with diabetes, which compounds the problems of tuberculosis; those with open cavities, which resist collapse therapy; and those with bronchostenosis, which eventually results in emphysematous, atelectatic, functionless pulmonary tissue.

Another indication for resection is a *tuberculoma,* an encapsulated mass of caseous material, which presents no symptoms but which is thought to have potentiality for activity. This lesion is usually discovered incidentally on x-ray, appearing as a tumor. Lobectomy or segmental resection is performed to confirm the diagnosis as well as to remove the lesion.

Collapse Therapy. Although collapse therapy is not used so freely as it was prior to the advent of antituberculosis chemotherapy and resection, it is used for those patients who cannot meet the criteria for resection.

Collapse procedures promote healing by placing the diseased tissues at rest, reducing both the respiratory and metabolic activity of the lung. Therapeutic collapse of lung tissue lessens the risk of reinfection by closing cavities and reducing blood and lymph flow.

Because the lung is an elastic, vascular, air-containing organ, it can be readily collapsed by compression. Collapse may be temporary or permanent, depending upon the method used.

The two methods of temporary collapse most commonly used are *pneumoperitoneum,* injection of air into the peritoneal cavity, and *phrenemphraxis,* crushing of a phrenic nerve. Both procedures cause the diaphragm to rise and compress pulmonary tissue. *Pneumothorax,* the injection of air into the pleural cavity, is occasionally used for temporary collapse of lung tissue.

The most commonly used method of permanent collapse is *thoracoplasty.* In this procedure short segments of ribs are removed to allow the thoracic wall to fall inward and compress lung tissue. Because the periosteum is not removed, the ribs regenerate in this new position and restore the stability of the thoracic wall, which is essential for effective respiratory excursions. Thoracoplasty is usually performed in two or three stages, with a total of five to seven ribs being partially resected. This procedure may be performed in conjunction with resection to prevent overdistention of a partially resected lung or to reduce the volume of the hemithorax when reexpansion is not desired or possible.

Another method of permanent collapse therapy sometimes used is *extraperiosteal plombage,* the insertion of a plombe, or synthetic sphere, beneath the ribs to compress a small area of pulmonary tissue. This procedure is used to close small cavities in patients with low respiratory reserves. Plombage may be combined with thoracoplasty. The plombe may erode through adjacent tissues and migrate, or may cause a foreign-body reaction; reoperation to remove the plombe then becomes necessary.

Empyema

In *empyema* a purulent exudate is formed in the pleural space. This condition may be secondary to tuberculosis or to pneumococcal or streptococcal pulmonary infections. It may follow trauma or may exist as a complication of pulmonary surgery.

The advent of antibiotic drug therapy has reduced the incidence, severity, and duration of empyema. The disease may be acute or chronic, chronicity developing when the organism is resistant to antibiotic drugs and the exudate becomes viscid.

Acute empyema is marked by toxicity. The patient runs a septic fever and experiences chills, sweats, tachycardia, weakness, cough, and pain on deep inspiration. The acute phase of empyema is treated by *closed thoracotomy drainage,* i.e., the insertion of an intercostal catheter into the empyema pocket to allow for irrigation and/or drainage. Sometimes intermittent aspirations are used in conjunction with the instillation of antibiotic drugs. Proteolytic drugs, such as trypsin, streptokinase, and streptodornase, may be instilled to lyse fibrin which is protecting the organism from action by the antibiotic drugs or to liquefy the exudate to facilitate drainage.

The chronic phase of empyema is treated by *open thoracotomy drainage.* If the process is localized, a short rib resection is performed and drains are inserted into the empyema pocket. During the prolonged period of drainage, these firm rubber tubes are changed weekly; progressively smaller drains are used as the empyema pocket diminishes in size. The drains should be well anchored.

If after drainage the underlying lung fails to expand and obliterate the cavity, or cavities, formed by empyema, additional surgical procedures will be necessary. The walls of the cavity may be excised. If the underlying lung is extensively diseased, the surgeon may perform a *pleuropneumonectomy,* removal of both pleurae, as a sac, together with the lung. When the lung is restricted by a thick fibrous peel, which may form over the visceral pleura in empyema, *decortication* will be performed to strip off this pseudomembrane. Thoracoplasty is indicated when the decorticated lung fails to expand satisfactorily.

Lung Abscess

An *abscess* is a localized collection of pus associated with cellular destruction. Organisms gain entrance into the lung by aspiration, hematogenous dissemination in septicemia, or by embolic spread from septic foci. The abscess may be secondary to primary respiratory infections, bronchogenic carcinoma, bronchiectasis, foreign-body aspiration, pulmonary infarction, or infection of congenital cysts.

The incidence of pulmonary abscess has been reduced markedly since the advent of antibiotic therapy. Although a rare entity, an abscess is serious because of the associated morbidity and possibility of complications, such as pleural effusion, empyema, and bronchopleural fistula; such an abscess may be fatal.

The most common symptoms are a cough which is productive of foul sputum, pleuritic pain, fever, malaise, and hemoptysis.

Lobectomy is the procedure of choice when antibiotic therapy and bronchial drainage fail to initiate a prompt response, although pneumonectomy may be necessary with extensive inflammatory reaction.

NURSING CARE AND TEACHING OF A PATIENT UNDERGOING THORACOTOMY

Preoperative Preparation

Thoracotomy (*thoraco,* chest + *otomy*), when employed in the treatment of the conditions described, is usually an elective procedure performed on a patient who is chronically ill. Therefore, a thorough preoperative evaluation and extensive preparation are necessary to reduce the surgical risk. The cardiovascular, renal, and respiratory systems especially must be brought to a state of optimal functioning. Exceptions to this include the patient who has empyema and must be operated on to establish drainage even though he may be acutely ill and the patient with an early primary pulmonary neoplasm who is in good condition and must be operated upon without delay.

Malnutrition and dehydration must be combated in a patient whose cough, sputum, and anorexia combine to result in hypoproteinemia, avitaminosis, secondary anemia, and weight loss. Infection must be controlled or eradicated by antimicrobial drug therapy. The volume of sputum must be reduced by encouraging expectoration and postural drainage and by administering the prescribed drugs. The patient who has pulmonary emphysema may require bronchodilators to increase the efficiency of his respiratory effort.

Usually the patient who is chronically ill is encouraged by the opportunity for surgical treatment as a means of recovering health. It is important that the patient be helped to view surgery as one phase of his medical treatment rather than as a cure-all for his illness. While it is true that surgery probably will restore the patient to health and useful activity, continued medical supervision and the use of sound hygienic practices will be necessary to maintain health and to prevent complications and recurrence of disease.

A Preoperative Nursing-care Plan for Mr. Thomas Jones

Description and History. The patient who will illustrate the immediate preoperative preparation and postoperative care for thoracotomy performed in the treatment of tuberculosis is Mr. Thomas Jones. He is 39 years of age, the father of sons, ages 10 and 15 years. He owns and operates an automobile repair shop where he works long hours. Mr. Jones is a member of the Roman Catholic Church.

One year ago Mr. Jones had a routine chest x-ray which showed evidences of active tuberculosis; studies of sputums confirmed this diagnosis. He was advised to enter a hospital immediately for treatment. He reacted with mixed feelings to being told suddenly that he had tuberculosis and would require long-term care. He was annoyed, frightened, and dubious, as his questions reveal:

I don't feel sick; how can I have such a serious disease?

How long will it be before I can come home and work again?

My sons need a father's guidance; will my wife be able to manage them alone?

Have I given this disease to my beloved family? my friends? my customers?

How can I afford hospitalization?

What will happen to my business?

My older son is so close to college now; will I not be able to give him this opportunity?

Maybe they made a mistake; perhaps they don't mean me after all.

Feeling that Mr. Jones needed more time to accept his situation, his physician allowed him to remain at home on bed rest and antituberculosis drug therapy. For 3 months the public health nurse visited Mr. Jones three times a week, helping him with his care and teaching both the patient and his family measures to prevent the spread of tuberculosis. With the encouragement and guidance of his physician, nurse, wife, and priest, Mr. Jones was helped to view his problems realistically and to consent to being admitted to a sanitarium for closer medical supervision and more adequate care. He was especially aided in making this decision by realizing that his family, who were being observed for the development of tuberculosis, were all still free from the disease. He was able to engage in a partnership which would allow him to leave his business without undue concern and which would reduce his working hours after recovery.

After 3 months of bed rest and antituberculosis drug therapy in the sanitarium, it became apparent that Mr. Jones would benefit by a lobectomy to remove the one cavity persisting in the left upper lobe.

Preoperative Teaching Plan. Preoperatively he was taught breathing exercises which would be necessary in the postoperative period to prevent complications and promote reexpansion of remaining lung tissue. He had learned the proper use and disposal of mouth wipes and was reminded that he should continue to use and dispose of them in this way. He was taught the importance of raising secretions postoperatively. Throughout his preoperative care, he was given ample opportunity to discuss his feelings about surgery and to have his questions answered.

Spiritual Reassurance. Mr. Jones was visited regularly by Father Burke, his parish priest, during the preoperative period. On the morning of surgery, prior to the administration of the preoperative sedative, Father Burke heard Mr. Jones's confession and administered Holy Communion. The preparation for confession and Communion is as follows:

1. Provide privacy.
2. Clear top of bedside table and cover with a clean scarf or towel.
3. Realize that the priest will want the following articles:

a. Linen napkin
b. Glass of water
c. Teaspoon, if the patient can not drink from the glass
d. Two candles
e. Crucifix

If the hospital does not provide the necessary articles, usually set up on a tray or in a box, the priest must be notified so that he can bring the candles and crucifix. He will bring the Host. Generally the Catholic patient is allowed fluids and necessary medications before Communion because during illness exceptions are permitted to the usual obligation of fasting before receiving this sacrament.

Non-Catholics too often feel uncomfortable because they do not know what to do in the presence of a priest wearing a Communion stole. Reverence is expected, but the nurse need only continue with her nursing duties and realize that she must refrain from talking to the priest while he wears the Communion stole. Catholic nurses and lay persons may kneel. True respect for other religions grows with more adequate understanding. The nurse will do well to learn all she can about her patient's religion in order to meet these needs more effectively.

Immediate Preparation for Thoracotomy. The same preoperative orders are carried out as described for general anesthesia and laparotomy (see Chapter 8), the only difference being the area of skin to prepare. One of several approaches may be used for pulmonary surgery: posterior, anterior, or lateral. Ribs may be retracted or resected, i.e., an *intercostal* (*inter*, between + *costa*, rib) or *transcostal* (*trans*, across + *costa*) incision may be used. The approach is frequently a combination, e.g., an anterolateral or posterolateral approach, and the incision is usually extensive. Therefore, the area to prepare includes the skin from the chin to the iliac crest, 3 in. past the midline on the anterior and posterior chest, and the axilla and shoulder on the affected side. The patient is commonly sent to the operating suite in his bed.

Operating Precautions

Thoracotomy is a major procedure which requires continuous, skilled attention on the part of every member of the operating-room team to prevent serious complications.

When the thorax is opened, atmospheric air immediately causes lung tissue to collapse. It is necessary, therefore, that respirations be controlled entirely by the anesthesiologist, who uses an endotracheal tube and a positive-pressure machine to administer the anesthetic and oxygen. The lungs are inflated and deflated by the anesthesiologist as directed by the surgeon throughout the operation.

Anoxia and *hypercapnia,* retention of carbon dioxide in the blood, can occur rather easily when respirations are so controlled and may result in ventricular fibrillation and cardiac arrest or standstill.

Cardiac arrest, or sudden circulatory failure, is a rare emergency which takes precedence over all other considerations. It may occur with any anesthetic or operation but is more likely in thoracotomy, especially when exposure and manipulation of the heart are necessary. The major signs of cardiac arrest are absence of pulse and blood pressure, cessation of bleeding, and mottling of the skin. The brain can withstand anoxia for only 3½ minutes without permanent impairment.[1] Therefore, the surgeon must immediately begin manual, rhythmic compression of the heart to initiate beating. Epinephrine 1:1,000 may be injected into the left ventricle to aid in initiating spontaneous contractions.[2] Calcium chloride in a 10 per cent solution may be used if the myocardium is atonic.[3] If the ventricle is fibrillating, an electrical defibrillator may be used to produce a complete arrest so that sinus rhythm can be reestablished by cardiac massage.[4] Procaine hydrochloride may be used to prevent and treat ventricular fibrillation. Atropine sulfate can also prevent fibrillation when administered in frequent, small doses. While the surgeon performs cardiac massage, the anesthesiologist gives oxygen and maintains artificial respiration. Cardiac arrest may occur on the clinical division. Necessary equipment should be ready.

A considerable amount of blood may be lost during pulmonary surgery. Transfusions approximating 1 to 1½ liters are commonly necessary during surgery to restore blood volume.

Nursing Care and Teaching in the Immediate Postoperative Period

Promotion of an Adequate Respiratory Exchange. The major emphasis of care in the early postoperative period is on promoting an adequate respiratory exchange. Several factors combine to make respiratory efforts difficult and often ineffective. Thoracotomy necessitates the cutting and stretching of neuromuscular fibers, reducing the capacity to breathe and causing pain. Pain is increased by respiratory activity, so that the patient

---

[1] E. Heckel and E. H. Fell, Cardiac Arrest during Surgical Operations, *S. Clin. North America,* vol. 35, no. 1, p. 243, February, 1955.

[2] *Ibid.,* p. 251.

[3] *Ibid.*

[4] *Ibid.*

attempts to minimize his discomfort by taking shallow breaths and by refraining from coughing. In addition, secretions, which may be excessive because of pulmonary disease and/or surgery, are easily aspirated or retained.

Therefore, to promote an adequate respiratory exchange, oxygen is administered early postoperatively, mild analgesia is used, and measures designed to clear the tracheobronchial tree are instituted. Narcotics must be used with caution following a thoracotomy. Pain must be minimized to allow coughing and deep breathing, but the cough center must not be depressed, nor should the sensorium be dulled. The patient must be kept alert enough to cooperate in his care and to permit accurate observations of his condition. Restlessness is one of the early signs of respiratory distress, hemorrhage, and shock, which might not be detected in a heavily sedated patient. Deep-breathing exercises are initiated when the surgeon indicates.

The patient is encouraged to cough at hourly intervals to clear the tracheobronchial tree. Coughing is more effective and easier to accomplish for the majority of patients if a sitting position is assumed and if the patient first takes two or three deep breaths. Firm support to the area operated on, anteriorly and posteriorly, should be provided by the nurse. The patient will require considerable persuasion but will usually cooperate if he has been adequately instructed preoperatively. Deep-breathing exercises are initiated when the surgeon feels that they are necessary. Frequent position change is essential.

If coughing is ineffective in clearing the tracheobronchial tree, nasotracheal aspirations may be necessary. This procedure is best performed by the surgeon, who is needed also for observing the condition of the patient who requires aspiration. However, the nurse may be asked to perform this procedure provided she has been taught how by an expert. She should hold her own breath while the catheter is in the trachea as a safeguard in timing the duration of occlusion of the airway. Insertion of the lightly lubricated catheter is facilitated by placing the patient in a semisitting position with his head and neck dorsally extended. The tongue is grasped with gauze and pulled forward. The trachea is entered as the patient takes a deep breath. When the catheter is well into the trachea, suction is applied at intervals of 10 to 15 seconds only, because the catheter is the patient's airway during this procedure. Oxygen should be available for administration between aspirations. If these measures fail to clear the airway, bronchoscopic aspiration may be required.

Steam inhalations or expectorant medications may be administered to loosen tenacious secretions and facilitate their removal by coughing or aspirating.

Any procedure requiring resection of ribs, such as thoracoplasty, may destroy the stability of the chest wall temporarily and allow *paradoxical respirations,* i.e., the unsupported portion of chest wall moves outward on expiration and inward on inspiration, a reverse of the normal pattern of respiratory excursions. Paradoxical respirations are ineffective in maintaining an adequate respiratory exchange and will, if not corrected, result in death. Treatment consists in applying a firm dressing and positioning the patient on the side that has been operated on with the area of paradoxical respirations splinted by a sandbag. Oxygen and a sedative may be administered.

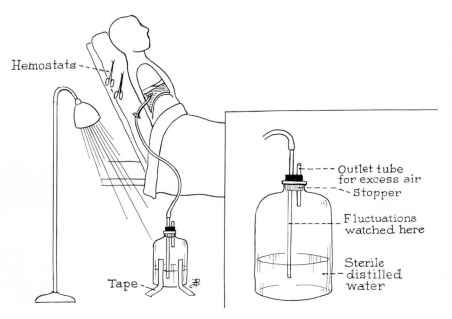

Fɪɢ. 45. Water-seal drainage. Note the tubing secured to the bed and the bottle taped to the floor. The lamp facilitates observation of the functioning of the system and the character of the drainage. The insert shows the water-seal bottle in detail.

Promotion of Lung Reexpansion. Another important consideration in the postoperative care of the patient who has had a thoracotomy is to keep the pleural space free from exudate and to promote reexpansion of the remaining lung tissue. To these ends closed drainage of the chest is usually initiated in the operating room and maintained for the first 48 hours or longer, except for patients who have had a thoracoplasty or a pneumonectomy. Closed, or water-seal, drainage, is accomplished by the use of one or more retention catheters inserted into the pleural space through separate small incisions. Each catheter is connected to tubing which leads to a glass tube, the end of which is submerged in sterile distilled water to prevent the entrance of air into the pleural space; hence the term *water-seal drainage*. (See Fig. 45.) The drainage bottle is placed well below the level of the patient's chest. This method of drainage by gravity is usually effective in promoting fairly rapid reexpansion of lung tissue. If a more active force is necessary, a pump which employs negative pressure may be added to the system. To prevent the pump from exerting too much negative pressure, a suction breaker may be installed between the water-seal bottle and the pump or wall suction. The suction breaker consists of a bottle partly filled with water in which is submerged one end of a glass tube, the other end of which is in communication with air. When the amount of suction present in the system exceeds that prescribed, air rushes in through the glass tube, raises the water level, and reduces the amount of suction. The distance that the glass tube is submerged in water determines the amount of negative or, more correctly, subatmospheric pressure exerted on the pleural space. Since the pressure in the pleural space is normally equal to —5 to —10 cm. water, —15 to —40 cm. pressure is employed to drain the pleural space and to reexpand the lung. The entire drainage system must be air-tight and handled with surgical aseptic technic to prevent the introduction of air or bacteria into the pleural space.

Mr. Jones is transported to the recovery unit with his two intercostal catheters clamped. This illustrates the first nursing responsibility for the safe and effective use of water-seal drainage of the chest. The catheter must be clamped during transportation of the patient, unless the bottle can be suspended at least 1 foot below the level of the chest, to prevent water from entering the pleural space. Once the patient is situated in the recovery unit or on the clinical division, the bottle is either suspended below the patient or taped to the floor. Taping the bottle to the floor not only ensures its remaining below the chest level but also guards against jarring. The nurse must be certain that no tension is exerted on the catheters, that they do not kink or twist, and that the patient does not lie on them. Another important nursing responsibility is the proper positioning of the patient. Usually the surgeon will order that the patient be placed in a sitting position when the blood pressure has stabilized at normal levels. This position facilitates the drainage of fluid into the dependent part of the pleural space where one catheter has been placed. Air rises to the superior part of the pleural space where the second catheter has been inserted.

Closed drainage of the chest requires frequent observations by the nurse to ensure continuous, effective functioning. With water-seal drainage the column of water in the glass tube should fluctuate with each inspiration. Its failure to do so may indicate obstruction of the catheter or tubing, most commonly by a blood clot from within or compression of the tubing from without; it may simply indicate that the lung has fully expanded. In either case the surgeon should be notified. The quantity and character of drainage must be closely observed. Drainage early postoperatively will be blood-tinged, gradually becoming clear and decreasing in amount. Sanguineous drainage in any appreciable amount requires the immediate attention of the surgeon. Although more air escapes through the superior catheter, air will be seen bubbling through the water in both bottles. The tubing should be "milked" or stripped in the direction of the water-seal bottle to prevent clots from occluding the tubing.

The nurse must be prepared for two possible emergencies, either one of which will cause a pneumothorax. The catheter may be pulled out of the chest wall, in which case the area must be firmly covered immediately with whatever is available until a snug dressing can be applied. If the tubing is disrupted, the bottle is broken, or the pump fails to function, the catheter must be clamped close to the patient's chest. One or two hemostats must therefore be kept at the bedside for this purpose. The surgeon will, of course, be notified immediately.

The intercostal catheters are usually removed within 48 to 72 hours but may be left in for a longer period if the lung is slow to reexpand. When the lung is reexpanded, as indicated by cessation of fluctuation of water in the water-seal bottle and by x-ray, the catheters are removed by the surgeon, who removes retaining sutures and quickly pulls each catheter from the pleural space. Simultaneously a compression dressing is applied to seal the opening and prevent pneumothorax.

Water-seal drainage is not used for the patient who has had a thoracoplasty, because diseased lung tissue is to be compressed, not reexpanded. After pneumonectomy, serous effusion is inevitable and helps to prevent overdistention of the remaining lung; water-seal drainage may or may not be employed.

Prevention and Detection of Complications. The patient undergoing thoracotomy is subject to all the complications described as a consequence of general anesthesia and major surgery (see Chapter 6). He is especially prone to hemorrhage, shock, atelectasis, and infection of the extensive incision. In addition, certain complications peculiar to pulmonary surgery may occur. A bronchopleural fistula may develop following pulmonary resections and result in pneumothorax (Fig. 46) and empyema. Lobectomy and segmental resections may be complicated by failure of remaining lung tissue to reexpand to fill the space created by surgery. Occasionally, after extensive resections, remaining lung tissue eventually overdistends and reduces pulmonary function. Both types of space-filling problems are treated by collapse procedures. The phrenic nerve may be crushed at the conclusion of a pneumonectomy, or pneumoperitoneum may be used. Thoracoplasty may be performed before, during, or after extensive pulmonary resections.

Proper positioning of the patient during the early postoperative period also helps to prevent complications. The nurse is responsible for

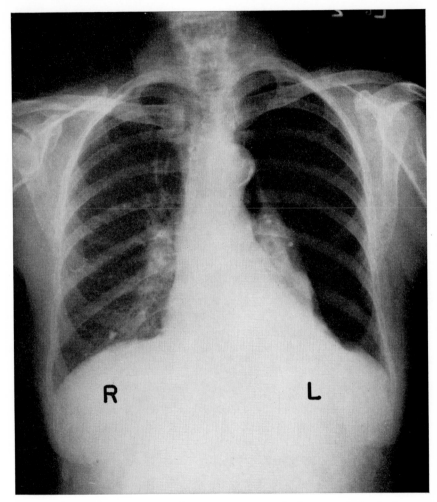

Fig. 46. Pneumothorax. Note in this roentgenogram the large amount of air compressing the left lung.

maintaining the patient comfortably in the positions ordered by the surgeon. There may be no restrictions regarding positioning, but usually following resections the patient is encouraged to lie either in the dorsal recumbent position or toward the side that has been operated on. Such positioning tends to improve respirations, facilitate drainage, reduce the risk of infectious secretions spilling over into the contralateral lung, and decrease the risk of having the remaining lung flooded by the fluid of pleural effusion which forms after pneumonectomy. When the patient is turned toward the side that has been operated on, he must be slightly propped with pillows to avoid compression of the drainage tubes. After subtotal resections for noninfectious conditions, the patient may be placed at intervals on the side that has not been operated on to encourage reexpansion of remaining lung tissue. Following thoracoplasty the patient is turned toward the side of the operation and a small pillow is placed in the axilla to enhance the collapse and to counteract the *scoliosis,* lateral curvature of the vertebral column, which may result. Paradoxical respirations are also counteracted when the patient is lying on the side of the operation against a firm pillow. With few exceptions the head of the bed is elevated to facilitate both respirations and drainage. The patient should be turned at hourly intervals and encouraged to cough and breathe deeply each time a different position is assumed.

The vital signs must be observed closely after thoracotomy. Almost all the complications which may occur may be detected early by noting a change or abnormality in the patient's blood pressure, pulse, and respirations. A rapid pulse is one of the first indications of respiratory distress; both the rate and quality must be noted at frequent intervals. The character of the respirations is very important. The nurse should note and record the rate, depth, and type of breathing, i.e., thoracic or abdominal. Dyspnea, cyanosis, noisy respirations, or a flapping chest wall, which is indicative of paradoxical respirations, must be noted and reported to the surgeon immediately. An increase in pulse and/or respiratory rate, elevation of temperature, and restlessness may indicate shock, hemorrhage, atelectasis, or infection. Dressings should be checked for evidence of bleeding, especially following thoracoplasty.

A portable x-ray film is usually taken daily to observe reexpansion of the lung and dryness of the pleural space, as well as to detect atelectasis and spread or reactivation of pulmonary tuberculosis.

For those patients whose surgery was necessitated by tuberculosis, antibiotic and antituberculosis drug therapy is continued postoperatively. Other patients may be treated by antibiotic drugs to prevent or combat infection.

To prevent overloading of the circulatory system, which imposes an additional strain on the heart and causes pulmonary congestion, fluids are administered sparingly in the early postoperative period. Oral fluids are allowed as soon as the patient has recovered from anesthesia. Thereafter his intake is increased to a full diet as tolerated. An accurate record of intake and output must be kept. Even though surgery has been performed on an area remote from the bladder, the patient may need to be catheterized because of retention due to the effects of general anesthesia.

Activation of the patient is initiated early postoperatively to combat circulatory stasis and other consequences of inactivity. Mr. Jones is allowed to stand to void the first postoperative day, is ambulated on the third day after his chest drainage is discontinued, and is encouraged in mild activity for a week or two. Thereafter he is returned to modified bed rest for 2 to 3 months or longer to complete his therapeutic program for tuberculosis. Some patients are ambulated prior to removal of intercostal catheters. The water-seal bottle must then be carried on a portable apparatus kept well below the level of the chest. When the patient is ambulated, it is important that he be encouraged to assume an erect position with the shoulders held level and with both arms swinging free to counteract postural deformity, which results primarily from the patient's attempt to splint the operated area.

Active and passive exercises are initiated early to prevent postural deformity and ankylosis of the shoulder joint. A physical therapist may be assigned to direct this part of the patient's rehabilitation. These exercises, when ordered, are started early postoperatively with rotation and flexion of the neck, extension and flexion of the fingers, wrist, and forearm, and rotation and elevation of the shoulder. They are gradually increased until the patient enjoys full range of motion in the affected arm. A tendency to scoliosis may require trunk-flexion exercises in the direction of the apex of the scoliotic curve. Leg and foot motion is also encouraged to prevent circulatory stasis, ankylosis and foot drop, and atony.

Another part of the patient's physical rehabilitation program designed to prevent complications by increasing pulmonary efficiency is diaphragmatic breathing. This exercise may be taught preoperatively, initiated early postoperatively, and continued following discharge from the hospital. The patient is taught to lie in dorsal recumbency with one hand on his abdomen and the other on his chest. He must practice breathing so that his abdomen protrudes with each inspiration. With each expiration the patient learns to press inward and upward on his abdomen until in time expiration is accomplished primarily by the abdominal muscles and diaphragm, with the thoracic cage remaining relatively immobile. This exercise is practiced several times daily while the patient is in bed and later while he is ambulatory.

Nursing Care and Teaching in Convalescence

Postoperatively Mr. Jones seemed apprehensive and irritable. He was reluctant to cough or to cooperate in his program of activation. He became very demanding, frequently calling the nurse to check his drainage tubes, to ask if his wife had called, and to request fresh drinking water.

Another nurse might have simply labeled this patient "difficult" and have responded accordingly. However, Mr. Jones's nurse recognized the behavior as a manifestation of extreme apprehension and sought to understand his feelings and possible reasons for them. Knowing that apprehension arises when needs are not being met adequately, the nurse reviewed the areas of human need in relation to this patient. First she considered the patient's physical condition. Difficult and painful respirations are in themselves frightening and tiring; she realized that Mr. Jones was probably reluctant to cough or move because of pain and fatigue. She further realized that his many requests were indications of his need to know that someone was alert to his needs and would take care of him until he could assume his own care.

The nurse revised her plan for the nursing care and teaching of this patient in order to meet his needs more adequately. She could not be with this patient all the time, because she had others in her care, yet she realized that Mr. Jones needed frequent nursing contacts. Therefore, rather than giving this patient his share of her time all at once, the nurse planned her work to allow frequent visits to his bedside. On these brief visits she would check his drainage tubing, change his drinking water or bring him a variety of fluids, and adjust his position. She encouraged him to cough while supporting his incision. Each time she left with a reminder that she would soon return. Frequent nursing contacts like this, even though brief, are reassuring to the patient, because they show him that his nurse is interested in his welfare and is not going to forget him. During the bath the nurse encouraged the patient to talk about his feelings at the level at which he was willing to discuss them. His comments did not lead her to probe, neither did she ignore them. For example, Mr. Jones frequently talked about children forgetting their parents when separated from them. The nurse realized that he was very much concerned lest his sons forget him, but to have asked Mr. Jones if he feared this would have been frightening and would have closed the channels of communication. Instead she repeated the patient's words, saying, "You feel that children forget their parents when separated from them?" This allows the patient to close the conversation or to continue as he desires, but even more important, it indicates the nurse's interest and willingness to listen. The patient may say many things in many ways. Mr. Jones is not really asking to be told that his sons will not forget him; he is asking that someone be interested in him and help him through this surgical experience.

Reassuring the patient is not limited to a few encouraging words. It takes considerable thought but not nearly so much time as many nurses would suppose. Reassurance is given more by the nurse's presence and by the gentle, considerate, kind manner with which she handles the patient than by any words she may speak. It implies empathy, which is conveyed by facial expression, by listening, and by the nurse's touch. The empathetic, reassuring nurse is, as one chaplain expresses it, "being human with another human being." [5]

A rather long convalescent period is usually necessary following pulmonary surgery for the treatment of conditions other than a neoplasm. For a patient like Mr. Jones the convalescent period may extend for many months to achieve arrest of his disease. The patient should be prepared for the fact that convalescence may be prolonged. He must be impressed with the need for maintaining his resistance at an optimal level. He must be helped to accept the need for gradually resuming full activity as his strength increases, for gearing his activity to his respiratory reserve, for maintaining an adequate intake of food and fluids, and for avoiding chilling, overexertion, and fatigue. He should avoid the inhalation of dust or smoke and contacts with persons who have upper respiratory infections. He must remain under close medical supervision and report promptly any symptoms of an upper respiratory infection. Deep-breathing and joint exercises may be continued.

A few patients may be required to change their occupations, especially to avoid heavy labor or undue stress. When this is anticipated, the patient's vocational rehabilitation should begin early in convalescence. Many times an avocation can become a vocation. All patients undergoing prolonged convalescence following pulmonary surgery should be helped to develop interests which provide them with worthwhile diversion without requiring undue exertion.

TRAUMATIC CONDITIONS OF THE THORAX

Injuries to the chest rank second only to those of the head as the leading cause of death due to automotive accidents. The major structures within the thoracic cavity which may be injured include, in addition to the respiratory organs, the contents of the mediastinum, i.e., the heart and great vessels, thoracic duct, and the esophagus. The confining borders of the thoracic cavity, i.e., the diaphragm and ribs, are also subject to trauma. Because of the intimate anatomic and functional relationship of these thoracic structures, a severe injury to one will affect the function of the others.

Types of Trauma

Thoracic contents may be injured by a force exerted from without or within. Perforation or penetration of the chest wall and underlying structures may be caused by a knife, bullet, or spicule of a fractured rib. A

[5] Quoted with permission from Chaplain Jackson Reed, Research and Educational Hospitals, University of Illinois, Chicago.

crushing injury may contuse, compress, tear, or lacerate. A blow to the chest wall may cause *contusion*, bruising, or even *avulsion*, i.e., disruption, of intrathoracic contents. Occasionally instrumentation, as with a bronchoscope or esophagoscope, may perforate the tract through which the instrument is passed. Rupture of the esophagus may result from violent retching, especially when that organ is diseased.

Consequences of Trauma and Treatment

Regardless of the type of injury sustained, the consequences of thoracic trauma usually include bleeding, shock, and decreased efficiency of respirations. Circulatory failure ensues when the heart and/or great vessels have been severely injured.

Hemorrhage. Bleeding may be mild or severe. If mild, bleeding usually subsides with rest; the clot which forms becomes organized and is usually absorbed. Blood in the pleural space, *hemothorax*, is usually aspirated prior to clotting. When a large thrombus forms and is not absorbed, the surgeon may instill streptokinase to lyse the fibrin and allow the blood to be aspirated. Occasionally decortication may be necessary to allow the lung to reexpand.

Even a slight amount of bleeding into the pericardial sac, *hemopericardium*, is serious, because the increasing pressure tamponades the heart and prevents adequate functioning. *Cardiac tamponade,* the restriction of heart action by pressure within the pericardium is evidenced by a decreasing *pulse pressure,* i.e., the difference between systolic and diastolic blood pressures, and by distention of the veins in the neck. Immediate aspiration is imperative.

Persistent or severe hemorrhage requires a thoracotomy to ligate the vessel and repair the wound. Rarely, a pneumonectomy is necessary when irrevocable pulmonary damage has occurred. If damage is not too extensive, the myocardium can be repaired. An injury to a blood vessel may require resection of the injured segment, followed by an end-to-end anastomosis or the insertion of a graft. Oxygen and blood transfusions are administered before, during, and after surgery as necessary.

Mediastinal Shift. An excessive amount of blood or air within the thorax crowds the mediastinal structures toward the side of lesser pressure. There are serious consequences of a mediastinal shift; the tracheobronchial passage may be compressed, closing the patient's airway; lung tissue may be collapsed; the great vessels may be kinked, reducing blood flow to and from the heart, resulting in circulatory collapse and heart failure. Treatment is immediate decompression and/or thoracotomy to ligate the bleeding vessels.

Reduced Efficiency of Respirations. The presence of blood or an exudate within the lung or pleural cavity mechanically hampers respirations. Usually spontaneous absorption occurs. If the fluid is in the pleural cavity, aspirations may be necessary. When the exudate within the pleural cavity is contaminated, the patient is treated as for empyema.

The efficiency of respirations is further decreased when the integrity of the chest wall is weakened, as by a rib fracture. Because immobilization of the chest wall is impossible, even a simple fracture of the rib causes a considerable amount of pain, which causes the patient to take shallow breaths and to ventilate his lungs inadequately. When a double fracture of a rib occurs, a flail chest with paradoxical respirations results. Cough is ineffective, and the resulting retention of secretions further limits the effectiveness of respiratory efforts. For very painful ribs fractures or for those which occur in patients who already have a decreased respiratory exchange, adhesive strapping or rest in bed with a sandbag support to the chest wall may diminish pain. A regional nerve block may be necessary. A flail chest may be treated by skeletal traction.

Traumatic pneumothorax is another condition which limits respiratory efficiency. Pneumothorax results whenever air gains access to the pleural space. This may occur through a torn bronchi or through an open wound. Therefore all open wounds of the chest require the immediate application of an occlusive dressing to prevent pneumothorax. When the wound has a flap acting as a valvular mechanism, air is sucked in faster than it can exit, and a *tension pneumothorax* results. The accumulating air causes collapse of the lung on the affected side and a mediastinal shift to the contralateral side; compression of the contralateral lung may occur. Tension pneumothorax is evidenced by shock, apprehension, rapid pulse and respirations, and cyanosis. Venous distention occurs with angulation of the heart and great vessels. Tension pneumothorax is incompatible with life and must be decompressed prior to transportation to a hospital. In the hospital shock is treated, water-seal drainage is instituted, and the wound is repaired.

Two other conditions which may limit respiratory functioning are emphysema and mediastinitis. *Pulmonary emphysema,* overdistention of the alveoli with air, does not lend itself to surgical treatment. However, *subcutaneous emphysema,* air in the connective tissue spaces under the skin, may require incisions to allow the air which is dissecting the tissues to escape if pressure is being exerted on the structures in the neck. This condition may result from trauma or from an air leak postoperatively. *Crepitation,* an audible sign of subcutaneous emphysema, should be reported to the surgeon promptly. If air is no longer gaining access to the subcutaneous tissues, the condition usually is self-limited and resolves spontaneously. However, a continuing air leak must be found and closed without delay.

Mediastinitis, inflammation of the mediastinal tissues, occurs when bacteria gain access through a wound. Esophageal injuries are especially prone to this complication. The patient is acutely ill with pain, fever, and rapid pulse and respirations. Antibiotic therapy is usually effective.

Gastrointestinal Complications. Symptoms referrable to the gastro-intestinal tract may follow thoracic injuries, because the intercostal nerves also supply a portion of the abdominal wall. The patient may experience abdominal spasm, gastric dilatation, or paralytic ileus. The nurse must report distention or abdominal pain promptly. The fact that gastro-intestinal complications may occur following thoracic injury or surgery should serve as a reminder that the patient functions as a whole. Although patients may be segregated for more efficient care and their conditions mentally compartmentalized for learning purposes, the nurse must realize that she serves the total person, whose needs and functions are inextricably interrelated.

Nursing Care

The principles of care already discussed for the patient undergoing a thoracotomy are applicable to the care of a patient with a chest injury. However, thoracic trauma requires emergency measures, which may include thoracotomy.

After the patient is out of shock he is usually more comfortable in a sitting position, alternating, of course, with periods of full extension. Measures to clear the tracheobronchial tree are instituted. Narcotics are administered in small doses. Oxygen is usually necessary, water-seal drainage may be used, and fluids adequate to meet needs without over-hydration are administered. Esophageal injury or associated gastro-intestinal complications will require, in addition, the use of decompression therapy. The patient requires the same type of close observation described for thoracotomy.

SURGICAL CONDITIONS OF THE ESOPHAGUS

Conditions of the esophagus which may require surgical treatment include obstructive lesions, such as benign stenosis and neoplasms, and diverticula. Stenosis due to cicatrization following trauma, peptic ulceration, or esophagitis is usually treated medically with periodic dilatations, dietary management with fluids and soft foods, and the administration of antispasmodic and antacid medications. If this treatment is ineffective, resection of the involved area is performed, provided the involved segment is not too extensive. Carcinoma of the esophagus is seldom detected early; resection may or may not be feasible. Benign neoplasms are usually resectable.

Symptoms associated with esophageal obstruction include dysphagia and regurgitation and distress after eating.

Esophageal obstruction may necessitate gastrostomy (see pages 91 to 93). If pathology is limited to a short segment, resection and an end-to-end anastomosis may be performed. If a large segment must be resected, various methods may be used to restore continuity. The stomach may be elevated into the thorax for anastomosis. A segment of colon or jejunum may be used as a graft, or synthetic material may be substituted. Sometimes the canal is exteriorized through a tubular skin graft or synthetic tube.

A diverticulum of the esophagus collects food particles, which are later regurgitated undigested. To prevent diverticulitis, perforation, and hemorrhage, diverticula are resected when feasible.

The nursing care of the patient who has had esophageal surgery employs the principles described for both thoracotomy and gastrointestinal surgery. Gastric decompression therapy is used to prevent regurgitation and keep the suture line clean, to encourage healing by splinting the area operated on, and to minimize gastric distress. Meticulous oral hygiene is necessary. Attention to the nutritional, fluid, and electrolytic levels is especially important. A gastrostomy or nasogastric feeding tube may be used. An external graft requires meticulous skin care during the stage of procedure when mucus and saliva drain through an exteriorized cervical esophagus. Catheter suction frequently is employed to collect secretions.

Another condition which involves the esophagus, although indirectly, is a *hiatal hernia*, protrusion of the stomach into the thorax; such protrusion is occasionally accompanied by that of other abdominal viscera, through the esophageal hiatus, or opening, in the diaphragm. The patient experiences regurgitation and respiratory distress in the reclining position, especially after meals. Dysphagia is common. The surgeon attempts to reduce the hernia when possible and to secure the stomach in place within the abdomen. The hiatus is surgically narrowed. Nursing care employs the principles described for thoracotomy, gastrointestinal surgery, and herniorrhaphy.

SUMMARY

Pulmonary surgery may be necessitated by primary neoplastic disease, infections, and injuries. Except for the patient who has an injury requiring emergency surgery, an extensive preoperative evaluation of the systemic and respiratory risk is necessary to establish the diagnosis, and to determine the extent of surgery necessary and possible to treat the disease without producing respiratory crippling. Roentgenographic, bronchoscopic, and pulmonary function studies are performed. The patient who has been chronically ill with tuberculosis or bronchiectasis requires a rather prolonged period of preoperative preparation. The immediate preparation for surgery is the same as that described for laparotomy except for the area of skin prepared and the usual need for antibiotic drug therapy.

Surgical procedures most commonly performed include wedge and segmental resections and lobectomy; pneumonectomy may be necessary. Other procedures performed include drainage of an abscess or empyema pocket, decortication, and thoracoplasty and other types of collapse measures.

Cardiac arrest is a rare surgical emergency which may occur with any surgery, but the incidence is greater with thoracotomy. Cardiac massage is immediately begun by the surgeon, while the anesthesiologist controls respirations. When the spontaneous heart beat is restored, fibrillation not uncommonly occurs and requires the use of an electrical defibrillator.

The postoperative care of a patient who has undergone a thoracotomy centers upon the promotion of an adequate respiratory exchange, the prevention and detection of complications, and the promotion of lung reexpansion except for those patients who have had a thoracoplasty or pneumonectomy. The most common complications include hemorrhage, shock, atelectasis, bronchopleural fistula, and underexpansion or overexpansion of the lung; following thoracoplasty, a planned program of exercises may be necessary to prevent postural deformity. Water-seal drainage is used to promote reexpansion of the lung by draining the pleural space. The nurse must observe the system frequently to ensure proper functioning. She must be familiar with emergency measures necessary should the catheter be dislodged or the drainage system be interrupted. Vital signs must be recorded at frequent intervals, and the character of the pulse and respirations must be noted. It is important that oversedation and overhydration be prevented. The activation regime is initiated early. Prior to discharge the patient must be taught hygienic measures necessary following pulmonary surgery.

Some of the serious consequences of pulmonary trauma are hemothorax, hemopericardium, pneumothorax, mediastinal shift, flail chest, and mediastinitis. Shock and hemorrhage must be treated promptly, followed by aspiration of air and blood, and restoration of the integrity of the chest wall. Thoracotomy may be necessary to control hemorrhage and repair the injury.

Esophageal surgery is performed in the treatment of neoplastic disease, diverticulum, or hiatal hernia. Principles of care required for gastrointestinal surgery and thoracotomy are employed.

BIBLIOGRAPHY

The Lungs

BASINGER, C., and W. E. ADAMS: Pneumonectomy, Lobectomy, and Segmental Resection, S. Clin. North America, vol. 35, no. 1, pp. 41–48, February, 1955.

BISHOP, C. A.: Cancer of the Lung, J. Thoracic Surg., vol. 33, no. 3, pp. 330–340, March, 1957.

BLADES, B., and O. GWATHMEY: The Thoracic Wall, Pleura, and Lungs, in "Christopher's Textbook of Surgery," 6th ed., L. Davis (ed.), W. B. Saunders Company, Philadelphia, 1956, chap. 16, pp. 414–428.

FARBER, S. M.: "Lung Cancer," Charles C Thomas, Publisher, Springfield, Ill., 1954.

FORSEE, J. H.: "The Surgery of Pulmonary Tuberculosis," Lea & Febiger, Philadelphia, 1954.

HECKEL, E., and E. H. FELL: Cardiac Arrest during Surgical Operations, S. Clin. North America, vol. 35, no. 1, pp. 243–252, February, 1955.

HINSHAW, H. C., and L. H. GARLAND: "Diseases of the Chest," W. B. Saunders Company, Philadelphia, 1956.

MERENDINO, K. A.: Lung, in "Surgery," J. G. Allen, H. N. Harkins, C. A. Moyer, and J. E. Rhoads (eds.), J. B. Lippincott Company, Philadelphia, 1957, chap. 42, pp. 1120–1163.

NACLERIO, E. A. (ed.): "Bronchopulmonary Diseases," Paul B. Hoeber, Inc., New York, 1957.

NOVAK, M. L.: Social and Emotional Problems of Patients with Tuberculosis, Nursing Outlook, vol. 6, no. 4, pp. 210–211, April, 1958.

OATWAY, W. H.: Aseptic Technic in the Care of Tuberculosis Patients, Am. J. Nursing, pp. 164–166, March, 1950.

Physical Therapy for Thoracic Surgery Patients, Veterans Administration Pamphlet 10–22, Dec. 31, 1947.

SLOAN, H., and M. E. BLACKBURN: The Patient with Bronchiectasis, Am. J. Nursing, pp. 561–564, May, 1955.

STEELE, J. D. (ed.): "The Surgical Management of Pulmonary Tuberculosis," Charles C Thomas, Publisher, Springfield, Ill., 1957.

SWEET, R. H.: "Thoracic Surgery," 2d ed., W. B. Saunders Company, Philadelphia, 1954.

"Thoracic Surgery Seminar," United States Army, Fitzsimmons Army Hospital, Denver, 1952.

WATERMAN, D. H., S. E. DOMM, and W. K. ROGERS: A Clinical Evaluation of Decortication, J. Thoracic Surg., vol. 33, no. 1, pp. 1–16, January, 1957.

WYLIE, R. H., and J. L. ANKENEY: Emergency Care of Chest Injuries, S. Clin. North America, vol. 35, no. 2, pp. 517–528, April, 1955.

The Esophagus

BERMAN, E. F.: Carcinoma of the Esophagus, a New Concept in Therapy, Surgery, vol. 35, no. 5, pp. 822–835, May, 1954.

BOYD, D. P., and L. D. HILL: Benign Tumors and Cysts of the Esophagus, Am. J. Surg., vol. 93, no. 2, pp. 252–257, February, 1957.

——— and B. F. WOOLDRIDGE: Congenital Diaphragmatic Hernia in Adults, Surg., Gynec. & Obst., vol. 101, no. 5, pp. 536–540, November, 1955.

CARSWELL, JR., J., R. P. HAYS, and W. N. VIAR: Notes on Conservation of Gastric and Duodenal Function in Palliative Esophageal Reconstruction, *Surgery*, vol. 37, no. 2, pp. 208–212, February, 1955.

DOBRUSHIN, D. J.: Diaphragmatic Hernia—Nursing Care, *Am. J. Nursing*, pp. 185–186, February, 1956.

HOLINGER, P. H., and K. C. JOHNSTON: Laryngology and Bronchoesophagology, in "The Recovery Room," M. S. Sadove and J. H. Cross (eds.), W. B. Saunders Company, Philadelphia, 1956, chap. 8, pp. 243–258.

HOLMES, G. W.: Diaphragmatic Hernia, *Am. J. Nursing*, pp. 183–184, February, 1956.

MAHONEY, E. B., and C. D. SHERMAN, JR.: Total Esophagoplasty Using Intrathoracic Right Colon, *Surgery*, vol. 35, no. 6, pp. 937–946, June, 1954.

MATHEWSON, JR., C., W. C. SCHAUPP, F. C. DIMOND, and S. W. FRENCH, III: Traumatic Rupture of the Esophagus, *Am. J. Surg.*, vol. 93, no. 4, pp. 616–621, April, 1957.

PUESTOW, C. B., and W. J. GILLESBY: Surgical Lesions of the Esophagus, *S. Clin. North America*, vol. 35, no. 1, pp. 67–78, February, 1955.

SOM, M. L., and L. M. ARNOLD: Esophagoscopy in the Diagnosis and Treatment of Esophageal Diseases, *Am. J. Surg.*, vol. 93, no. 2, pp. 183–195, February, 1957.

STOREY, C. F., and W. C. ADAMS, JR.: Leiomyoma of the Esophagus, *Am. J. Surg.*, vol. 91, no. 1, pp. 3–22, January, 1956.

SWEET, R. H.: Esophagus, in "Christopher's Textbook of Surgery," 6th ed., L. Davis (ed.), W. B. Saunders Company, Philadelphia, 1956, chap. 20, The Alimentary Canal, pp. 577–589.

WATSON, W. L., and J. T. GOODNER: Carcinoma of the Esophagus, *Am. J. Surg.*, vol. 93, no. 2, pp. 259–265, February, 1957.

WOODWARD, F. D.: Diseases of the Esophagus, *Clinical Symposia*, Ciba Pharmaceutical Products, Inc., Summit, N.J., vol. 8, no. 1, pp. 3–29, January–February, 1956.

17

SURGERY OF THE MEDIASTINUM, II; THE SURGICAL CARDIAC PATIENT

Patients who are referred for heart surgery are those suspected of having operable congenital or acquired conditions which are interfering with the normal flow of blood through the heart and great vessels to such a degree that the patient's activity is markedly limited or his health and life are endangered. The development of technics which permit detection and surgical correction of congenital and acquired conditions of the heart and great vessels (Fig. 47) has improved the prognosis for life and usefulness for great numbers of patients. Cardiac surgery is a newly developing field which holds promise for removing heart disease from its place as the greatest single cause of death among all age groups.

PREOPERATIVE EVALUATION

Under most circumstances a surgeon and internist or cardiologist usually work together, particularly in the area of preoperative evaluation and postoperative care. Through this teamwork the diagnosis, operability, and preparation of the patient are worked out. The preoperative status of the patient must be thoroughly evaluated, not only to detect deficiencies which must be corrected to bring the patient to his optimal condition but also to determine whether the cardiovascular lesion is operable and whether the patient can withstand cardiac surgery.

Medical History and Physical Examination

An evaluation of the duration and degree of disability due to heart disease is important in the determination of the risk of surgery. It is important, therefore, that the surgeon know of any history of rheumatic fever, bacterial endocarditis, or repeated pneumonia. He must know how many attacks of congestive heart failure the patient may have had and when, what treatment he has received, and how well he has compensated after each attack. The patient may not volunteer this information when the history is taken, because it is difficult to recall such details under the stress of a physical evaluation conducted by a surgeon who may not have been known previously by the patient. However, in the course of close nursing contacts, the patient may recall important facts, which the nurse must relay to the surgeon.

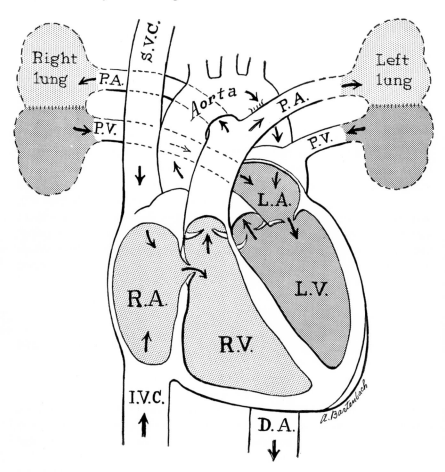

FIG. 47. Schematic representation of the heart and great vessels in section, viewed from the front.

Since the amount of cardiac reserve can be approximated by the patient's response to exercise, the surgeon will be especially interested in the patient's ability to exert himself without experiencing dyspnea. He will ask the number of stairs that can be climbed easily and how far the patient can walk on a flat plane without undue fatigue or difficult breathing. Exercise-tolerance tests may be conducted to note the amount of activity necessary to produce dyspnea.

In his physical examination of the patient the physician will determine the size and position of the heart as well as the rate and rhythm of its beat. Evidences of dyspnea and edema may indicate congestive heart failure. Valvular dysfunction produces characteristic murmurs. In some conditions, blood pressure studies are very important. For example, *coarctation of the aorta*, an abnormal localized narrowing of the aorta, may be detected by a higher blood pressure in the arms than in the legs, a reverse of the normal pattern. Therefore, pressure readings may be taken on both arms and one leg.

Laboratory Tests

As a part of the total evaluation, urinalyses, complete blood counts, determinations of hemoglobin content, and blood chemistry analyses are usually ordered. Bleeding and coagulation times in addition to pro-thrombin times may be determined to detect bleeding tendencies that might be troublesome during surgery. Blood serum tests are ordered to detect syphilis, which may be present and which can cause serious cardiac abnormalities. Sedimentation rates and blood cultures may be studied to note the presence and activity of infection. Basal metabolic rate determinations may be ordered to rule out hyperthyroidism as the cause of the cardiac condition.

Circulation Time. A determination of the time taken by blood to pass from one point to another in the circulatory system is a valuable aid in diagnosing certain cardiac lesions and in evaluating their severity. The time taken for a substance to travel from the antecubital vein through the heart and lungs to the pharyngeal arteries is called the *arm-to-tongue* time. Decholin, a 20 per cent solution of sodium dehydrocholate, is commonly used. This solution is injected into the antecubital vein, with the patient lying supine, and the time taken to reach the tongue to produce a bitter taste is noted. The average normal arm-to-tongue time is between 10 and 20 seconds. If a longer period of time is taken, an obstruction may be indicated; a shorter time suggests an over-riding aorta or abnormal communication. The *arm-to-lung* time is measured, commonly, with ether in saline solution. This solution is injected into the antecubital vein, and the ether vapor is normally noted in expired air in approximately 3 to 8 seconds. Both circulation times may be measured simultaneously and the findings compared.

Roentgenologic Diagnostic Procedures. Roentgenographic and fluoroscopic examinations are used to delineate the size, position, and shape of the heart. Lesions of the heart and great vessels produce characteristic roentgenologic findings which can be appreciated by taking several different views of the chest. The usual views employed are posteroanterior, left lateral, and left and right anterior oblique. These views are usually taken with barium in the esophagus to note the presence of an anomalous vessel constricting the esophagus or displacement of the esophagus by an enlarged heart chamber.

Angiocardiography. Visualization of blood flow through the heart can be accomplished by injecting a radiopaque substance into a peripheral vein and making a rapid series of x-ray exposures. This procedure helps in the detection of abnormal communications and obstructions. To permit a heavier concentration of the contrast medium within the heart local angiocardiography is used. In this procedure, a catheter is introduced, under aseptic precautions, into the right or left side of the heart, and the contrast medium is injected directly into the chamber being studied. Simultaneously, serial x-ray films record the progress of the flow of the contrast medium and reveal abnormal communications and obstructions. The patient is prepared for this procedure by premedication with a sedative or narcotic. The preceding meal is omitted, and fluids are withheld for 2 hours prior to the procedure. Following the procedure, vomiting and urticaria are occasionally noted.

Aortography. This procedure is similar to angiocardiography. The patient is prepared in a similar manner. Postoperatively, occasionally, the same problems will follow. A catheter is threaded into the thoracic aorta by way of the radial or femoral artery, and the contrast medium is injected. Aortography is useful in detecting the exact location of an aneurysm, abnormal communication, or obstruction.

Cardiac Catheterization. In this procedure, a radiopaque catheter is threaded, under fluoroscopic control and with strict aseptic technic, into the great vessels and chambers of the heart by way of a peripheral vein. At times, abnormal communication, such as an atrial septal defect, may be noted when the catheter passes into the left atrium from the right. Pressure measurements are taken within the various areas of the heart, and blood samples are withdrawn for oxygen determinations. These determinations and similar ones made in the peripheral vessels and aorta are compared with normal ones, permitting more accurate diagnoses. The left atrium may be reached by direct needle puncture from behind through the main-stem bronchus by way of a bronchoscope. The left ventricle is entered by needle puncture anteriorly.

In preparation for cardiac catheterization, the preceding meal is omitted, and a mild sedative is administered. Sufficient explanation must be given to allow the patient to be relaxed and cooperative. However, many of these patients are extremely apprehensive, and some may be in a precarious condition with regard to their cardiac status; detailed explanation may be more frightening than reassuring for such patients.

Therefore, the nurse must confer with the surgeon to learn how much explanation he has given the patient; the nurse must not overstep the limits of this instruction. Following cardiac catheterization, the vital signs must be observed and recorded at frequent intervals.

Other Specialized Diagnostic Procedures. Many specialized procedures are used to investigate cardiac function. For a more complete list and for greater detail, the reader is referred to the bibliography.

Electrocardiography. The electrocardiogram is a record of electrical changes associated with the heart beat. As the electrical impulse spreads out over the heart, characteristic waves are recorded on the electrocardiogram. Interference with the conduction of this impulse can be detected, and abnormal rhythms can be recognized. The efficiency of coronary circulation can be evaluated by performing functional tests along with electrocardiography. The most common of these is the Master's two-step test, in which the patient is asked to walk up and down a two-step stool; electrocardiographic tracings precede and follow this activity.

Phonocardiography. The phonocardiogram is an electronic phonetic representation of the sounds produced by the heart. This record enables a more accurate determination of the timing of sounds referable to systole and diastole.

Ballistocardiography. A ballistocardiogram is a record of the recoil of the body in response to the ejection of blood from the heart into the pulmonary artery and aorta. These movements are magnified, recorded, and calibrated. The ballistocardiogram permits a rough calculation of cardiac output and stroke volume.

PREOPERATIVE PREPARATION

All patients require considerable reassurance and support in their decision to undergo elective surgery. The majority of adult patients undergoing heart surgery are aware of the limitations imposed by their condition and are eager to have treatment which well may restore them to a fuller life. However, they are also aware of the risk of surgery, which has been dramatically presented in current means of public communication. Actually, for the well-selected, noncomplicated candidate, the risk is comparable to that associated with gastrectomy, pneumonectomy, and other procedures of similar magnitude. In addition, the nurse must realize that the heart is regarded by many as the seat of the soul, which also influences the patient's concern. The nurse must encourage free channels of communication for the patient to aid him in expressing his concerns. Spiritual therapy must be obtained when requested.

Some patients may require digitalization, restriction of sodium and fluid intake, and the administration of diuretic drugs. Antibiotic drugs may be ordered prior to surgery. The immediate preparation is as described for thoracotomy in the preceding chapter. The incision is usually extensive. A bilateral thoracotomy may be necessary. The skin preparation will vary, and the nurse should consult with the surgeon to learn the area that must be prepared.

METHODS OF ANESTHESIA AND OPERATIVE TECHNICS

The immediate preparation of the patient for surgery of the heart or great vessels includes the placement of infusion cannulas to allow for the administration of fluids and medications and the placement of electrocardiographic leads to permit constant observation of cardiac functioning. Endotracheal intubation is necessary, not only to ensure a patent airway but also to permit the anesthesiologist to manage respiratory functioning for the patient when the thorax is open. Light general inhalation or intravenous anesthesia is used. Surgery is performed using either the closed or open technic.

The Closed Technic for Intracardiac Surgery

In the closed technic, repair is made without direct visualization of the defect or valve. A purse-string suture is applied at the base of the auricular appendage. As the appendage is opened and the surgeon introduces his finger through this incision, the purse string is drawn snug to prevent bleeding.

Intracardiac Surgery under Direct Vision

Open cardiotomy, which permits the correction of acquired and congenital defects under direct vision, is being used with greater frequency as the risks involved with this method are being reduced. To achieve a dry operative field one of the following methods is used: inflow occlusion, hypothermia, or cardiopulmonary bypass. Inflow occlusion, the clamping of the venae cavae, is feasible for a 3-minute period without risking severe ischemic changes. The use of *hypothermia*, the induction of a significant reduction in body temperature, lowers the metabolic demands for oxygen and permits inflow occlusion for a maximum period of 6 minutes. Cardiac defects which require longer than this to repair necessitate the use of some method of bypassing the heart and lungs while maintaining circulation to the rest of the body.

Hypothermia. The therapeutic reduction of body temperature to between 29 and 34°C. (84.2 and 93.2°F.) can be achieved by one of several methods. Surface-cooling measures include immersing the patient in a tub of ice water or using a refrigeration blanket. Direct cooling of blood

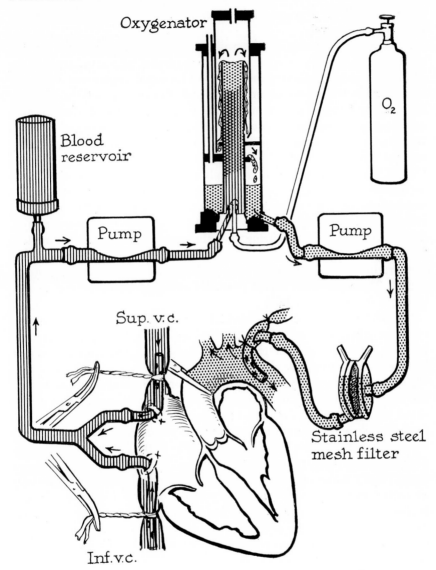

FIG. 48. Diagrammatic representation of a heart-lung machine.

is another way to induce hypothermia. Venous blood is diverted through a cooling coil in a mechanical pump and returned to the patient's venous system.

Hypothermia requires the use of a special temperature-recording device to permit constant observation of temperature changes. The thermistor is placed in the esophagus or rectosigmoid prior to the induction of hypothermia and is left in place until the temperature has stabilized at normal levels postoperatively.

Rewarming following hypothermia is generally accomplished by the same devices used to cool the patient except that heat is substituted for cold. Short-wave diathermy may be used for rapid rewarming. Profound alterations in physiology occur during both the cooling and the rewarming periods. Cardiac arrhythmias, especially ventricular fibrillation, may occasionally occur. Electrolyte and acid-base balance is disturbed. The temperature may overshoot in either direction. Drugs used during surgery are not detoxified readily and may prolong the period of anesthesia. During the crucial period immediately postoperatively the patient must be constantly attended. The nurse must observe the temperature, pulse, respirations, and blood pressure at 5-minute intervals until circulatory sufficiency and stability are assured. She must watch for hemorrhage, shock, and atelectasis, realizing that the usual signs of these complications may be disguised by the effects of hypothermia, i.e., pallor, elevated temperature, increased pulse rate, and depressed respirations are expected. The nurse must report promptly any evidence of a burn or disturbance in sensory function.

Hypothermia has real value especially for the adult patient undergoing repair of a limited number of congenital anomalies. This procedure may be used for either open or closed intracardiac surgery, with or without the use of a heart-lung machine. (See Fig. 48.)

Cardiopulmonary Bypass. Two methods are commonly used to bypass the heart and lungs. In one procedure, blood flow is intercepted at the venae cavae, rerouted through a mechanical pump-oxygenator, and returned to the aorta. Depending upon which vessels are cannulated, selective bypassing of either the right or left side of the heart can be accomplished. Safety features are incorporated within the pump-oxygenator to control the volume and rate of blood being circulated and to prevent air embolism and clotting. The other method of cardiopulmonary bypass is that of continuous arterial reservoir perfusion. Arterial blood, which has been collected from several donors preoperatively, is pumped into the patient's arterial system while venous blood is collected from the cannulated venae cavae.

OPERABLE ACQUIRED CONDITIONS OF THE HEART AND GREAT VESSELS

Mitral Stenosis

One of the most common of the acquired conditions of the heart is *mitral stenosis*, a narrowing of the valve which separates the left atrium from the left ventricle. This condition is due to rheumatic fever valvulitis with subsequent cicatrization of the valvular leaflets.

Obstruction of blood flow from the left atrium results in a reduced cardiac output. As the degree of stenosis becomes more severe, the pressure within the left atrium increases and is transmitted back through the pulmonary bed and thence to the right ventricle. This is an insidious process with symptoms gradually increasing in severity. The patient will experience fatigue and exertional dyspnea. Many of the patients will have experienced episodes of palpitation, pulmonary edema, paroxysmal nocturnal dyspnea, cough, and hemoptysis. If the obstruction is not relieved, pressure is transmitted to the right ventricle and atrium, and right heart failure occurs, evidenced by peripheral edema, venous dis-

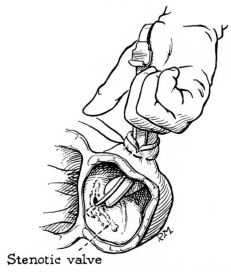

Stenotic valve

Fig. 49. Valvulotomy used in the treatment of a stenotic valve.

tention, ascites, and hepatomegaly. With marked mitral stenosis, life expectancy is greatly foreshortened. In the absence of active rheumatic carditis, severe disease of the valves, marked mitral regurgitation, or intractable heart failure, surgery can improve the patient's chances for a longer, more active life.

Mitral stenosis is identified on the basis of characteristic heart sounds, including a diastolic murmur, and roentgenographic evidence of enlargement of the left atrium and right ventricle. The electrocardiogram usually reveals right ventricular hypertrophy, but may be normal; auricular fibrillation may be detected. If cardiac catheterization is performed, the pressures within the pulmonary artery and capillaries are found to be increased; cardiac output is reduced.

Surgery is designed to open the valve as much as possible to permit an adequate blood flow without producing an incompetent valve with mitral regurgitation. (See Fig. 49.) *Commissurotomy,* separation along the lines of fusion between the valvular leaflets, is performed without direct vision under general anesthesia. The commissures may be separated by pressure as the surgeon forces his finger through the valve, or the lines of fusion may be cut by a specially designed scalpel which is attached to the surgeon's operating finger.

Peripheral arterial embolism is not uncommon during surgery of the mitral valve. Episodes of auricular fibrillation are conducive to the formation of thrombi in the left auricular appendage. The auricular appendage is flushed out at the beginning of surgery and is commonly amputated at the close of the operation to remove this source of emboli. Postoperatively the nurse must be particularly observant for evidences of arterial embolism. The patient may have signs of a cerebral vascular accident. Peripheral arterial embolism is manifested most commonly by sharp excruciating pain in an extremity, followed by pallor, coldness, numbness, and absence of pulses distad to the site.

Mitral Insufficiency

The competency of the mitral valve may be destroyed by left ventricular hypertrophy, rheumatic valvulitis, with or without mitral stenosis, and by calcification of the valvular leaflets. The consequent retraction of the leaflets, shortening of the chordae tendinae, or dilatation of the mitral annulus, the ring supporting the leaflets, prevents the leaflets from contacting each other during systole. Therefore, with each contraction of the left ventricle, blood is regurgitated into the left atrium, markedly reducing the volume of ventricular output and causing aneurysmal dilatation of the atrium. The left ventricle undergoes hypertrophy and dilatation. Symptoms of severe mitral insufficiency are similar to those of mitral stenosis. Unrelieved severe mitral insufficiency eventuates in heart failure and death. One method of correcting mitral insufficiency is by placing approximating sutures around the incompetent pole of the mitral annulus. This procedure draws the leaflets closer together and permits more normal leaflet action. (See Fig. 50.)

Aortic Stenosis

Aortic stenosis is most commonly the result of rheumatic fever valvulitis or atherosclerosis. Symptoms are similar to those produced by mitral stenosis but more severe because of the strain imposed upon the left ventricle. The thickened cusps of the aortic valve obstruct the systolic discharge of blood from the left ventricle, which undergoes hypertrophy. As resistance to outflow increases, the adequacy of both systemic and coronary circulation is reduced. Coronary insufficiency causes anginal pain and even sudden death. Severe conduction disturbances are common. Unrelieved severe aortic stenosis eventuates in left ventricular failure.

If the degree of stenosis is mild, the patient may live a normal span of years. However, a stenosis which seems to be becoming progressively more severe requires surgical intervention.

Aortic commissurotomy is performed by using the finger, dilator, or scalpel. The approach is through the ventricle or the aorta. The risk is higher than in mitral disease because of the basic strain imposed upon the left ventricle.

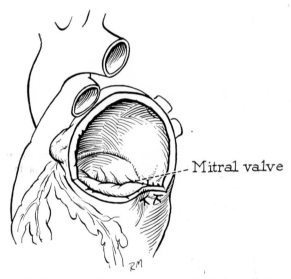

Mitral valve

Fig. 50. Cross polar fusion used in the treatment of mitral insufficiency. Note in this diagram the sutures approximating one end of the mitral annulus.

Aortic Insufficiency

Aortic insufficiency is most commonly the result of rheumatic fever valvulitis or syphilitic aortitis. Incompetence of the valve permits regurgitation of blood, resulting in dilatation of the left ventricle. The left ventricle hypertrophies in an attempt to maintain an adequate circulation. In time, however, the systolic discharge is markedly reduced, resulting in coronary insufficiency. Left ventricular failure occurs eventually when a severe degree of aortic insufficiency is not relieved.

Direct approaches to repairing the aortic valve are still experimental. The most universal method of reducing aortic regurgitation is by the insertion of a synthetic valve into the descending aorta, just distad to the left subclavian artery. Hufnagel's valve is essentially a modified tube with a ball-type valve. (See Fig. 51.) During systole the ball moves away from the proximal opening, permitting blood flow, and returns to its seat in diastole, preventing backflow. The insertion of the valve is performed under general anesthesia and requires brief occlusion of the aorta by noncrushing clamps. The results from this surgery have been promising. Symptoms are relieved, further damage from regurgitation is halted, and the patient gains strength. This valve does create a continuous click-

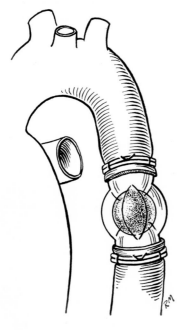

FIG. 51. Diagram showing the Hufnagel valve placed in the aorta to relieve aortic insufficiency.

ing sound, as the ball moves back and forth with each ejection of blood from the left ventricle. This sound is audible, but the patient learns to accept this.

Coronary Occlusion

Occlusion of a coronary artery, most commonly by a thrombus superimposed upon atherosclerosis, results in an area of myocardial ischemia followed by infarction, death of the tissues supplied by the involved artery. Death may occur with the initial attack. However, the majority of patients survive and return to their previous occupations after a prolonged period of rest and gradual resumption of activity.

During the period of rest, a collateral circulation develops to substitute for the occluded artery. However, if an adequate collateral circulation fails to develop, as evidenced by continued episodes of pain with exertion and prolonged physical incapacity, or if repeated attacks of arterial occlusion occur, surgical intervention is indicated.

The aim of surgery is to establish an efficient collateral blood supply. This may be accomplished by one of several methods. A chronic inflammatory pericarditis may be produced by dusting the visceral pericardium with sterile magnesium silicate powder. The granulation tissue which forms is the source of fine capillaries which penetrate into the myocardium to enrich the blood supply. Another method of stimulating collateral circulation is that of grafting a highly vascular structure to the heart. When coronary angiography demonstrates segmental atherosclerotic occlusion of one major vessel, *endarterectomy* may be performed using a cardiopulmonary bypass. In this procedure an instrument called a stripper is introduced into the vessel and is withdrawn with the avulsed atherosclerotic placque and lining. Heparinization prevents thrombosis.

Pericarditis

Inflammation of the pericardium may be secondary to trauma, tuberculosis, rheumatic fever, or septicemia. Two types of pericarditis are treated surgically, namely, acute pericarditis with purulent effusion and chronic constrictive pericarditis.

An accumulation of fluid within the pericardial space causes cardiac compression with failing heart action, rising venous pressure, and the development of ascites and peripheral edema. A purulent effusion, which will not subside with medical management nor respond adequately to pericardicentesis, requires pericardiostomy to permit irrigation and the instillation of antibiotic solutions.

In chronic constrictive pericarditis the formation of fibrous scar tissue restricts the movements of the heart. Symptoms depend upon the extent and location of fibrosis. Pericardectomy is performed to permit unembarrassed cardiac activity.

OPERABLE CONGENITAL ANOMALIES IN ADULTS

Congenital anomalies of the heart and great vessels are far less common than acquired conditions. They comprise less than 3 per cent of all organic heart lesions. They are usually corrected more easily in childhood prior to the onset of repeated attacks of decompensation, atherosclerosis, and associated changes. However, surgery is successfully performed in adulthood.

Patent Ductus Arteriosus

The ductus arteriosus is a communicating vessel between the fetal pulmonary artery and aorta. The fetal lungs require only enough blood circulation to sustain their growth, since the placenta performs the function of oxygen, nutrient, and waste exchange between fetal and maternal circulation. Consequently, the greater volume of blood is shunted from the pulmonary artery directly into the aorta through the ductus arteriosus for immediate systemic circulation. After birth, when the lungs expand and assume their function, this shunt is no longer necessary, and the duct normally closes within the first few weeks of postnatal life. Failure of the duct to close results in a shunting of blood from the aorta back into the pulmonary circulation, because the pressure of blood in the aorta exceeds that in the pulmonary artery after birth and causes a reversal of the direction of the prenatal flow. Blood is then rerouted through the pulmonary circuit in amounts proportionate to the size of the shunt. The additional volume of blood being recirculated increases the work of the left ventricle, which in turn increases the size, output, and work of the left side of the heart. Heart failure may develop. Subacute bacterial endarteritis, inflammation of the inner arterial coat, may be superimposed but usually responds well to antibiotic drug therapy.

The majority of patients have no symptoms. However, if the shunt is large, the patient may experience easy fatigability and exertional dyspnea.

The diagnosis is made on the basis of clinical findings. There is a harsh "machinery-like" murmur, and frequently a wide pulse pressure is found when the shunt is large. The diagnosis may be confirmed by cardiac catheterization when an increased oxygenation is detected in the pulmonary artery. Angiocardiography or retrograde aortography may be necessary to demonstrate the ductus.

The treatment is surgical division of the ductus with suturing of the severed ends or multiple ligation. (See Fig. 52.)

Coarctation of the Aorta

Congenital stenosis, *coarctation*, of the aorta occurs either immediately proximal or distad to the ductus arteriosus, which may be open or closed. Blood flow distad to the coarctation is maintained by an extensive *collateral circulation*, i.e., smaller vessels dilate to assume the function of the larger vessel which they accompany.

Coarctation of the aorta produces no symptoms early. In time, a fixed hypertension of the upper extremities develops, and the patient may experience headaches, dizziness, palpitation, and dyspnea. In some patients the legs may be underdeveloped in comparison to the arms because of lesser blood supply. Diminished blood flow to the lower extremities results in absent or negligible femoral pulses and cold feet.

The diagnosis can frequently be made on the basis of blood pressure studies on the arms and legs. As has been stated, the blood pressure is higher in the arms. A systolic murmur is usually heard. X-ray may reveal erosion of the ribs by the collateral circulation. When the extent and size of the lesion can not be determined with accuracy, angiocardiography or aortography may be necessary to demonstrate the lesion. The prognosis for these patients is grave. Cerebral hemorrhage may result from the proximal hypertension. Left ventricular failure or rupture of the left ventricle and/or aorta may occur. Without surgical intervention, over one-third of these patients will die before the age of thirty years; the

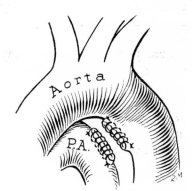

Fig. 52. Diagram showing the treatment of patent ductus by surgical division.

other two-thirds will probably be invalids throughout the remainder of their shortened life span. Surgery is performed most satisfactorily in childhood or adolescence prior to the development of irreversible cardiovascular degenerative changes.

At surgery, noncrushing clamps are applied proximad and distad to the site of the coarctation, and the segment is resected. Aortic continuity is reestablished by an end-to-end anastomosis, or, if the segment is long, by a graft. A synthetic material, such as nylon, orlon, dacron, or teflon, may be used to fashion a graft. Sometimes an *arterial homograft* is used. This homograft is prepared from the aorta of a person who died free from infection or arterial disease, is subjected to lyophilization, i.e., freeze-drying, and then is stored for future use.

Pulmonary Stenosis

Stenosis of the valve between the main trunk of the pulmonary artery and the right ventricle may occur as a separate entity or may be associated with other anomalies, such as narrowing of the ventricular outlet, i.e., the infundibulum, and/or interatrial or interventricular septal defects.

Pure pulmonary stenosis is well tolerated by many patients; some may never be symptomatic. However, a marked degree of stenosis imposes upon the right ventricle a greater work load in order to eject blood through the small opening into the pulmonary circuit. Cardiac output, therefore, tends to be reduced, and the patient may experience fatigue and dyspnea with exertion. Right heart failure may occur.

The diagnosis is made on the basis of a characteristic systolic murmur, electrocardiographic evidence of right ventricular hypertrophy, and post-stenotic dilatation of the pulmonary artery, as well as poor vascularity in the lung fields as revealed by x-ray. To confirm the diagnosis, it may be necessary to perform cardiac catheterization, which reveals increased systolic pressures within the right ventricle and decreased systolic pressure within the pulmonary artery. Angiocardiography may visualize the obstruction.

Pure pulmonary stenosis may be corrected without direct vision by passing a specially designed scalpel through an incision in the right ventricle and then through the pulmonary valve. Some surgeons prefer to open the valve under direct vision using hypothermia or some method of artificial circulation. Infundibular pulmonary stenosis requires surgery under direct vision to remove a portion of the muscular septum; a plastic repair may be necessary.

Atrial Septal Defect

A direct communication existing between the atria most commonly results in a *left-to-right shunt*, i.e., some of the oxygenated blood returns to the right atrium to be recirculated through the right ventricle, pulmonary arteries, and lungs. If the volume of blood thus shunted is large, a strain is imposed upon the right ventricle.

The patient may be asymptomatic, but if the defect is large, signs and symptoms of cardiac failure develop. X-ray and fluoroscopy commonly reveal an enlarged pulmonary artery and increased vascularity in the lung fields. A characteristic murmur may be detected. Cardiac catheterization is used to make the definitive diagnosis. In this procedure the catheter may pass through the defect. An immediate increase in arterial saturation is noted as the catheter enters the right atrium; no further increase is noted as the catheter passes through the right ventricle and into the pulmonary artery. The systolic pressure is the same in both the right ventricle and the pulmonary artery.

The defect may be repaired without direct vision by suturing part of the atrial wall as a patch. Open cardiotomy with direct visualization of the defect permits suturing the edges of the opening together or inserting a graft of compressed polyvinyl sponge to close the opening.

Tetralogy of Fallot

The prefix *tetra-* means "four." Tetralogy of Fallot is a complex anomaly composed of pulmonary stenosis, hypertrophy of the right ventricle, a ventricular septal defect, and an overriding aorta which arises from both ventricles. (See Fig. 53.)

Primarily this condition results in a right-to-left shunt. Blood from the right ventricle is shunted directly into the aorta in amounts proportionate

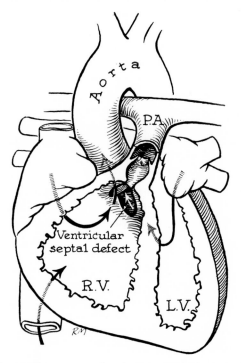

FIG. 53. Tetralogy of Fallot. Note in this diagram of the heart in frontal section the hypertrophied right ventricle, over-riding aorta, atrial septal defect, and pulmonary stenosis.

to the size of the shunt and the degree of pulmonary stenosis, which combine to prevent an adequate amount of blood from passing through the lungs. The oxygen content of systemic arterial blood is seriously reduced by the mixing. In an attempt to compensate for the decreased oxygen content of arterial blood, a compensatory polycythemia develops.

The patient shows evidence of oxygen deficiency, with easy fatigability, exertional dyspnea, cyanosis, clubbing of the fingers and toes, and underdevelopment. A murmur may be detected. A squatting posture is commonly assumed by the patient when overactivity has increased his dyspnea and exhaustion.

Early surgery can restore the patient's chances for a reasonably normally long and useful life. Without surgical intervention, death occurs for the majority of patients before twenty-five years of age and follows a life of invalidism due to congestive heart failure, subacute bacterial endocarditis, and cerebral thrombosis due to polycythemia.

The diagnosis is made on the basis of the findings from physical examination, x-ray and fluoroscopy, and special studies, such as blood circulation time, electrocardiography, angiocardiography, and cardiac catheterization. X-ray and fluoroscopy reveal decreased vascularity in the lung fields and a "boot-shaped" heart. Because of the over-riding aorta, a substance injected into a peripheral vein passes directly into the systemic circulation so that the arm-to-tongue time is markedly reduced and may equal the arm-to-lung time. Angiocardiography reveals filling of the aorta and pulmonary artery with the contrast medium almost simultaneously before the medium enters the left side of the heart. In cardiac catheterization a lower pressure is found in the pulmonary artery than in the right ventricle. The catheter may be passed occasionally into the over-riding aorta.

The majority of patients with tetralogy of Fallot are treated by open-heart surgery, utilizing a cardiopulmonary bypass while the pulmonic stenosis is corrected and the ventricular septal defect is closed. When definitive surgery is not feasible, considerable relief is obtained by an anastomosis of the left branch of the pulmonary artery to either the descending aorta or a branch of the left subclavian artery. These last two procedures create an artificial patent ductus arteriosus and permit blood to be shunted from the systemic to the pulmonary circulation.

POSTOPERATIVE CARE AND TEACHING

The plan for nursing care following surgery of the heart and great vessels is very similar to that described in the preceding chapter for the patient who has had a thoracotomy for pulmonary resection. Because the lungs must be retracted and/or collapsed to permit an adequate exposure of the operative field, water-seal drainage is necessary to promote reexpansion. The airway must be kept patent. The management of water-seal drainage and maintenance of a clear airway have been described in the preceding chapter; the reader is urged to review this material on pages 232 to 234.

Oxygen is usually administered in the early postoperative period and should be readily available. Fluids are limited to prevent overloading the circulatory system. An accurate intake-and-output record is essential. If the urinary output falls below that volume usually excreted by the patient, the surgeon must be notified promptly. Oliguria may be an indication of incipient renal failure, shock, and/or fluid retention. Mild analgesia is used. Oversedation, with its depressing effect upon the sensorium, cough center, and activity, is to be avoided. The patient must be kept alert enough to cooperate in coughing, moving, and taking limited amounts of fluids at regular intervals. The activation regime is instituted early in moderation. This is particularly important, since certain types of cardiac lesions predispose to pulmonary complications, particularly atelectasis. After vital signs have stabilized, the head of the bed is usually raised to a 20° angle to facilitate respirations.

The patient must be constantly attended early postoperatively. The nurse's observations are essential in helping the surgeon to detect complications and to evaluate the adequacy of cardiorespiratory function. Vital signs are observed and recorded at least every 15 minutes until stable, then every hour for 8 hours, and then every 4 hours for the next 2 days. The temperature is taken every 10 minutes until the normal is reached in patients who have had hypothermia. The surgeon may order a different schedule for recording of vital signs, but they must be taken frequently. A falling blood pressure may indicate shock, hemorrhage, or heart failure. A falling pulse pressure suggests cardiac tamponade due to bleeding into the pericardium. The quality of the pulse may indicate shock, hemorrhage, or conduction disturbances. A rising pulse rate suggests respiratory difficulty or early hemorrhage. The color of the patient is watched closely for pallor or cyanosis. Venous congestion, evidenced by distention of the veins in the neck, may be expected with straining, coughing, or chest pain but should be reported promptly because venous distention may also occur with heart failure, obstruction of vena cava, herniation of the heart through the pericardium, and pressure pneumothorax with massive atelectasis. Central nervous system disturbances, such as paralysis, numbness, or changes in the sensorium, may result from prolonged occlusion of circulation or from embolization. The nurse should make frequent observations of the equality and size of the pupils until the patient is awake; she should note the state of alertness regularly thereafter to detect a cerebral vascular accident. Arterial embolization may occur, especially following surgery of the mitral valve, and may be manifested by an absent peripheral pulse or a painful, cold, blanched extremity; pulmonary embolism is accompanied by chest pain and cyanosis. The carotid, femoral, and dorsalis pedis pulses should be checked frequently to detect obstructing emboli.

Excessive coughing, vomiting, and constipation must be avoided to prevent hemorrhage due to strain. Abdominal distention interferes with respirations and cardiac function and must be avoided.

Quinidine may be administered postoperatively to establish a sinus rhythm. Digitalis may be necessary to slow and strengthen the heart beat. A low sodium intake is usually continued.

The amount of rest depends upon the type of surgery performed and the patient's preoperative condition. Generally, frequent rest periods are prescribed until the patient has regained strength and can undertake activity without dyspnea or undue fatigue.

The results of heart surgery tend to be dramatic. The majority of patients are operated upon after a more or less prolonged period of cardiac invalidism, having experienced considerable discomfort, fear, and discouragement. Once the discomfort associated with surgery is over, they suddenly realize that they have survived the operation, which they may have elected with considerable trepidation, and that they now have a future in which they can be comfortably active. Two extremes in reaction must be watched for; the patient may be overly optimistic and exercise no caution in resuming full activity, or she may be overly cautious about her heart and continue to be a cardiac invalid. Both reactions require careful explanation by the surgeon, reinforced in his absence by the nurse, to help the patient to understand and to accept her true capabilities and limitations. Surgery of the heart is palliative more often than curative and usually requires moderation in all areas, gradual resumption of activity, and continued medical supervision.

SUMMARY

The extensive preoperative evaluation necessary for the cardiac patient includes a complete history and physical examination, including chest x-ray and blood tests. One or more of the following specialized diagnostic tests may be necessary: angiocardiography, aortography, cardiac catheterization, electrocardiography, phonocardiography, and ballistocardiography.

The patient is prepared for surgery as described for thoracotomy. Cardiac compensation is necessary before the patient can be safely operated upon for the correction of congenital and acquired lesions.

Surgery is performed under general anesthesia, using the closed or open operative technic. Open cardiotomy requires the use of either hypothermia or cardiac bypass to achieve a dry field. Hypothermia may also be used with the closed operative technic.

Operable acquired conditions of the heart and great vessels include mitral stenosis, mitral insufficiency, aortic stenosis, aortic insufficiency, coronary insufficiency, and pericarditis.

Congenital anomalies which may be treated surgically in adulthood include patent ductus arteriosus, coarctation of the aorta, pulmonary stenosis, atrial septal defects, and tetralogy of Fallot.

Postoperatively the plan for care is similar to that described for a patient undergoing thoracotomy. The nurse must be particularly vigilant for signs of hemorrhage, shock, cardiac failure, and disturbances of the central nervous system. Quinidine or digitalis may be administered postoperatively. The patient must be helped to plan and live a life of moderation.

BIBLIOGRAPHY

BAILEY, C. P.: "Surgery of the Heart," Lea & Febiger, Philadelphia, 1955.

───── and D. P. MORSE: Mitral Commissurotomy Performed from the Right Side, *J. Thoracic Surg.*, vol. 33, no. 4, pp. 427–484, April, 1957.

BLAIR, E., R. R. AUSTIN, S. G. BLOUNT, JR., and H. SWAN: A Study of the Cardiovascular Changes during Cooling and Rewarming in Human Subjects Undergoing Total Circulatory Occlusion, *J. Thoracic Surg.*, vol. 33, no. 6, pp. 707–718, June, 1957.

CLAGETT, O. T., J. W. KIRKLIN, and F. H. ELLIS, JR.: Surgical Treatment of Coarctation of the Aorta, *S. Clin. North America*, vol. 35, no. 4, pp. 937–946, August, 1955.

─────, ─────, and J. C. COOLEY: Surgical Treatment of Patent Ductus Arteriosus, *S. Clin. North America*, vol. 35, no. 4, pp. 965–973, August, 1955.

Congenital Heart Disease and Surgery of Cardiovascular Anomalies, *Scope*, The Upjohn Company, Kalamazoo, Mich., vol. 11, no. 12, pp. 2–11, March, 1950.

COOLEY, R. N., and R. D. SLOAN: "Radiology of the Heart and Great Vessels," The Williams & Wilkins Company, Baltimore, 1956.

CREIGHTON, H., and C. A. HUFNAGEL: Aortic Insufficiency, *Am. J. Nursing*, pp. 547–550, April, 1958.

DEXTER, L.: Pathologic Physiology of Mitral Stenosis and Its Surgical Implications, in "Disorders of the Circulatory System," R. L. Craig (ed.), The Macmillan Company, New York, 1952, chap. 8, pp. 104–118.

DODRILL, F. D., N. MARSHALL, J. NYBOER, C. H. HUGHES, A. J. DERBYSHIRE, and A. B. STEARNS: The Use of the Heart-Lung Apparatus in Human Cardiac Surgery, *J. Thoracic Surg.*, vol. 33, no. 1, pp. 60–73, January, 1957.

DRIPPS, R. D. (ed.): "The Physiology of Induced Hypothermia," National Academy of Sciences, National Research Council, Washington, 1956.

DYE, W. S., and O. C. JULIAN: Vascular Surgery, in "The Recovery Room," M. S. Sadove and J. H. Cross (eds.), W. B. Saunders Company, Philadelphia, 1956, chap. 18, pp. 463–476.

ELLIS, JR., F. H., and J. W. KIRKLIN: Aortic Insufficiency, *S. Clin. North America*, vol. 35, no. 4, pp. 1035–1039, August, 1955.

─────, ───── and O. T. CLAGETT: Tetralogy of Fallot, *S. Clin. North America*, vol. 35, no. 4, pp. 1013–1021, August, 1955.

GOLDBERGER, E.: "Heart Disease," Lea & Febiger, Philadelphia, 1951, pp. 25–96.

HENDERSON, L.: Nursing Care of the Patient with a Mitral Valvulotomy, *Am. J. Nursing*, pp. 424–428, April, 1954.

Henry Ford Hospital: "International Symposium on Cardiovascular Surgery," C. R. Lam (ed.), W. B. Saunders Company, Philadelphia, 1955.

HUFNAGEL, C. A.: The Heart and Pericardium, in "Christopher's Textbook of Surgery," 6th ed., L. Davis (ed.), W. B. Saunders Company, Philadelphia, 1956, chap. 17, pp. 437–471.

HUMPHREYS, II, G. H.: Surgical Revision in Congenital Cardiovascular Disease, in
    "Disorders of the Circulatory System," R. L. Craig (ed.), The Macmillan Company,
    New York, 1952, chap. 10, pp. 134–149.
JOHNSON, J.: Cardiac Surgery in "Surgery," J. G. Allen, H. N. Harkins, C. A. Moyer,
    and J. E. Rhoads (eds.), J. B. Lippincott Company, Philadelphia, 1957, chap. 41,
    pp. 1081–1118.
———— and C. KIRBY: "Surgery of the Chest," 2d ed., Year Book Publishers, Inc.,
    Chicago, 1958.
KIRKLIN, J. W., O. T. CLAGETT, and F. H. ELLIS, JR.: Chronic Constrictive Peri-
    carditis, S. Clin. North America, vol. 35, no. 4, pp. 1023–1027, August, 1955.
———— and F. H. ELLIS, JR.: Atrial Septal Defect, S. Clin. North America, vol. 35,
    no. 4, pp. 989–996, August, 1955.
———— and ————: Mitral Stenosis, S. Clin. North America, vol. 35, no. 4, pp. 1041–
    1049, August, 1955.
———— and ————: Pulmonary Stenosis with Intact Ventricular Septum, S. Clin.
    North America, vol. 35, no. 4, pp. 1005–1011, August, 1955.
————, ———— and B. G. BARRATT-BOYES: Technique for Repair of Atrial Septal
    Defect Using the Atrial Well, Surg., Gynec., & Obst., vol. 103, no. 5, pp. 646–649,
    November, 1956.
————, H. G. HARSHBARGER, D. E. DONALD, and J. E. EDWARDS: Surgical Correction
    of Ventricular Septal Defect, J. Thoracic Surg., vol. 33, no. 1, pp. 45–57, January,
    1957.
LUISADA, A. A.: "The Heart Beat," 2d ed., Paul B. Hoeber, Inc., New York, 1953.
NICHOLS, H. T.: Mitral Insufficiency, Treatment by Polar Cross-fusion of the Mitral
    Annulus Fibrosus, J. Thoracic Surg., vol. 33, no. 1, pp. 102–116, January, 1957.
PRATT, G. H.: "Cardiovascular Surgery," Lea & Febiger, Philadelphia, 1954, chaps.
    7–13 incl., pp. 57–156.
PRICE, C. G.: Mitral Stenosis, Am. J. Nursing, pp. 72–74, February, 1951.
SCHWEITZER, R. J.: Purulent Pericarditis, Am. J. Surg., vol. 91, no. 6, pp. 906–910,
    June, 1956.
VIRTUE, R. W.: "Hypothermic Anesthesia," J. Adriani (ed.), Charles C Thomas, Pub-
    lisher, Springfield, Ill., 1955.
World Congress of Cardiology, 2d: "World Trends in Cardiology—Cardiovascular
    Surgery," H. B. Taussig and A. S. Cain (eds.), Paul B. Hoeber, Inc., New York,
    1956.

STUDY GUIDE FOR PART THREE

1. What are the most common conditions which require thyroidectomy?
2. Describe four special diagnostic procedures which may be performed prior to thyroidectomy. What is the purpose of each?
3. Why is an understanding of the anatomic relationships of the structures in the neck important to rendering effective nursing care following thyroidectomy?
4. You have been assigned to the care of a patient who is to undergo a radical neck dissection.
    a. Describe the care and teaching necessary in the preoperative and postoperative periods.

    b. What additional nursing measures and rehabilitation would be necessary if this patient required a permanent tracheostomy?

5. Assume that you are a senior student on an affiliation experience in a rural hospital. You have been asked to address a women's group from a local church on the subject of self-examination of the breast.

    a. Outline the essential information to be conveyed. How would you attempt to impress these women with the need for self-examination without stimulating fear?

    b. How should this information be applied to yourself?

6. What are some of the psychologic implications of mastectomy?

7. Outline a program of rehabilitation for the patient who must have an extensive mastectomy.

8. How does the preoperative preparation of the patient undergoing a lobectomy for tuberculosis differ from that required for the patient undergoing the same surgery for carcinoma? In what ways is the preparation identical?

9. What preparation is necessary for bronchography? What are the nursing responsibilities following this procedure?

10. In the hospital in which you gain your medical and surgical nursing experience, what plans have been made for the emergency treatment of cardiac arrest?

11. While on affiliation in a large tuberculosis sanitarium, you are assigned to Mr. Smith, who has had a thoracoplasty, and Mr. White, who has had a segmentectomy. In what ways would your plans for the care and teaching of these patients be similar? What are the major dissimilarities in the postoperative clinical needs of these patients?

12. Identify the principles of physics, anatomy, and physiology which underlie water-seal drainage of the chest. Describe the nursing responsibilities associated with this procedure.

13. What instructions should be given to a patient prior to discharge following a lobectomy for bronchiectasis?

14. What two methods are used to achieve a dry field for open cardiotomy? What are the nursing responsibilities associated with each method?

15. Describe some of the congenital conditions of the heart and great vessels which may be treated surgically in adulthood.

16. Miss Allens has been admitted to the hospital with the diagnosis of mitral stenosis.

    a. Describe some of the special diagnostic procedures which might be performed to determine operability, and state the major nursing responsibilities each entails.

    b. Outline a plan for the care and teaching necessary for this patient following mitral commissurotomy.

Part Four

CARE OF THE PATIENT WITH SURGICAL CONDITIONS OF THE PERIPHERAL VASCULAR AND INTEGUMENTARY SYSTEMS

18

SURGERY OF THE ARTERIES, VEINS, AND NERVES AFFECTING PERIPHERAL BLOOD FLOW

Conditions affecting the peripheral blood flow have marked physiologic, psychologic, and socioeconomic significance. The cardiovascular and renal systems function as a whole. Arterial insufficiency may be the cause or result of cardiac or renal disease. Increased resistance to arterial blood flow resulting in hypertension adversely affects the heart and kidneys. In addition, these conditions are often chronically painful and disabling. The patient may be unable to continue in a gainful occupation. His medical expenses may be considerable, as prolonged care is necessary.

Surgery is generally palliative, since the effect of the disease, not the underlying cause, is usually remedial. Nevertheless, combined medical-surgical efforts can contribute years of more comfortable, active living for the majority of patients.

SURGICAL INTERVENTION IN ESSENTIAL HYPERTENSION

Essential hypertension is a familial disease marked by a significant elevation of blood pressure, particularly the diastolic. The cause is unknown, but hypersensitivity of the autonomic nervous system and increased resistance to peripheral blood flow are known contributing factors. A persistently high blood pressure may result in cardiovascular and renal disease, causing death at an early age.

Surgical intervention is indicated for those patients under forty years of age who fail to respond adequately to medical treatment and in whom it can be demonstrated that the blood pressure is not fixed, i.e., it is reducible. If the blood pressure can be reduced significantly by a period of bed rest and by sedation with sodium amytal, surgery probably will be effective in relieving the hypertension, at least temporarily.

At surgery, sympathetic nerve fibers, which carry vasoconstrictor im-

273

pulses to the abdominal viscera, or splanchnic bed, and lower extremities, are interrupted, permitting vasodilatation and a consequent reduction in blood pressure.

Sympathectomies are commonly performed bilaterally in two stages, spaced several days apart. The approach is usually posterolateral.

The least extensive procedure is a *subdiaphragmatic splanchnicectomy* and *upper lumbar sympathectomy,* which involves resection of part of the celiac ganglion and two upper lumbar sympathetic ganglia. More commonly, *Smithwick's thoracolumbar sympathectomy with splanchnicectomy* is performed. In this procedure the splanchnic nerves are removed, together with the chain of sympathetic ganglia extending from the eighth thoracic to the second lumbar vertebrae. This procedure can be extended upward to the fourth thoracic ganglion to relieve angina pectoris which may be associated with hypertension. Thoracic ganglionectomy requires a rib resection to permit an adequate exposure.

Postoperatively, the patient requires nursing measures described for both laparotomy and thoracotomy. Oxygen and water-seal drainage may be used early postoperatively. Intravenous neo-synephrine may be necessary to counteract a precipitous fall in blood pressure until stabilization of circulation has occurred at adequate levels. The blood pressure should be taken every 15 minutes in the immediate postoperative period, and every 4 hours thereafter. Since ambulation is practiced early and may result in syncope, the blood pressure should be taken with the patient sitting erect immediately prior to walking. Intake-output records are necessary to help determine adequacy of renal function. Complications which may develop include cerebral thrombosis or paraplegia caused by a precipitous drop in blood pressure, intrapleural or extrapleural effusion, and intercostal neuritis.

The full benefits of sympathectomy may not be noted for some time, and once achieved are not necessarily permanent. It takes the patient a month or more to become readjusted to the marked physiologic consequences of sympathectomy. A persistent postural hypotension is often one of the most troublesome situations with which the patient must cope. Syncope when erect must be avoided by ambulating the patient early, but not suddenly, and by applying an abdominal support and elastic stockings, which prevent pooling of blood in these denervated parts, until circulation has become stabilized. The undenervated portions of the body may undergo a compensatory hyperactivity, resulting in profuse sweating in summer and excessive cold in winter, which must be met by adjustment of clothing and adequate explanation and reassurance. Splanchnic sensation is lost, although parietal sensation is retained, which may confuse and delay the diagnosis of acute abdominal conditions, because pain is absent. The patient should remain under close medical surveillance.

ARTERIAL ANEURYSM

An *aneurysm* is a saccular or fusiform dilatation of an artery which develops at a point already weakened by disease or trauma. The containing wall of the aneurysm is composed only of the fibrous adventitia. A thrombus forms within the aneurysm and undergoes organization and calcification in an attempt to reinforce the wall of the artery. However, in time, the constant pulsation of arterial blood results in liquefaction necrosis of the thrombus, further dilatation and thinning of the adventitia, and finally rupture of the aneurysm and consequent exsanguination.

The aorta is the most common site, but an aneurysm can form in any artery. The symptoms produced are due to erosion or compression of adjacent structures. An aneurysm of the thoracic aorta may compress the esophagus, trachea, or superior vena cava, producing dysphagia, dyspnea or cough, and venous distention. Erosion of the bony confines of the thorax produces severe pain. A pulsating tumefaction of the anterior thoracic wall may be palpable or visible. The diagnosis may be confirmed by x-ray, aortography, or exploratory thoracotomy. An abdominal aortic aneurysm, commonly secondary to atherosclerosis, produces pain with very rapid expansion or with retroperitoneal bleeding. The patient may experience a sensation of abdominal fullness. A pulsating mass in the midabdomen may be palpable. The diagnosis is usually made on physical examination and confirmed by x-ray, but an exploratory laparotomy may be necessary for confirmation.

Preparation for Surgery

The patient is prepared for resection of an aneurysm as described for thoracotomy or laparotomy, depending upon the site. The incision made for resection of a thoracic aneurysm requires that the skin preparation include the entire anterior chest and both axillae. For resection of an abdominal aneurysm, the skin is prepared on the anterior surface from the neck to and including the upper thighs. If the aneurysm is in a peripheral artery, the entire extremity is prepared.

If an aortic aneurysm has ruptured, the patient will be moribund, and surgery is truly emergent. The patient is then prepared as rapidly as possible for general anesthesia and the incision. The salvage rate is high enough to justify operating upon such a sick patient, but shock must be vigorously combated.

Surgical Technic

The surgical correction of a saccular aneurysm involves occlusion of arterial blood flow, resection of the sac, and *arteriorrhaphy*, repair of the defect in the wall. Excision of a *fusiform aneurysm*, which is a longitudinal dilatation, requires a more extensive resection and reestablishment of arterial continuity by the use of a homograft or synthetic graft. A fusiform aneurysm of the abdominal aorta usually is located between the renal arteries and the aortic bifurcation. Occlusion of arterial blood flow by the application of noncrushing clamps can usually be tolerated for the period of time required for resection and grafting. However, resection of a fusiform aneurysm above the level of the renal arteries requires the use of hypothermia to reduce metabolic demands and to permit occlusion of arterial blood supply without producing ischemic paraplegia or renal shutdown. If the aneurysm involves the aortic arch, safe occlusion of blood flow is not possible, and a temporary bypass must be created by suturing a synthetic tube to the aorta, proximad and distad to the aneurysm and anastomosing the limbs of the shunt to the carotid arteries. This tube is then removed after the aneurysm has been resected and the permanent graft has been sutured into place.

Nursing Care

The plan for the care of the patient who has undergone resection of an aneurysm depends largely upon the site of surgery. A patient who has had resection of a thoracic aneurysm requires the care described for one who has undergone thoracotomy. The abdominal aorta lies retroperitoneally; therefore, resection of an aneurysm in this portion of the artery requires considerable manipulation and prolonged retraction of abdominal viscera. Nursing care, therefore, includes postlaparotomy measures, decompression therapy because of the resultant paralytic ileus, and the insertion of an indwelling catheter to relieve urinary retention. If the aneurysm was in a peripheral artery, the most important part of the nursing care is the protection of the extremity from trauma and observation for evidence of arterial insufficiency, once the patient has recovered from anesthesia and shock.

For all these patients an accurate intake-and-output record is necessary to detect renal shutdown resulting from diminished blood flow during surgery. This record also aids the surgeon to meet the needs for parenteral fluid administration without overloading circulation.

Vital signs must be checked at frequent intervals. The nurse must realize that hemorrhage is most likely to occur after the blood pressure has stabilized at normal levels, although this complication is not common. To help evaluate the adequacy of blood flow through the site of the operation, the quality of the femoral, popliteal, and dorsalis pedis pulses must be recorded at hourly intervals. Pallor or cyanosis of the extremities, coldness, or the patient's report of numbness or tingling must be brought to the surgeon's attention immediately. Neurogenic damage due to temporary occlusion of blood flow during surgery will be evidenced by motor and sensory disturbances below the level of the operative site; such symptoms must be reported promptly.

These patients are kept flat in bed for 24 to 48 hours, although turning from side to side is encouraged. Ambulation is initiated on the third postoperative day if the patient's condition permits. Resumption of oral intake depends upon the site of surgery; no restrictions are necessary following recovery from resection of an aneurysm in the thoracic aorta or a peripheral artery; oral intake is gradually resumed when peristalsis has returned following resection of an aneurysm of the abdominal aorta. Skin sutures are removed in 7 days, after which no dressing is necessary. Analgesic drugs will be necessary in the early postoperative period; addiction must be avoided. Anticoagulant and antibiotic drugs may be administered.

OCCLUSIVE DISEASE OF THE ARTERIES

Arterial occlusion may develop gradually or suddenly. The seriousness of arterial occlusion depends upon the rapidity and completeness of closure, the ability of the collateral vessels to dilate, the size and number of vessels involved, the site of occlusion, and the presence of infection.

If the lumen is gradually occluded, as by atheromatous deposits, symptoms of progressive arterial insufficiency with ischemia commonly develop, although symptoms may be minimal or absent. However, with gradual occlusion, collateral circulation has time to develop to maintain viability of the affected limb, provided collateral vessels are able to dilate.

Sudden occlusion of a major artery by an embolus or by spasm associated with thromboembolic phenomena or trauma produces an uncompensated ischemia, which immediately threatens the viability of the extremity.

Diagnostic Procedures

In the treatment of a patient with arterial insufficiency, the underlying disease must be diagnosed and controlled, if possible. Specific diagnostic procedures are performed primarily to determine the level and extent of occlusion. *Oscillometry,* measurement of arterial pulsations, and recording of skin temperatures can be performed easily on all patients. If the patient is not moribund, aortography under general or spinal anesthesia may be performed. Arteriograms are helpful in evaluating the level of occlusion and in demonstrating patency of vessels distal to the site. Occasionally biopsy study of the affected arteries may be necessary to establish the diagnosis.

Chronic Arterial Insufficiency

Symptoms. Early in the development of arterial insufficiency, the patient experiences *intermittent claudication,* cramping pain located in the muscles of the feet, legs, thighs, and buttocks, occurring with activity and subsiding with rest. Inadequate arterial blood supply to other parts of the body may produce this same type of pain. Claudication indicates that the muscles are not being supplied with an adequate amount of oxygen. In time, pain may become continuous and is then termed *rest pain.* Trophic changes occur, manifested by smooth shiny skin, loss of hair, thickened nails, and superficial ulcerations. Skin temperature is reduced. Ankle pulses are feeble or absent. Ischemic neuropathy produces numbness or sensations of tingling and burning in the parts supplied by the involved arteries. Severe arterial insufficiency eventually produces ischemic necrosis, owing either to a rapidly progressing infection in an ulcerated area or interdigital fissure or to complete occlusion of an artery, or more than one. A thrombus of the aortic bifurcation commonly propagates upward to encroach upon the renal arteries, eventually producing uremia.

Treatment and Nursing Care. The patient's cooperation in adhering to hygienic measures designed to promote collateral circulation and to prevent vasoconstriction, trauma, and infection is essential. Walking and swimming are helpful in promoting collateral circulation, provided the activity is stopped prior to the development of intermittent claudication or fatigue. The use of drugs which produce vasoconstriction, such as nicotine, ergot, and epinephrine, must be scrupulously avoided. The patient who smokes will relinquish this habit reluctantly. He must be made to understand that continued smoking will nullify all therapeutic efforts and may cost him a limb.

Wearing constricting garments and assuming positions of flexion for prolonged periods interfere with circulation to and from the extremity and encourage thrombosis; therefore, both must be avoided. The physician may require the patient to take frequent rest periods lying down. He may instruct the patient to exercise his legs by elevating them until pallor appears, then hanging them in a dependent position until rubor appears. These positions must not be maintained after the appearance of pallor or rubor. The patient will prefer to sit with legs dependent, a position which relieves pain by promoting arterial blood supply. However, this position is to be avoided because the resulting venous congestion and edema compound the patient's problem; amputation may be necessary.

Foot care is especially important in the presence of arterial insufficiency, because healing is delayed and infections progress rapidly, predisposing the extremity to gangrene. The patient must keep his feet and hose clean and dry. He must be taught to wash his feet with a bland soap solution once or twice daily and to be gentle in drying them. Dry skin should be lubricated with a bland lotion. Shoes must fit well and be kept dry. Barefoot walking is to be discouraged because of the danger of trauma. Injuries to the feet, interdigital fissures, and mycotic infections demand the attention of the physician. The patient should apply no strong antiseptics or heat to his extremities. He should relinquish the care of corns, calluses, and nails to a *podiatrist*, one skilled in foot care.

Finally, the patient should have a liberal fluid intake to prevent the blood from becoming viscid, thereby promoting circulation and preventing thrombosis. He must build his general resistance by living a life of moderation, avoiding exposures to extremes of temperature and moisture, and by eating a nourishing diet.

Vasodilator drugs may be ordered. The patient should know that vasodilators will cause prickling sensations and flushing of the face and scalp; otherwise this reaction, when initially experienced, will be alarming. In some patients the surgeon may perform a *thromboendarterectomy*, removal of an obstructing clot together with the intimal and medial layers of the artery, with anastomosis of the adventitia. If the involved segment is not resectable without sacrificing the collateral blood supply, a bypass graft may be used to circumvent the area, the ends of the graft being sutured to the side of the artery proximad and distad to the site of occlusion. Sympathectomy, as a last resort, may be performed when arterial insufficiency is threatening ischemia; this procedure produces vasodilatation.

Acute Arterial Occulsion

Symptoms. Acute complete occlusion of a major artery occurs suddenly and is frequently accompanied by shock. Marked pain, coldness, and pallor of the extremity are present. Pulses distad to the obstruction are absent. Later, anesthesia and paralysis may develop. When venous return is also affected, mottling and edema are present.

Treatment. Therapeutic measures to promote an adequate arterial blood flow and to prevent trauma and infection must be instituted prior to the development of irreversible *ischemic necrosis*, or gangrene, and toxemia.

The patient is placed on bed rest, and a cradle without heat is placed over the affected extremity to protect it from the weight of bedding and to prevent trauma. Shock, if present, must be treated promptly.

Sympatholytic drugs, sympathetic nerve blocks, and spinal anesthesia are used in an attempt to improve circulation by vasodilatation. Anticoagulant drug therapy is instituted to prevent extension of a blood clot and to promote dissolution. Arteriospasm may be relieved by blocking sympathetic ganglia and by administering alcohol orally or intravenously.

If these measures fail to relieve the occlusion, surgical intervention is indicated within 3 to 6 hours following onset. Surgery consists of embolectomy. This procedure may be performed under local anesthesia if the patient is moribund. Spinal anesthesia may be used because it has the added advantage of promoting vasodilatation.

Occlusion due to arteriospasm may be relieved by the direct application of warm saline solution or packs to the artery. The direct application of papaverine solution may permit relaxation of the vessel. Resection and anastomosis may be necessary if a localized arterial segment persists in spasm.

Frequently these procedures are preceded or followed by lumbar sympathectomy to prevent stimuli for vasoconstriction from reaching the occluded artery and collateral vessels. When vasoconstrictor impulses are removed, vasodilatation occurs, provided the vessels are not bound by arteriosclerosis.

Nursing Care of the Patient Undergoing Surgery for Arterial Occlusion

The preparation for surgery and the postoperative care are the same as described for the patient undergoing resection of an aneurysm. In addition, the care described for sympathectomy may be necessary.

All measures described for the care of a patient with arterial insufficiency are resumed postoperatively. The patient must be helped to understand why these measures are necessary and how to apply them at home.

Gangrene

All the therapeutic measures just described for the care of the patient with occlusive disease of the arteries are designed to prevent gangrene, which may produce pain, toxemia, and loss of an extremity.

Pathology and Symptomatology. Death of tissues, *gangrene*, results from occlusion of arterial blood supply. The area of necrosis starts in the distal portion of an extremity, progresses upward through the ischemic tissues, and stops at the level where the blood supply is adequate to support the inflammatory process. This level is described as the *line of demarcation*. Ferric sulfide formed in the tissues is responsible for the characteristic black appearance of a gangrenous area. In the absence of infection, gangrene is a dry, mummifying process in which the affected parts, usually the toes, may spontaneously amputate themselves. Infection produces moist gangrene due to mycotic and bacterial activity. This type of gangrene progresses rapidly and is associated with a putrefactive odor and marked toxemia. Pain usually accompanies gangrene due to atherosclerosis, but when the neuritis of diabetes mellitus is superimposed pain is singularly absent.

Diabetic gangrene may be considered to be more serious than gangrene due to atherosclerosis alone, because the patient tends to underestimate the seriousness of an ulcer which is not painful and to delay seeking treatment. In addition, he has a low resistance to infection, coupled with retarded healing powers. The patient and/or a member of his family should be taught to inspect his feet daily and to seek medical attention immediately should an ulcer, interdigital fissure, or area of discoloration be noted.

A Nursing Care Plan for a Patient with Gangrene. The plan for the nursing care and teaching of a patient with gangrene will be illustrated by Mr. Aaron Rosenberg. This 52-year-old patient owns and operates a large delicatessen shop in partnership with his oldest son. He is a member of the Jewish Orthodox Church. Mr. Rosenberg has been known to have diabetes for 20 years; it has been well controlled by insulin and diet. For the past 18 months he has experienced intermittent claudication, which is particularly severe in his left leg. During the past 2 months he has had to walk more slowly and to take frequent rest periods during the three-block walk to his delicatessen shop. A few days ago he stubbed his left foot; within a few hours his third and fourth toes were inflamed. Last night he noticed that both toes were turning a purplish hue and that there was a black spot in the center of an ulcer on his third toe.

The physician who examines Mr. Rosenberg makes the diagnosis of arteriosclerotic gangrene with diabetes mellitus; the gangrene is described as moist.

A program of conservative therapy is instituted to prevent trauma, combat infection, and hasten the process of demarcation. Mr. Rosenberg is placed on bed rest, and he is instructed to keep his legs level with his body. The gangrenous area is protected from trauma by the placement of a bed cradle. Daily foot soaks are ordered for cleansing purposes, to be followed by the application of a light porous dressing which neither retains heat nor constricts the area. Sometimes exposure to air is used instead of a dressing. Antibiotic drugs are administered.

For patients with atherosclerotic gangrene, narcotics may be necessary during the process of demarcation, which usually is accompanied by intense pain; addiction must be avoided.

Mr. Rosenberg was able to accept his treatments fairly well, but he complained rather bitterly about the food which was served to him and ate very little. In order to help Mr. Rosenberg with his dietary problem, the nurse consulted his rabbi to learn what modifications should be made. She learned that the laws governing food practices are given in Leviticus 11.[1] She learned that pork, sea food with shells, and fish without scales are forbidden, and that meat and dairy products are not served at the same meal. The rabbi talked with Mr. Rosenberg and reminded him that his religion, in common with all others, imposes no restrictions during an acute illness. Because Mr. Rosenberg enjoyed foods he was used to, arrangements were made for his wife to bring him Kosher foods, which are prepared in a manner prescribed by Hebrew law. The dietitian then calculated the diabetic diet to include these foods.

With conservative therapy, Mr. Rosenberg's gangrene demarcated at the proximal phalanges. The surgeon debrided the toes, and healing progressed uneventfully. During convalescence, Mr. Rosenberg was taught all the hygienic measures described for patients with arterial insufficiency.

Amputation of the gangrenous extremity is necessary when the process of ischemic necrosis can not be halted by conservative measures.

The patient is prepared as for laparotomy. He may be given gas gangrene antitoxin, since the anaerobic organisms which cause this disease commonly contaminate necrotic areas. Because surgery extends through bone, which has a low resistance to invading organisms, skin preparation is more thorough. Twenty-four hours or more before surgery, the extremity is shaved and cleansed from the line of demarcation well above the intended site of amputation, and sterile wrappings are applied. The cleansing is repeated once or twice prior to surgery.

Most commonly, spinal or general anesthesia is used. Refrigeration of the extremity may be used when the patient is toxic and moribund. Enclosing the limb in an ice tent, ice pack, or refrigeration blanket, with or without the high application of a tourniquet, reduces the temperature and rate of metabolism in the extremity, retards circulation of toxic products from the area, anesthetizes nerve endings, and inhibits the growth of microorganisms. Refrigeration therapy thus combats shock, toxemia, pain, and infection. The response to this treatment is usually dramatic: the hyperpyrexic, delirious, moribund patient is rapidly converted into a candidate for surgery which is designed to save his life, if not his limb. The patient and his family must understand that the extremity when packed in ice is consigned to amputation.

The most important aspect of the nursing care of a patient whose extremity is being refrigerated is that of maintaining hypothermia. Under no circumstances should the extremity be allowed to rewarm prior to surgery. Sedation may be administered during the cooling process. The

[1] "The Holy Bible," Leviticus 11:1–47.

use of an ice pack requires nursing skill to avoid a wet bed, which predisposes to chilling, decubitus formation, and general discomfort. The ice pack must be well insulated and applied snugly, but without causing added pressure; the bed should be elevated at the head to encourage drainage of melting ice by gravity; the drainage system must be patent.

Amputation is performed well above the line of demarcation in viable tissues which have an adequate blood supply. Too low an amputation may result in spreading gangrene, necessitating subsequent higher amputations. General or spinal anesthesia is commonly used.

Postoperatively, the nurse must be alert to the signs of shock and hemorrhage, although these complications are not common. Flexion contractures of the knee and/or hip must be prevented by full extension of these joints several times daily. Occasionally slight elevation of the stump is ordered early postoperatively, but this elevation must not be maintained continuously. An extension apparatus with 2 to 4 lb. traction may be used, not only to prevent contracture but also to prevent retraction of tissues and thus prepare the stump for the application of a prosthesis. The patient is ambulated early in a walker or on crutches and is fitted for a prosthesis within 6 to 12 weeks. An elastic bandage is commonly applied in the operating room to promote smooth healing over the stump and to prevent edema and hemorrhage. Unless infection is suspected, the dressing is not changed for a week or more. The detailed care and rehabilitation of a patient with an amputation are not within the scope of this textbook; the student should consult an orthopedic nursing reference for this information.

Arterial Trauma

An artery may be injured by contusion, compression, or stretching. Although the integrity of the arterial wall may be preserved, these injuries produce arteriospasm, which occludes blood flow. Collateral vessels may also be in spasm. Loss of arterial continuity occurs with penetration, perforation, and laceration and causes blood loss, which may be severe. Thrombosis may develop at the site of injury or in the distal arteries unless circulation can be restored promptly. An arteriovenous fistula or arterial aneurysm may develop later at the site of the injury.

In the treatment of arterial trauma, consideration is first given to the control of hemorrhage, which can exsanguinate the patient. Bleeding is best controlled by direct pressure, but a tourniquet may be necessary. The tourniquet itself jeopardizes circulation and should be used as a last resort. It is applied between the heart and the site of injury to control arterial bleeding. It should be constructed of wide material, applied tightly enough to stop the bleeding and should be labeled with the exact time of administration. Once applied, a tourniquet should not be loosened, but other measures to control bleeding must be available within an hour's time, for a tourniquet left on beyond this time limit risks irreversible ischemic changes. Transfusions of whole blood or plasma are administered as soon as possible to combat shock, which in itself predisposes to thrombosis. When the patient's condition permits, operative repair is made. Compression may be relieved by evacuating a hematoma. Sometimes a rent in the arterial wall can be repaired by suture. More often, resection of the injured segment with an end-to-end anastomosis or insertion of a graft is necessary. Ligation of an injured artery is performed safely only when the vessel is of minor importance. Arteriospasm must be relieved by measures already described.

VARICOSE VEINS

A *varix* is a vein which is segmentally dilated, elongated, and tortuous. (See Fig. 54.) This condition is due primarily to valvular incompetence, which permits pooling and some retrograde flow of blood in dependent parts of the body, most commonly in the legs. There are two basic causes for varicosities: a congenital weakness, aggravated by man's upright posture, and injury to the vein due to thrombophlebitis.

Symptomatology

Symptoms usually do not appear until adulthood, after years of heavy labor, prolonged standing, or repeated pregnancies have imposed a chronic strain on the venous system. Venous blood normally flows from the superficial saphenous network, through short communicating or perforating veins, into the deep femoral vein, propelled in the direction of the heart primarily by muscular activity and the arterial and capillary blood pressures which exceed that in the veins; competent valvular action prevents a retrograde flow of blood. Incompetence of the valves permits blood to flow in both directions when the vein is compressed by muscular activity, resulting in dilatation of the veins and an increased venous pressure in the legs when the patient is erect. The superficial saphenous veins lack a firm musculofascial support; therefore, they are first affected by varicose vein formation and appear as lumpy clusters along the course of the veins. Moderate pooling of blood in the lower extremities causes aching fatigue, which is particularly aggravated by erect posture with inactivity and is relieved by recumbency; nocturnal muscle cramping may occur. When the valves in the femoral vein are also incompetent, or absent, venous return is markedly reduced. Nutrient fluid escaping from the capillaries is prevented from reentering the circulatory system because of the increased capillary pressure, and edema results.

The complications of untreated severe varicose veins are frequently chronic and may be serious. Edema and venous stasis devitalize tissues, especially in the ankle area. The skin undergoes trophic changes and is pigmented by numerous minute hemorrhages; it is common for eczema and/or ulceration to develop.

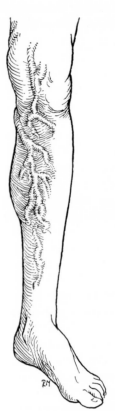

FIG. 54. Varicose veins of the leg.

Diagnostic Methods

The diagnosis can be made by palpation of the extremities while the patient is standing. Another useful method of evaluating valvular competence is that of the *Trendelenburg test*. With the patient lying supine, one leg at a time is elevated to a 65° angle to promote drainage of the superficial saphenous network. A tourniquet is then applied to the thigh to occlude only the superficial veins, and the patient is placed in an upright position. If the varicosities do not reappear for 20 seconds, the valves in the communicating veins are adequate and the test result is negative. Incompetence of the valves in the communicating veins is demonstrated by the rapid reappearance of the varicosities, even with the tourniquet in place. Rapid filling of the varicose veins from above when the tourniquet is released indicates incompetence of the valves in the saphenous veins. When valvular incompetence is demonstrated, the test result is positive.

Rarely, phlebography is necessary to clarify the extent of the pathologic process and to determine the presence of a previous thrombophlebitis. However, as with arteriography, reactions may be severe.

Surgical Treatment

When the Trendelenburg test result is positive, the involved veins should be removed by subcutaneous stripping under general anesthesia. The patient is prepared for this procedure as for laparotomy. The skin is prepared from the umbilicus to and including the perineum and the entire leg and foot. The patient is placed in shock position for surgery, to aid in preventing blood loss and the formation of a hematoma. An incision is made into the groin, the saphenous vein is ligated close to the saphenofemoral junction, all tributaries are ligated and divided, an incision is made into the saphenous vein to permit the introduction of the stripper, ligatures distad to the incision are tightened, and the vein is divided. The stripper is a long, flexible, rodlike instrument with a cup at one end. As the instrument is passed through the vein the vessel is stripped from its attachments and is folded into the cup. An incision made below the knee permits the stripper with the superficial saphenous vein from the thigh to be removed. The lower portion of the vein is removed by passing the stripper through an incision made below the ankle and out through the incision previously made below the knee. The lesser saphenous vein which courses upward posteriorly is removed in a similar manner. Bleeding from the tributaries occurs as the stripper is passed, and is controlled by pressure; innocuous thrombosis of these minute vessels later occurs. The subsequent formation of varices in some of the larger tributaries is treated by sclerotherapy. Following recovery from this operation, stripping of the other leg is performed as necessary.

Postoperative Care and Rehabilitation

Postoperatively a compression bandage is worn for several days to prevent bleeding and to aid venous return. The nurse must reapply the elastic stocking once or twice daily to ensure that even compression is being exerted. The dressing is changed by the surgeon when sutures are removed, usually on the seventh postoperative day. The nurse should watch for evidence of hemorrhage, wound infection, or deep thrombophlebitis and report symptoms immediately.

Late on the operative day, or on the first postoperative day, a program of alternating ambulation and elevation is initiated, as directed by the surgeon. Generally, the patient is instructed to walk for 10 minutes of each hour for 10 to 12 hours, returning to bed for elevation of the extremity between periods of ambulation. This program encourages venous flow from the lower extremities by muscular action. Mild analgesia may be necessary early postoperatively. Oral intake is in no way restricted. A liberal fluid intake is encouraged.

Since varicose veins usually develop in both lower extremities, bilateral stripping is commonly performed. This may be performed in one stage, but more often the more severely affected leg is stripped, and after a period of a few days or weeks, surgery is performed on the other leg.

Prior to discharge the patient must be taught that she will have to wear elastic hose continuously, except when bathing and at night when in bed, until the surgeon directs removal, which is usually accomplished gradually. If the patient can be made to understand the importance of wearing elastic hose to prevent further disability, she will usually cooperate in this measure. Two stockings are needed for each affected leg to permit a change. With care, the stockings retain their elasticity for several months. The patient should be taught to wash the hose, without rubbing or stretching, in lukewarm soapsuds, rinse well, and lay them flat on an absorbent towel to dry. New hose must be purchased when elasticity is gone. The patient must also be taught to take three or more half-hour rest periods daily, lying with legs elevated. Prolonged standing is to be avoided. When sitting, the patient should elevate her legs on a chair placed well up under the knees for adequate support. If the patient is obese, she will be placed on a reduction diet, since weight adds to the strain already placed on the venous system. She must understand her diet and the need for it before she is discharged.

Stasis Ulceration

Ulceration due to venous stasis may be a delayed sequela to neglected varicosities or deep thrombophlebitis [2] and usually represents irreparable damage to the deep venous system. Mild trauma usually is the factor initiating ulceration.

All the measures described in the teaching plan for the patient with varicose veins must be practiced for the lifetime of the patient with a stasis ulcer to prevent recurrence.

Healing of the ulcer may be accomplished by a period of bed rest, the use of warm, moist compresses, and the administration of antibiotic drugs during the acute phase of infection. When the wound is clean, debriding and grafting may be performed, or the ulcer may heal with several applications of the Unna boot. The boot is applied much like a

[2] The prevention and treatment of thrombophlebitis have been presented on pp. 50 to 52.

cast. Each layer of gauze is painted with warm Unna paste, which is composed of zinc oxide, glycerin, gelatin, and water; the boot hardens as it dries.

Following healing of the ulcer, which may require several months, definitive surgical measures, such as stripping, must be performed to ensure permanent healing.

SUMMARY

Surgical treatment is frequently indicated to prevent or to relieve the serious, disabling effects of conditions affecting the peripheral vascular system.

Essential hypertension related to increased resistance to peripheral blood flow may sometimes be relieved, at least temporarily, by sympathectomy. The patient is prepared for thoracotomy or laparotomy, depending upon the extensiveness of the proposed procedure. Postoperatively, frequent blood pressure readings and an accurate intake-output record are especially important. The patient is ambulated early, but with caution to avoid syncope due to postural hypotension.

An arterial aneurysm, which most commonly develops in the aorta, is excised, if possible, to prevent eventual rupture and exsanguination. Postoperatively, thoracotomy or laparotomy nursing measures are necessary, depending upon the site. Following resection of an abdominal aortic aneurysm, paralytic ileus and urinary retention are common. The nurse must observe vital signs closely, keep an accurate intake-output record, and note signs of arterial insufficiency in the parts distad to the site of resection.

Arterial occlusion may develop gradually or suddenly, the seriousness of the occlusion depending primarily upon the adequacy of collateral circulation. Chronic arterial insufficiency imposes the need for adherence to certain hygienic practices designed to promote collateral circulation, to avoid chemical and physical causes of vasoconstriction, and to maintain resistance to infection. Care must be taken to avoid trauma. An occluded segment may be treated by excision or the insertion of a bypass graft.

Acute arterial occlusion requires prompt treatment to restore blood flow and prevent ischemic necrosis. Therapeutic measures include bed rest; the use of sympatholytic drugs, sympathetic nerve blocks, and spinal anesthesia to promote vasodilatation; and anticoagulant drug therapy. If, after a few hours, treatment fails to restore arterial blood flow, embolectomy is indicated; sympathectomy may be performed. The postoperative plan for care depends upon the site of surgery, which may have been in the thoracic or abdominal aorta, or in a peripheral artery. The nurse must be particularly observant for evidence of arterial insufficiency in the parts supplied by the involved artery. Hygienic measures described as necessary for a patient with chronic arterial insufficiency are resumed postoperatively.

Therapeutic measures described for the care of a patient with arterial insufficiency and occlusion are designed to prevent gangrene, which may be self-limited or may require amputation. The conservative treatment of a patient with gangrene is designed to promote adequate circulation and to combat infection. Amputation is performed above the line of demarcation in viable tissues. Spinal or general anesthesia is used. Preoperative refrigeration of the gangrenous extremity may be necessary to improve the chances of the toxic patient for successful surgery. The patient must be helped to accept the need for amputation and must be assisted in full postoperative rehabilitation.

Arterial trauma may require operative repair following treatment for hemorrhage and shock. Nursing care is the same as that described for the patient undergoing surgery for arterial occlusion.

Incompetence of the valves in the superficial saphenous system may result in varicose veins which require surgical treatment to prevent circulatory impairment and stasis ulceration. Provided the valves in the deep veins are competent, varicose veins are treated most effectively by vein stripping, followed by the wearing of elastic hose and by ambulation alternated with periods of elevation of the extremities.

Stasis ulceration, which may be a sequela to neglected varicosities or deep thrombophlebitis, is treated by debriding and grafting of the ulcer or by the application of an Unna boot. To ensure permanence of healing, the varicosities must be treated directly.

BIBLIOGRAPHY

Abramson, D. I.: "Peripheral Vascular Disorders," Paul B. Hoeber, Inc., New York, 1956.

Barrow, D. W.: "The Clinical Management of Varicose Veins," 2d ed., Paul B. Hoeber, Inc., New York, 1957.

Conn, J. H., and K. Sparkuhl: Arterial Homografts, Am. J. Surg., vol. 94, no. 5, pp. 695–704, November, 1957.

DeBakey, M. E., D. A. Cooley, and O. Creech, Jr.: Surgery of the Aorta, Clinical Symposia, Ciba Pharmaceutical Products, Inc., Summit, N.J., vol. 8, no. 2, March–April, 1956.

DeTakats, G.: Acute Arterial Occlusion, S. Clin. North America, vol. 35, no. 1, pp. 265–272, February, 1955.

Dye, Jr., W. S., and O. C. Julian: Vascular Surgery, in "The Recovery Room," M. S. Sadove and J. H. Cross (eds.), W. B. Saunders Company, Philadelphia, 1956, chap. 18, pp. 436–476.

Ellis, Jr., F. H., O. T. Clagett, and J. W. Kirklin: Aneurysms of the Aorta, S. Clin. North America, vol. 35, no. 4, pp. 953–963, August, 1955.

GILMAN, R. A., and C. P. BAILEY: Surgical Treatment of Dissecting Aneurysm, *J. Thoracic Surg.*, vol. 33, no. 5, pp. 670–678, May, 1957.

GLOVER, J. R.: The Major Amputations, *Am. J. Nursing*, pp. 544–550, September, 1950.

GRAHAM, E. A.: The Aorta and Peripheral Arteries, in "The Year Book of General Surgery," Year Book Publishers, Inc., Chicago, 1955, pp. 283–335.

GREEN, H. D.: Pharmacology of Antihypertensive Drugs, *Clinical Symposia*, Ciba Pharmaceutical Products, Inc., Summit, N.J., vol. 9, no. 4, pp. 139–147, September–October, 1957.

HOLDEN, W. D.: "Acute Peripheral Arterial Occlusion," Charles C Thomas, Publisher, Springfield, Ill., 1952.

HOLMAN, E.: "New Concepts in Surgery of the Vascular System," Charles C Thomas, Publisher, Springfield, Ill., 1955.

JANES, J. M., and J. C. IVINS: Surgery of Peripheral Arterial Disease, *S. Clin. North America*, vol. 35, no. 4, pp. 1133–1144, August, 1955.

JULIAN, O. C., and W. S. DYE: Peripheral Vascular Surgery, in "Surgery," J. G. Allen, H. N. Harkins, C. A. Moyer, and J. E. Rhoads (eds.), J. B. Lippincott Company, Philadelphia, 1957, chap. 40, pp. 1032–1077.

KANTROWITZ, A.: The Management of Cardiovascular Surgical Emergencies, *S. Clin. North America*, vol. 35, no. 2, pp. 531–540, April, 1955.

KIRKLIN, J. W., and F. H. ELLIS, JR.: Occlusive Disease of the Terminal Aorta, *S. Clin. North America*, vol. 35, no. 4, pp. 947–951, August, 1955.

LUKE, J. C.: Venous Disorders of the Lower Extremity, *Clinical Symposia*, Ciba Pharmaceutical Products, Inc., Summit, N.J., vol. 5, no. 4, July–August, 1953.

MOSKOPP, M. E., and J. SLOAN: Nursing Care for the Amputee, *Am. J. Nursing*, pp. 550–555, September, 1950.

MYERS, T. T.: Management of Varicose Veins with Special Reference to the Stripping Operation, *S. Clin. North America*, vol. 35, no. 4, pp. 1147–1173, August, 1955.

PRATT, G. H.: "Cardiovascular Surgery," Lea & Febiger, Philadelphia, 1954, chaps. 14–37, incl., pp. 159–713.

RUGGIERO, W. F., and FEY CHU: The Management of Peripheral Vascular Emergencies, *S. Clin. North America*, vol. 35, no. 2, pp. 543–550, April, 1955.

SAMUELS, S. S.: "Diagnosis and Treatment of Vascular Disorders," The Williams & Wilkins Company, Baltimore, 1956.

STEWART, H. J.: "Cardiac Therapy," Paul B. Hoeber, Inc., New York, 1952, chap. 9, pp. 259–263. (Reprinted with corrections, 1953.)

VERBRUGGHEN, A.: "Neurosurgery in General Practice," Charles C Thomas, Publisher, Springfield, Ill., 1952, chap. 21, pp. 492–497.

VORIS, H. C.: Thoracolumbar Sympathectomy for Hypertension, *S. Clin. North America*, vol. 35, no. 1, pp. 255–263, February, 1955.

WILKINS, R. W.: The Treatment of Hypertension, *Clinical Symposia*, Ciba Pharmaceutical Products, Inc., Summit, N.J., vol. 9, no. 4, pp. 115–133, September–October, 1957.

19

BURNS AND SKIN GRAFTS

Knowledge of burns and their treatment is tremendously important to the nurse, both in her personal life and in the care of patients. Few persons grow to adulthood without having experienced a burn of some nature. Since burns are sudden and accidental, they may entail great emotional shock and economic disruption. They may be severe enough to cause death. They will surely involve pain and some degree of disability, in addition to possible prolonged, expensive hospitalization and even disfigurement.

FIRST–AID TREATMENT OF BURNS

Nurses are often called upon to administer or teach the first-aid care of burns. Such treatment should be directed toward allaying apprehension, treating shock, and preventing infection. The wound should be covered with a dressing, preferably sterile, to alleviate pain and prevent infection. Shock is treated by keeping the patient lying quietly in dorsal recumbency with feet elevated. Fluid intake, preferably of normal saline solution,[1] should be encouraged if the patient is not unconscious. Medical attention must be obtained promptly.

PATHOLOGY

Regardless of the causative agent, the pathologic effects of a burn are the same. A sunburn, for example, initiates the same pathologic changes and is no less serious than a burn acquired by contact with other forms of heat.

---

[1] Normal saline solution is made by adding one level teaspoonful of table salt to 1 pt. water.

Burns are commonly classified on the basis of degree of tissue destruction. The least severe burns initiate erythema with inflammation of the superficial layers of skin; these are called *first-degree. Second-degree* burns involve the deeper layers and are marked by erythema with vesicle formation. The most severe involve the total thickness of skin and are characterized by necrosis and slough of the nonviable tissues; these are called *third-degree.* Many burns involve all three stages of tissue destruction.

When tissues are destroyed by a burn, certain pathologic changes are initiated. In the inflammatory reaction which occurs, fluids are allowed to escape from the vascular tree into the tissues, causing local edema, dehydration, and shock. If the burn has been severe enough to denude the area, this exudate, which contains water, electrolytes, and protein, escapes to the external environment.

All burns produce some toxemia when toxic products formed by death of tissues are absorbed. Uremia due to kidney failure may ensue if the patient has a severe burn with marked toxemia and deep irreversible shock.

PROGNOSIS

A burned area has both depth and width, and both factors are considered in evaluating the seriousness of a burn. A third-degree burn usually produces more toxemia, deeper scar-tissue formation, and greater local disability. Moist heat penetrates deeper into the tissues than dry heat; therefore, scalds are usually more serious than a burn due to contact with a hot object. On the other hand, all burns destroy the ability of the skin to function in heat control, protection, and excretion of water and salts; therefore, the extent of surface area involved may be more important than the depth of the burn. A small third-degree burn, for example, might conceivably be less serious than an extensive first-degree burn. The extent of the burned area seldom can be judged accurately until demarcation and slough of necrotic tissue occur. Therefore, all burns are considered serious initially and are treated accordingly.

The condition of the patient also determines the seriousness of a burn. A patient already weakened by disease, age, or malnutrition will be more seriously affected and will be less able to heal effectively. The area involved is also to be considered, as some areas carry the risk of greater disability. For example, a severe burn of the face may involve the eyes, with loss of vision. The edema which results from a severe burn of the face and neck may obstruct respirations so much that a tracheostomy may be necessary. Burns of the flexor surfaces are difficult to treat because contractures are likely to develop.

TREATMENT AND NURSING CARE

The therapeutic program is designed to assist the patient safely through the crucial period immediately following the burn, to prevent or minimize disability, and to achieve maximum rehabilitation. Therefore, therapy is directed toward counteracting the systemic and local effects of a burn.

General Therapeutic Measures

In addition to local therapy, general therapeutic measures are instituted to combat shock, to alleviate pain, and to prevent infection, anemia, and prolonged disability.

In the treatment of a patient with shock due to a severe burn, glucose, then saline solutions are the fluids of choice to restore blood volume. These solutions may be followed by plasma. When blood concentration is revealed by a high hematocrit reading, 5 per cent glucose or normal saline solution supplies the needed water which lessens the concentration of the blood and improves circulation.[2] The glucose also helps the liver combat toxemia due to tissue destruction. The patient with extensive burns and severe shock will not have many veins readily accessible for infusion; he may require a phlebotomy for the purpose of administering fluids. Therefore, once fluids are started the nurse must be vigilant to keep the infusion running without incident. Oxygen may be indicated, especially for patients with inhalation burns or for those with severe anoxia due to shock.

A narcotic is usually administered to alleviate pain due to the burn and initial dressing. Barbiturates may also be used to allay apprehension and to control restlessness initially. Once the dressing is applied or encrustations form, pain is usually minimal and can be controlled by analgesics. The cerebral anoxia caused by shock produces a dulling of sensation, especially with third-degree burns, which usually are not painful until slough of necrotic tissue occurs several days after the burn. Occasionally it is necessary to administer an anesthetic for subsequent dressings, but by then the patient is out of shock and is a better candidate for anesthesia.

Infection is combated by the use of antibiotic drugs. Tetanus antitoxin or toxoid is administered as soon as possible after the burn is sustained. ACTH or cortisone may be administered to aid in reparation.

The fluid-electrolyte balance and serum-protein level must be restored promptly. The protein supplies are rapidly depleted in a patient who has

[2] A. G. Bettman, Contraindications for Plasma as the First Fluid in Severe Shock after Burns, *Am. J. Surg.*, vol. 91, no. 6, p. 937, June, 1956.

a severe burn because urinary excretion of nitrogenous products is increased, protein is lost in the exudate, and anorexia limits the patient's intake. Protein is essential for repairing tissues, combating anemia, and restoring health and strength. Therefore, a high-caloric, high-protein diet is given, with supplementary feedings between meals. Frequent, small feedings, attractively served, help to combat anorexia. The diet early may be liquid, increased to full as soon as tolerated. A liberal oral intake of fluids is encouraged.

An accurate intake-output record and frequent urine specific gravity determinations are necessary to evaluate the adequacy of renal function and the intake needs. They also help in the recognition of the period of diuresis, which occurs 3 to 4 days after the burn has been sustained and which is due to absorption of the fluid of edema; fluids are given sparingly during this period.

Local Therapeutic Measures

The primary aim of local therapy is to convert the open, moist wound into a clean, dry area to arrest further loss of protein-rich exudate, control shock, prevent infection, and promote comfort. This can be achieved by several methods; by the application of voluminous pressure dressings, by exposure to air to facilitate drying, or by early skin grafting.

All three methods of treatment are preceded by thorough but gentle cleansing of the area with a bland soap and sterile water. Detached, devitalized tissue is excised, because its presence deters healing. If the wound presents a clean, granulating surface, the patient is prepared for immediate skin grafting. The strictly aseptic conditions of an operating room are necessary for the initial cleansing and subsequent dressings. All persons in the room, including the patient, should be capped and masked.

Pressure Dressings. With or without grafting, voluminous pressure dressings may be applied over sterile gauze which has been lightly impregnated with petroleum jelly to prevent adherence of the dressings to the granulating area. The pressure helps prevent loss of exudate and encourages smoother repair. These dressings are left undisturbed for a week or longer. They are then changed by the surgeon at regular intervals until healing is complete. The initial petroleum-jelly mesh is not removed early unless infection occurs.

When pressure dressings are used, the nurse must be particularly watchful for symptoms of infection, such as fever, restlessness, and odor. These dressings are circumferential and may, therefore, interfere with respirations and/or circulation. If the dressing involves the thorax, the nurse must watch for cyanosis, rapid pulse, and dyspnea. If an extremity is wrapped, the nurse must observe for color and temperature changes, edema, or reports of paresthesias or numbness. Such symptoms must be reported promptly.

Dressings must be kept clean and dry. It may be necessary to reinforce areas where drainage has saturated dressings to prevent infection by capillary attraction. If the dressings extend close to the perineal area, they should be reinforced with a waterproof material to prevent soilage from excretion. A retention catheter may be necessary to keep dressings dry.

Because these voluminous dressings limit activity, the nurse must be alert to meet the patient's needs, especially with regard to intake, output, and position change. The patient should be lightly covered because these dressings retain body heat. Skin care of all exposed surfaces is important to promote functioning of intact skin, prevent decubiti, and control odor. Room deodorants are often helpful, especially if the patient has an infected burn.

Exposure Therapy. Some burns heal well with the exposure method of treatment, which allows the air to dry moist surfaces and permits the plasma to form a protective encrustation. This method is used to treat areas which are difficult to dress and which can be adequately exposed and kept at rest. The patient is placed on sterile sheets of double thickness. A cradle is used to keep bedding off the burned surfaces. Care must be taken to prevent chilling by regulating room temperature and preventing drafts, because the burned surfaces have lost their ability to aid in the regulation of body temperature. If a heat lamp is used to prevent chilling and/or to aid in the drying process, caution must be exercised to prevent further burning.

Treatment of Burns of Special Areas. Some areas require special attention when burned. The face is highly vascular, and burns of this area promptly produce edema. The patient with a burn of the face and neck may have respiratory difficulty because of edema or direct inhalation of fumes. He may need a tracheostomy and oxygen. He will need meticulous oral hygiene; a hydrogen peroxide solution is excellent. Facial burns respond well to the exposure method of treatment, followed when necessary by skin grafting. Eye irrigations followed by the instillation of a sterile ointment are often necessary to keep the cornea moist and to prevent ulceration. If pressure dressings are used, care is taken to avoid pressure upon the cornea and to pad burned ears well.

A burn of the hand may be treated by the exposure method or by pressure dressings. Both methods require that the fingers be separated to prevent raw surfaces from adhering to each other as healing ensues. The hand should be splinted or supported during the healing process in the position which minimizes disability should ankylosis occur, i.e., with the fingers slightly flexed over a ball. A burn involving the palm of the hand or plantar surface of the foot requires the immediate application of split-thickness grafts, followed later, if necessary, by a full-thickness graft.

Burns of the perineum are treated by the exposure method. A retention catheter is used to keep the area dry. After the protective encrustations have formed, perineal irrigations may be ordered to promote cleanliness.

Use of Wet Dressings. Continuous wet packs may be used to hasten demarcation and sloughing of necrotic tissue, especially if the wound is infected, in preparation for skin grafting. If the exposure method is to be followed by skin grafting, these packs may be used to remove the encrustations. Cold, moist compresses are sometimes used in the treatment of burns. They effectively reduce the temperature of the part, relieve pain, and minimize the amount of exudation and swelling by vasoconstriction.

Rehabilitation

The activity of the patient is limited by the burn, massive dressings, and sedation. Therefore, the activation regime is necessary to prevent pulmonary and vascular stasis, atony, and ankylosis. The patient must be encouraged to exercise unaffected parts regularly and frequently. He must be correctly aligned and properly supported. If possible, the patient should not lie on the affected areas. However, if burns are extensive and involve both the anterior and posterior surfaces, frequent turning without disruption of the healing areas can be accomplished by the use of a Stryker frame or Foster bed.

Contractures constitute one of the most common causes of disability following the healing of a burn. A contracture may be due to tightening of scar tissue or to shortening of muscles, which may occur when the patient is allowed to maintain a position of prolonged flexion. This disability is more easily prevented than remedied. A splint, or occasionally a cast, may be applied early to prevent a flexion contracture. Exercise of the affected part is initiated as soon as healing has progressed sufficiently to permit activity without disruption. If a contracture does develop, surgical correction is necessary.

Physical therapy is especially important in the rehabilitation of the patient who has sustained a severe burn. The therapist can direct the exercising and positioning of the patient. Hydrotherapy is a useful adjunct early to remove encrustations and later to facilitate exercise.

The patient who has been severely burned requires a great deal of emotional support and encouragement. His initial experience was painful and shocking. Emergency conditions such as a burn always tear a patient from his responsibilities and social ties without warning, and, consequently, without preparation. A prolonged period of hospitalization with many operative procedures is usually necessary. In addition, the patient fears disfigurement and disability. He needs the reassuring knowledge of progress in plastic surgery so that he can hope for eventual recovery with minimal disfigurement and optimal function. Faith in his recovery must be stimulated from the beginning to prevent undue discouragement. The nurse may be taxed to provide much-needed diversional therapy for the patient whose burns prevent the use of his hands. She may encourage visitors to read to the patient, to write notes for him, and to keep him in touch with the outside world. Radio is useful, provided someone assumes responsibility for tuning to the programs the patient wants to hear.

The family members must also be considered in planning the rehabilitation program for a patient who has sustained a severe burn. Their lives, too, have been disrupted by the emergency which has removed their loved one from the home for a prolonged period of treatment. They, too, are concerned about possible disfigurement. They must be helped to understand that scarring may be extensive but that plastic surgery can do much to restore normal appearance and function. They are the ones whom the patient has learned to depend upon and to whom he will probably return for convalescent care. Their optimism and acceptance, regardless of the outcome of the burn, will be conveyed to the patient; to be helped to accept himself the patient must realize that his family still finds him acceptable. However, if the family members are to be able to lend such support, they must first be helped to talk out and work through their feelings.

SKIN GRAFTS

Skin grafting is one method of covering a severely burned area. This is the procedure of transplanting skin from an unaffected part of the body to the involved area. Grafts will grow on perichondrium, periosteum, bone, tendon, fascia, fat, muscle, or healthy granulation tissue.[3] They serve three major purposes: (1) to protect a large, denuded area, such as a third-degree burn or ulcer, (2) to improve appearance, as may be necessary when fibrous scar tissue has contracted, distorting a person's appearance, and (3) to improve function when scar tissue has caused limitation of motion. The transplant may be permanent, or it may serve as an emergency measure only, to allow healing before the graft sloughs off or until a thin graft is replaced with a thicker, more functional transplant.

Essentially two types of free skin grafts are used for these purposes. One of the most commonly used is a *split-thickness graft*, which corre-

[3] P. W. Greeley and J. W. Curtin, Clinical Application of Skin Grafting Procedures, S. Clin. North America, vol. 35, no. 1, p. 203, February, 1955.

sponds to the epidermis and part of the corium. The other type is a *full-thickness transplant*, corresponding to epidermis and all of the corium. (See Fig. 55.) The type of graft selected depends upon the purpose it must serve and the area to be covered. Thin, split-thickness grafts grow the most rapidly and "take" most completely. Full-thickness grafts are more functional and produce a better cosmetic effect, especially for grafts on the face and flexor areas of the hands. The *donor site*, the area from which intact skin is taken, is selected to approximate the skin of the re-

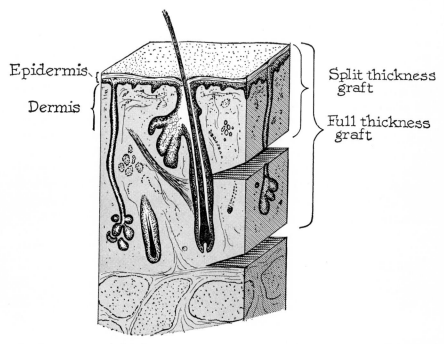

Fig. 55. Diagram of the skin in cross section to show the depth of grafts taken from a donor site.

cipient area as much as possible in appearance and function. For example, hair-bearing skin would not be grafted to an area usually devoid of hair.

The graft may be taken in one piece. If donor sites are at a premium, as with an extensive burn, small multiple grafts are taken and planted like islands in the area to be covered. Secondary healing occurs between these *pinch* or *stamp grafts*. Healing is less smooth than with a graft of one piece, because extensive fibrosis may occur. Since scarring of the donor site may occur, areas are selected which will be covered with clothes, such as the abdomen, chest, back, or thighs.

Preoperatively the patient is prepared for general anesthesia, and the donor area is surgically prepared. Preparation of the recipient site will be ordered by the surgeon. The patient must know enough about a skin graft to understand why he will have another area healing postoperatively in addition to his original wound. Postoperatively the grafted area will have a pressure dressing for 2 to 3 weeks to promote smooth healing. The patient may have nonabsorbable sutures in both sites, especially with full-thickness grafts. Split-thickness grafts may need trimming when first dressed, because they are not cut to the exact size and shape of the area, as is a full-thickness graft.

The general care for a patient with a skin graft closely resembles that for a burned patient. Depending upon the area involved, he may need assistance with eating, turning, and activation. He will need diversion and encouragement. To prevent ankylosis and muscle atony the surgeon may prescribe exercises for the grafted area at a time when he feels the graft has anchored itself safely. A grafted area needs a good blood supply; therefore, the nurse must guard against undue pressure or constriction of the grafted site. The patient should be turned frequently but should not lie on the sites of operation.

SUMMARY

The most important aspects of the initial care of a patient with an extensive burn are the treatment of shock and the prevention of infection.

Burns are classified on the basis of degree of tissue destruction as first-, second-, and third-degree. The extent of tissue destruction must also be considered, since an extensive first-degree burn might conceivably result in greater loss of skin function than a small third-degree burn. The basic pathologic processes involved in a burn are inflammation, tissue destruction, and toxemia.

Burns may be treated by application of pressure dressings, by exposure to air, or by skin grafting. All three methods are preceded by gentle but thorough cleansing. Antibiotic drugs may be administered.

A skin graft may be used to cover an area denuded by a burn, by ulceration, or by extensive surgery. They are also used to improve appearance and/or function following extensive cicatrization.

A graft is a *split-thickness* or *full-thickness* graft, depending upon whether part or all of the corium is included. The graft may be transplanted in one piece, or stamp grafts may be used.

The care of the patient following a graft is similar to that described for the convalescent care of the patient with a burn. Motion in the site of the operation is discouraged until the graft is secure; thereafter positioning and exercise are depended upon for the prevention of contractures.

Long-term treatment may be necessary following a burn or extensive grafting. The patient and his family require much encouragement and support.

BIBLIOGRAPHY

ALLEN, H. S.: Thermal and Irradiation Injuries, in "Christopher's Textbook of Surgery," 6th ed., L. Davis (ed.), W. B. Saunders Company, Philadelphia, 1956, chap. 10, pp. 210–239.

ARTZ, C. P., and B. G. MACMILLAN: Treatment of Burns of Difficult Areas, *Am. J. Surg.*, vol. 91, no. 4, pp. 517–520, April, 1956.

————, E. REISS, J. H. DAVIS, and W. H. AMSPACHER: The Treatment of Burns by the Exposure Method, *Postgrad. Med.*, vol. 13, pp. 535–546, June, 1953.

BELL, J. L.: The Local Care of Burn Wounds, *S. Clin. North America*, vol. 35, no. 1, pp. 195–201, February, 1955.

BROWN, J. B., and M. P. FRYER: Principles of General Plastic Surgery, in "Surgery," J. G. Allen, H. N. Harkins, C. A. Moyer, and J. E. Rhoads (eds.), J. B. Lippincott Company, Philadelphia, 1957, chap. 45, pp. 1165–1210.

GREELEY, P. W., and J. W. CURTIN: Clinical Application of Skin Grafting Procedures, *S. Clin. North America*, vol. 35, no. 1, pp. 203–209, February, 1955.

MILLER, C. W.: Nursing Care of Severely Burned Patients, *Am. J. Nursing*, pp. 456–459, April, 1954.

MOORE, F. D.: Burns, *M. Clin. North America*, vol. 36, no. 5, pp. 1201–1213, September, 1952.

MOYER, C. A.: Burns, in "Surgery," J. G. Allen, H. N. Harkins, C. A. Moyer, and J. E. Rhoads (eds.), J. B. Lippincott Company, Philadelphia, 1957, chap. 16, pp. 274–308.

The Problem of Sunburn, *Therapeutic Notes*, Parke, Davis and Company, Detroit, vol. 63, no. 6, pp. 151–155, June, 1956.

SARVAJEC, J.: Basic Principles in the Treatment of Burns, *Nursing Outlook*, vol. 5, pp. 21–22, May, 1957.

STOKES, R. F.: (1) Plastic Surgery, and (2) The Treatment of Burns, in "The Recovery Room," M. S. Sadove and J. H. Cross (eds.), W. B. Saunders Company, Philadelphia, 1956, chap. 14, pp. 373–393, and chap. 15, pp. 393–403.

STUDY GUIDE FOR PART FOUR

1. In vascular clinic you are assigned to teach a small group of patients who have arteriosclerosis. Each has mild symptoms of arterial insufficiency. Outline a plan for teaching these patients the hygienic measures necessary for their well-being.

2. Many months later one of these patients is admitted to the hospital with sudden occlusion of the left popliteal artery. What is the probable cause of the obstruction? Describe the appearance of the leg. What surgical procedures might be used to relieve the acute condition?

3. Another patient is admitted to the same clinical division with moist gangrene of the right foot. What factors predispose to gangrene?

What are the principles of care for a gangrenous extremity? When is the use of refrigeration indicated, and what are the responsibilities of the nurse during this therapy?

4. List the members of the health team who would be involved with the rehabilitation of an amputee patient in the hospital in which you are studying.

5. How does a thoracolumbar sympathectomy relieve essential hypertension? Outline the plan for the postoperative care and teaching of a patient undergoing this operation.

6. Nurses not uncommonly develop varicose veins in the lower extremities. What factors predispose to this condition? What are the hygienic practices which should be started by the student in nursing to prevent or delay the onset of this condition?

7. You are assigned to the care of a patient who is to undergo vein stripping. What is the purpose of this procedure? What nursing measures are necessary postoperatively?

8. Although a sunburn is considered lightly by many persons who willfully overexpose themselves to intense sunlight year after year in the interest of obtaining a tan, this is a very dangerous practice which may eventuate fatally. Describe the pathologic consequences of a severe burn. What general therapeutic measures are necessary in the care of a patient with an extensive burn? Describe the local measures used in the treatment of the burned area and the nursing responsibilities necessary with each.

9. What are the purposes for which skin grafts are used? How are skin grafts classified? In what ways is the care of a patient with a skin graft similar to the care of a patient with a burn?

INDEX